D1351517

Sister Dora

THE LIFE OF DOROTHY PATTISON

by the same author

ELIZABETH GARRETT ANDERSON

For children
THE STORY OF ALBERT SCHWEITZER
A PORTRAIT OF BACH

with Robert Gittings
THE STORY OF JOHN KEATS

Sister Dora

THE LIFE OF DOROTHY PATTISON

by JO MANTON

METHUEN & CO LTD

11 NEW FETTER LANE · LONDON EC4

First published in 1971
by Methuen & Co Ltd
Copyright © 1971 by Jo Manton
Printed in Great Britain
by Ebenezer Baylis & Son Ltd
The Trinity Press, Worcester, and London

SBN 416 10900 4

To

ROGER and ELIZABETH FISKE

'I wish less of our piety were spent on imaginary perfect goodness, and more given to real imperfect goodness.'

George Eliot

Contents

❋

Illustrations

❀

A*

Illustrations

Abbreviations used
in the Notes

Pattison, plus volume and folio number – Collection of Pattison MSS., Bodleian Library, Oxford

C.H.R. – Collection of MSS. at the Convent of the Holy Rood, Middlesbrough

W.C.H.A.R. plus date – Walsall Cottage Hospital Annual Reports 1863–1886

W.C.H. MS. plus date – Minute books in MS. of Walsall Cottage Hospital Committee of Management 1863–1878

Memoirs – Mark Pattison, *Memoirs*, 1885

Lonsdale – Margaret Lonsdale, *Sister Dora*, 1880

Ridsdale – E. M. M. Ridsdale, *Sister Dora*, 1880

Reprints – Articles and correspondence on Sister Dora reprinted from the *Walsall Observer*, 1886

W.P.L. Album – Collection of un-named or dated press cuttings in the local history room of Walsall Public Library

Acknowledgments

❊

'I wish,' wrote George Eliot, 'less of our piety were spent on imaginary perfect goodness and more given to real, imperfect goodness.' Few mid-Victorians would have agreed with their great contemporary; as the biographies they read and wrote plainly reveal, they wanted the good to be perfect, even if this meant softening the outlines of a personality or tidying away unacceptable facts. Sister Dora was not one of them. 'Let there be no vain eulogy of me after my death,' she said, conscious of the legend which had gathered round her, even in her lifetime. In search of the living human being behind this legend, I have attempted to visit every place and see every known document connected with her life, and it is a pleasure to thank many institutions and individuals for making this possible.

My first thanks must be for the Leverhulme Research Award, which allowed me to undertake the book. It also owes much to the kindness of friends, among whom I should particularly like to thank Dr and Mrs Roger Fiske for the generous loan of their house at Oxford. I owe thanks for much help to the staffs of libraries, record offices and institutions which have made collections or individual documents available. The Keeper and staff of the Department of Western Manuscripts at the Bodleian Library, Oxford allowed me to look through the volumes of the great Pattison collection and transcribe Dorothy Pattison's unpublished letters to her brother Mark. It is a pleasure to thank the Librarian and staff of Walsall Public Library, as it was a pleasure to work among the documents, press cuttings, photographs and paintings in their local history room. The Secretary and staff of Walsall Group Hospital Management Committee produced not only a complete set of printed Annual Reports but the unique manuscript Minute books of their hospital from its foundation, all of which they allowed me to take home and study at leisure. The

Editor of the *Walsall Observer* has given me permission to draw extensively on its early files and to quote from two sets of Sister Dora's letters in the possession of the West Midlands Press. The Reverend Mother Superior and Community of the Holy Rood, Middlesbrough, made their earliest records and photographs available and generously placed no restriction on their use. The North Riding County Record Office and the Chester Diocesan Archives provided documentation on the parishes of Hauxwell, Bellerby and Aysgarth and on the Pattison, Winn and Stirk families. The Rector of Edgbaston and the Vicars of Spennithorne and Aysgarth kindly searched their parish registers for further information.

Librarians and curators of specialized collections frequently directed me to valuable secondary sources, which I might otherwise have missed: among them the library staffs of the Royal College of Nursing, the Wellcome Institute of the History of Medicine, the Birmingham Public Library and University Library, the Manchester Public Library, the Royal Society of Medicine and the Institute of Historical Research. My thanks are also due to the Librarians and staffs of London University Library, Cambridge University Library, the British Museum and the Newspaper Library, and the excellent Reference Section of the West Sussex County Library. Among many individuals who answered personal inquiries I should like to thank the Rev Dr V. H. H. Green of Lincoln College, Mrs A. Bailey of Hauxwell, Mrs J. E. Howard, Mrs J. Harker and Clement Redfern Davies, Esq.

For illustrations I must thank Mrs Bailey, the Rev Dr V. H. H. Green, John Sparrow, Esq., the Community of the Holy Rood, the Trustees of the British Museum, the Walsall Public Library and Clare Gittings, who also made the rubbing of the Pattison tombstone. I am grateful to E. S. Peacock, A.I.B.P., for technical assistance with photographs and A. Pamela Taylor and Kathleen Sale for much skill and patience in typing the manuscript. My husband's insight and interest helped every stage of the work. Finally, I am greatly indebted to Dr E. J. L. Lowbury, M.A., D.M., F.R.C.Path., Hon. Director, Hospital Infection Research Laboratory, Birmingham, for his kindness in reading the typescript.

Jo Manton
Chichester, 1970

A Day in 1878

December 28th, the first Saturday after Christmas, 1878, was a day of drizzling rain in the Black Country. Snow had fallen on the town of Walsall, briefly veiling the dense rows of houses; it had been pock-marked by soot and flying cinders, and was now melting into a grimy slush. The town, usually raucous with the shouts of market people and the distant thud of steam hammers, was strangely quiet. The shops were closed. Houses stood silent, with drawn blinds. From St Matthew's Gothic spire, crowning the steep and winding high street of the old borough, the bells rang a 'muffled peal, as they had each day since Christmas Eve. The sound, said a hearer, struck a dull chill into every heart.[1]

At two o'clock in the afternoon a procession called at a small house in Wednesbury Road. Eighteen railwaymen, engine drivers, porters and guards, in their working uniform, bore a plain wooden coffin from the door to a plain hearse. Behind it followed a choir, strangely composed for that period of sectarian strife; robed choristers from the Parish Churches walked with singers from the Dissenting chapels, from Roman Catholic churches, from the Unitarian meeting house. After them came clergy of every denomination in the town, with two bishops on foot. The Mayor and Corporation of Walsall were there, a representative of the Member of Parliament, the Magistrates and members of the Hospital Committee.[2] Yet this was not the funeral of some borough dignitary who had lived rich and successful, died full of honours and was now being escorted to an official grave. They were following the body of a woman who had come among them as a stranger, member of an Anglican religious order, only fourteen years before and who had died at forty-six, poor as the day

she came. She had been beautiful and fascinating, gay and courageous, the friend of all present, yet separated by an invisible
barrier from the values and conventions of their society. How far
she stood outside appeared as they wound a circuitous route
between gutters of grey slush, through crowded streets towards
the Walsall Cottage Hospital for casualties from the mines and
iron-works of the district.

The invitation to the funeral had been to official bodies only.[3]
Yet now from every turning came working men and women in
Sunday clothes, to fall in behind the procession. For four days
they had been knocking at the door of the house in the Wednesbury Road, demanding to see the dead woman for the last time.
The same answer was given to each one; she had given orders that
no one should be admitted. Nor did she wish for an elaborate
funeral. 'Let there be no vain eulogy passed upon me when I am
gone and no reference to my former life. Quietly I came among
you and quietly let me go', she had said.[4] Only by their presence,
marching silently through the rain, could they show their affection, the traditional loyalty of the working-classes, strongest in
death. From slums, courtyards and back alleys came the really
poor, the unemployed, the drunkards, the Irish tinkers, ragged
men with blackened faces and fierce white eyes, women with half-
starved children dragging at their skirts. 'She was the best friend
we ever had', said one of these, looking with tears towards the
coffin. In the open space outside the gates of the hospital a dense
crowd of men stood silently waiting under the lowering sky.
They were rough, often scarred; some were crippled and mutilated, but they too joined the march. All were patients, whom the
dead woman had nursed in her life as Sister-in-Charge. Here, too,
waited the Governors of the Grammar School, the Poor Law
Guardians, the School Board, the Sunday School children, and
the Workmen's Friendly Societies. They followed the coffin down
Bradford Street and Park Street, till it looked, said an onlooker, as
though the whole town was moving towards the cemetery. There
were no carriages; all went on foot.

Beyond the hospital a short cut across the railway line led
directly to the gates of the burying-ground. Hundreds of onlookers, who had lined the streets, swarmed over the rails and met,
head on, a police guard at the cemetery gates. The gates were shut

after the official procession and the crowd told to wait outside. There was an angry mutter, 'We've as good a right to be there as them', and a sharp hand-to-hand struggle. The police had no chance against the pressure of the crowd. The gates were forced open, the cordon swept away, and the people poured into the graveyard.⁵ There they waited, so dense the very tombstones were hidden, for the white-robed choir and the railwaymen, now moving with slow and heavy tread as bearers of the coffin. They set it down in the porch of the mortuary chapel. Swaying and shifting, those nearest pressed round to read and repeat to others further back, till the whole gathering murmured the words, 'Sister Dora entered into rest 24th December 1878'. Sister Dora was the only name by which most of them had ever known their friend.⁶

The procession was late. Four other coffins were already waiting in the chapel. They had been sent from Walsall Union Workhouse for a pauper funeral. They would have been set aside to wait, but for a nurse from the hospital. 'Just what Sister Dora herself would have wished', she said. 'Not to be divided even in death from the poor people she loved so well.'⁷ The funeral service was read over all five coffins together. The choirs sang a favourite Victorian hymn:

Father, in thy gracious keeping
Leave we now thy servant sleeping

After all was over, the nurses took flowers from Sister Dora's coffin to lay on the graves of these nameless poor. The official party left; the huge crowd dispersed, taking orderly turns to look into the open grave. To the manifest surprise of an onlooker: 'Nothing could be more reverent than the behaviour of these dense masses, belonging to the lowest grade of society.' Slowly they went home. 28th December 1878 was a quiet Saturday night in Walsall. Next day the parish church was crowded to hear a memorial sermon, called simply 'A Princess among Nurses'.

It was an extraordinary achievement for one woman to have crossed the barriers of sectarianism and social class, so much more menacing a hundred years ago than now, still more remarkable to have subdued a tough and combative industrial society to

17

single-minded love and grief at her going. In the years after her death an extraordinary cult of Sister Dora grew not only among the working people of the Black Country who had known her, but by hearsay far beyond. 'Hundreds of thousands', wrote a reviewer of the memoir published in 1880, 'knew vaguely that there was something wonderful about the sway exercised by a beautiful and fascinating woman, and submitted to alike by radical mayors and evangelical vicars, by the surgeons of the hospital in which she nursed, and the colliers and puddlers who filled its beds.'[8]

The cult of Sister Dora grew in a world of pious enthusiasms and religious romanticism. In this world an admired figure must be presented as nothing less than perfection, and a loved leader claimed as the exclusive possession of a number of rival devotees. So it was with Dorothy Pattison, known as Sister Dora. An atmosphere of unreality surrounds her. Every group, every individual, drawn by her strangely compelling personality, claimed a particular understanding of her secret, till the living woman was shrouded in a curtain of legend. It was inevitable that her reputation should be caught in the crossfire of ecclesiastical party warfare, which raged through most of the nineteenth century. High Church enthusiasts pointed out that Sister Dora fasted in Lent and read prayers from the Prayer Book at eight in the morning, noon, and eight at night, every day without fail, that she went to confession and prayed with equal fidelity for the dying and the dead. Evangelicals countered by claiming with equal truth that she enjoyed not only the hymns of Charles Wesley, but the rousing revivalist jingles of Moody and Sankey, that the hospital services were in the nature of family prayers, and that her love for her roughest patients was shot through with an ardour for 'winning souls'. Even the agnostics laid claim to this unconventional Anglican nun. 'Her moderate Anglicanism was scarcely a part of Sister Dora's nature,' wrote the same reviewer. 'There was more of nature than of grace in her devotion, as well as in her wilfulness and inarticulate passion, which sought an escape from sadness in the triumphs of despair.' There were other prejudiced parties, among them Florence Nightingale, always ready to demonstrate the miraculous benefits of trained nursing. 'May every nurse,' she wrote, 'though not gifted with Sister Dora's genius, grow in training and care of her patients, that none but may be better for

18

her care, whether for life or death. May she remember courage and obedience and that men patients especially are critical of religion nowadays and look sharp to see if she is acting up to her profession. Such are some of the lessons taught by Sister Dora's life.'[9] The medical profession, reasonably enough, saw the nursing sister as a valuable servant to their own superior skill. 'A most patient, skilful and devoted nurse,' wrote a Midland doctor. 'She possessed to a remarkable extent that rare quality of inspiring confidence,'[10] in patients whom she could persuade to accept treatment where the surgeon, alien in speech and manner, aroused fear or distrust. Under her care the death rate in an accident hospital receiving desperate injuries had been lower than the average for the most progressive surgical departments in London teaching hospitals.[11]

Sister Dora cast a spell over every chance acquaintance, leaving each convinced that he or she had enjoyed a unique relationship. Their portraits of her revealed their own prejudices. To her first biographer, Margaret Lonsdale, grand-daughter of a former Bishop of Lichfield and a vivid writer in the style of the period, Sister Dora was a creature of high romance. Her background in the remote North Riding of Yorkshire was impeccably county, she rode to hounds, visited a distinguished brother at Oxford and played Lady Bountiful to a chorus of grateful villagers. Her chosen work in the Black Country was represented as a great personal sacrifice, for 'her life would be spent among people inferior to herself in education and position and her singular talents would be wasted'.[12] She was depicted as condescending to a hospital committee of 'men actively engaged in trade or retired tradesmen.' Her life up to the age of thirty is dismissed in fifteen pages. Moreover, in deference to the etiquette of the day, essential facts were often suppressed, while names, dates and places were shrouded in a fog of anonymity, still difficult to penetrate. For dramatic effect the background was blackened in order to make the figure of Sister Dora appear more bright. Not surprisingly, this approach infuriated many readers in the Black Country and beyond.[13] They complained that the working men and women Sister Dora had loved were presented as unlovely, the town, for which she had such deep affection that she chose to live and die there, was described as a dark wilderness, and the woman herself as lacking ordinary friendship. This bitterly offended the people of Walsall. 'We could not have loved her more,' wrote a Walsall correspondent simply. 'There was little we could ever do – there was nothing she would let us do – to relieve the self-imposed rigours of her life. But we loved her in all sincerity.'[14] Another party of Sister Dora's admirers was equally shocked by the idea that their idol might have worldly interests or ambitions. 'We have read with pain much that has been written about her,' wrote a pious and impressionable young Methodist minister's daughter, Eliza Ridsdale, in a sort of anti-memoir. 'Writers have attributed to restlessness or something like ambition her longings after and efforts to enter upon a life of consecrating herself to the services of suffering humanity.' Her Sister Dora was a 'loving, patient spirit full of sweet glad joyous self-forgetfulness and supreme devotion' who 'heard the master's voice in early life, inclining to the work which he had marked out for her and rejoicing to obey it'.[15]

Those nearest to Dorothy Pattison in her youth, the members of her own family, hinted at conflicts in her life concealed from the admiring public. 'I wish she could marry some of these doctors who seem so fond of her,' wrote her sister Rachel soon after Dorothy had entered her Order and become Sister Dora. 'Then she might live a safer life for her character.'[16] Sister Dora's most distinguished relation, Mark Pattison, Rector of Lincoln College and owner of the finest private scholar's library in Oxford, paid her an ironic compliment. 'She spent a faculty of invention which would have placed her in the front rank as a novelist in embellishing the everyday occurrences of her own life. A very faint reflection of Dorothy's powers of self-glorification is preserved in Miss Lonsdale's romance *Sister Dora*',[17] he wrote.

He did not attend Sister Dora's funeral, nor did any of her eight surviving sisters, some of whom had tried to visit her in her last illness and been sent away because 'there was nothing they could do'. In the vast crowd of mourners there was only one representative of her own family, none from the Anglican convent in the north where she had developed her nursing vocation, very few who could claim any close relationship with the woman whom a whole region mourned. She had passed her life, first in a crowded Rectory house, then in a series of institutions, school, convent, hospital, yet when she was dying she sent away her watchers. 'I have lived alone,' she said, 'let me die alone, oh let me die alone!' These were the last words she was heard to speak.

NOTES

1. *Walsall Observer*, 28th December 1878.
2. Ibid., 4th January 1879.
3. Ibid., 28th December 1878.
4. Ibid., 28th December 1878.
5. Ibid., 4th January 1879.
6. Ibid., 28th December 1878.
7. Lonsdale, 244.
8. Edith Simcox reviewing *Sister Dora* by Margaret Lonsdale. *Fortnightly Review*, XXVII, 656.
9. Florence Nightingale in Reprints, p. 10.
10. F. W. Willmore, *History of Walsall*, p. 431.
11. W.C.H.A.R., 1870.
12. Lonsdale, 41.
13. Two medical men, who had known the original, objected to 'Miss Lonsdale's work of imagination' as 'a somewhat vapid story of Sister Dora'.
14. Reprints, 31.
15. Ridsdale.
16. Pattison, 56, ff. 424–5.
17. *Memoirs*, 61.

PART ONE

Dorothy Pattison

CHAPTER ONE

Hauxwell Rectory
1821–1834

On 1st January 1821, Jane, the wife of the Reverend Mark James Pattison, celebrated the New Year by composing a prayer for her husband and children. She was in every way a pious and blameless young woman, but so ingrained was her sense of her own failings and her dread of 'back-sliding' that she began with an abject appeal for God's mercy.

> Oh Lord God Almighty, who hearest and answerest prayer, unworthy though I am to approach thy footstool, yet trusting to thy gracious promise that thou wilt hear those who call upon thee and knowing that we have a great high priest passed into the heavens, I come boldly to the throne of Grace entreating thee for the sake of thy beloved son to grant my prayers, so far as thou mayest see fitting.
>
> Lord I would humbly pray thee to bless my beloved husband and children. I ask not for temporal blessings, for I know that they who fear God will lack nothing that is good. But Lord, I beseech thee, grant them the richer blessings of thy grace. May thy Servant be daily growing in holiness, may he devote himself to his Master's business, and oh, be thou with him and make him the humble instrument of turning many from the error of their ways. And oh may *we* be heirs together of eternal life. Be with us Lord in the education of our children and whilst we endeavour to fit them for useful members of society, let our first concern be to teach them that the fear of the Lord is the beginning of wisdom. Shed thine Holy Spirit upon their infant hearts and may they *all* be thy children by adoption and grace.[1]

She finished copying the prayer and carefully pasted it into the back cover of her commonplace book, to be read and pondered over. She never doubted, though much conspired to make her doubt, that Providence watched over the smallest details of her family life. Perhaps she was right to do so, for her children, departing far from her in faith and practice, kept all their lives the imprint of this intense personal dedication.

Their father was less malleable. Mrs Pattison adored her husband with all the deference due to God's ordained minister and his own formidable character. He was a large, imposing figure, urbanely overbearing in manner, handsome when his features were not darkened and distorted by one of the sudden rages to which he had been subject since childhood. He was a passionate and devout snob. In the mid-eighteenth century his family had owned and worked a farm at Portrack on the River Tees near Stockton. This consisted of eighty acres of low-lying 'holms', liable to flood in winter. The total income from the land was only one hundred and five pounds a year and it was a continual struggle to keep down the expenses on dykes, jetties and a bridge.[2] His grandfather, Mark Pattison, gave up the struggle and entered the navy, selling the farm in 1787. A son, also Mark Pattison, born in 1763, stayed with relations in York to attend a day-school there. The family was not well off, and the schoolboy received parcels of shirts and worn clothing from a wealthier godmother. He was handsome and intelligent; through the patronage of Lord Townshend, he was presented to a place at the Royal Military Academy, Woolwich, from which he was commissioned into the Royal Artillery. He served in Quebec, rose to the rank of Captain, and was posted to Plymouth, where in 1787, his son Mark James Pattison was born.[3] The family had thus risen in the social scale during the course of half a century and this seems to have affected Mark James powerfully. Both father and grandfather died before he was ten. His early schooling is not mentioned but he went up in 1806 to Brasenose College, Oxford, which, he said, 'numbered among its members many gentlemen commoners of wealthy and noble families.' Scholars he spoke of with disdain as 'charity boys' not gentlemen, 'a low set and having low tastes.' Twenty years later he was still dwelling on his college days with a glow of nostalgic pride. His social advancement was assured when in 1811 and 1812 he was ordained deacon and priest in Exeter Cathedral. Mr Pattison's self-regard as a gentleman and a clergyman was prodigious, and it was to play a fatal part in his daughters' lives. At the outset the career of this self-assured young cleric looked promising. He was appointed curate of Hornby near Bedale in the North Riding of Yorkshire and in the absence of the rector served as curate in charge. His widowed mother settled nearby at Ainderby Steeple, where she shared a house with his widowed sister, Mary Meadows. A second sister, Eleanor Miller Sairey, had married an army officer, Captain Seward.[4]

At the age of twenty-four, the Reverend Mark James Pattison married a girl of nineteen, Jane Winn of Prior House in the ancient and beautiful Swaledale town of Richmond. Her father had been Mayor of the Borough and owner of the town's small private bank. By local standards Jane was an heiress, with a dowry secured to her under Deed of Trust. She had been well educated for a girl of her time at a reputable boarding-school in Doncaster; her family background was of the utmost middle-class respectability. She was small and fragile, pretty in her youth but always delicate in health and timid by temperament. Her ruling passion, apart from admiration and fear of her husband, was an intense, rigid, profoundly arid Evangelical faith, which was never to waver, though tried to the utmost by the experiences of her married life. The young couple moved into the parsonage house of Hornby, which stood within the grounds of Hornby Castle, seat of the Duke of Leeds and centre of an exquisite landscape, painted by Turner. Mr Pattison found himself, at a still impressionable age, serving as chaplain to the Duke, dining at his table, and addressed with ducal affability by the aristocratic nickname of 'Chancellor'. This was the origin, thought Mark Pattison, his eldest son, of his father's 'social aspirations which he continued to nourish . . . he liked to live with gentlemen and to know what was going on in the upper world. His acquaintance with the peerage was accurate; he must have read Debrett at that time more than the Bible'.[5]

Jane Pattison played little part in these aspirations apart from giving birth in 1813 to Mark, who, it was assumed from the cradle upwards, should go to Oxford and become fellow of a college frequented by the sons of gentlemen.[6] Thereafter her repeated pregnancies and confinements ended in the births of Jane Eleanor, Frances, Grace and Mary, all destined for a humbler, more sub-servient role in life. In 1815 her husband removed to a parish. He had no hope of the living at Hornby, which remained for three generations in the influential Alderson family, connections of Baron Alderson. He was therefore persuaded to exchange his curacy for the rectorship of Hauxwell a few miles away. There his wife further gave birth to Anna, Elizabeth, Sarah, Rachel, and, when she was forty, at nine o'clock in the morning of 16th January 1832 to Dorothy Wyndlow Pattison.[7]

Hauxwell was a parish of about three hundred people, living in hamlets and farms scattered over the high ground between lower Swaledale and Wensleydale. Leyburn was a five-mile walk away and Richmond about eight miles over a moorland road. It is still a lonely place. A hundred years ago it was isolated. A Yorkshire topographer wrote: 'A long and dreary tract of sloping ground is interposed between the valleys of the Swale and the Ure. The general declination of this tract is eastward; in traversing it a black or purple expanse of heath sheds its sombre hues far and wide. . . . To the right of this elevated road the prospect is wide and diversified, towns, villages, woods, lying in a mass before the eye. On the confine of this tract is Hauxwell, of which the principle feature is a deep and winding dell hung with oak. . . . The church and vicarage stand at some distance from this obscure place.'[8] Mark, who loved the freedom and solitude of Hauxwell, remembered, 'living on the borderland of oakwoods, with green lanes before me and an expanse of wild heather and moorland extending into Northumberland behind.'[9] Winter froze the streams into silence, blotted out sky and hills in a bitter whirl of snowflakes and filled up Hauxwell's single winding lane with snow; the village could remain cut off from the rest of the world for weeks at a time. The strange story of the Pattisons is bound up with this remoteness. The journey to London by coach took three days; the railway did not extend up Wensleydale to Hawes until the year of Sister Dora's death. While the West Riding of York-shire was exporting broadcloth to half the globe, the North Riding still lived in the world of Dotheboys Hall and Wuthering Heights. This sets the scene for the first thirty years of Dorothy Pattison's life.

A family of this size was necessarily widespread in age. Dorothy was only three months old when her elder brother Mark went up to Oriel College, Oxford, proud to ride on the box-seat in the rain with a friendly coachman, but thinking regretfully what a fine fishing day was going to waste. Nine sisters of all ages from three years to eighteen were delighted to dangle toys over her cradle, for it was noted from the first that she was an exceptionally pretty, intelligent and engaging child. Her father christened her himself when she was six months old. Just after her first birthday the last of the family, Frank Pattison was born. Their father sent affectionate news to Mark at Oxford of 'the object of your kind anxiety, your Mother and her young charge. But the former does not regain her strength with the rapidity of former times'.[10]

The buried, but all important, years of Dorothy's earliest childhood were happy, and survived in an enduring zest for life, which no hard experiences could destroy. Her mother was ailing and weary with household cares, but she was surrounded by 'a bevy of sisters'. She was taken, wrapped-up in shawls, to watch the older skating and the younger sliding on the ice. There were horses in the stable, cats in the kitchen and dogs all spoken of affectionately as members of the family. Life at the Rectory was 'cosy and patriarchal'. Her father, though alarmingly large, was benevolent in an august way. 'I spent a very happy afternoon yesterday', he reported, 'with your mother and five of my girls in Swinton grounds. We ate a cold veal pie and drank of the water of the pond by which we sat reclined.'[11] He was hospitable. 'You may of course invite whom you please to that which is your own home,' he wrote to Mark at Oxford. 'As far as I can consistently with the retired habits of a very retired country priest, I will do my little possible to render your guests comfortable.'[12] He was generous with bills and Christmas boxes and the bow-windowed Georgian rectory under the beech-trees was filled with warmth and comfort; Mark later recalled with bitter nostalgia the spell of the unbroken family circle in this country home.

It was not to remain unbroken for long. The years were passing; the Reverend Mark Pattison was now forty-five, yet preferment showed no signs of coming his way. At Hauxwell he was doubly isolated. Many of the working farmers and dalesmen were Methodists; some indeed had been converted by Wesley from the unchanged Roman Catholicism of their ancestors. The surrounding clergy, on the other hand, were often younger sons of county families. They were closely intermarried and formed a rich, powerful fox-hunting cousinage, which Mr Pattison had no hope of entering on equal terms. He might have lived a happy and useful life in his parish if he had possessed any strong vocation for pastoral work, but this he lacked. He was a man of vigorous but totally undisciplined powers, increasingly bored and contemptuous of the farming society which surrounded him. Partly from pride, partly from laziness, he chose to live without seeing anyone but 'a few like-minded evangelical clergy of the neighbourhood'. His elder children had already felt the lack of companionship, especially the girls, who were not allowed to play with the cottage children in the village. For some years Mr Pattison had the education of his son to distract him; Mark did not go to school and together they ploughed their way through Greek and Latin authors with the help of a dictionary and a crib. Then came the choosing of a College, with much resort on the Rector's part to 'my Vade Mecum', the Oxford Calendar, and the pleasure of seeking advice from the private tutor of Lord Conyers Osborne, son of the Duke of Leeds. Once Mark had gone up to Oriel, this distraction faded, the education of girls being of no interest. Mr Pattison sat for hours before the blazing fire in his little book-room, reading and re-reading the obituaries in an old volume of the *Gentleman's Magazine*. He brooded over the unjust fate which had carried him from Hornby Castle, its towers and terraces, the peacocks, the picture gallery and the conversation of noblemen, to this village stagnation. He continued to cherish social aspirations, though there was no hope at Hauxwell of achieving them.[13] Frustration gathered with the years and projected itself in angry resentment. His black moods came faster and blacker. In June 1834 he suffered a total mental breakdown.

It is not clear how much of this terrifying spectacle the younger children now saw, though they were later to see all too much. The case was clearly beyond the family doctor, Richard Bowes of Richmond. Mrs Pattison, who was caring for a baby less than six months old, and who had never taken an independent decision in her life, turned for help to her husband's brother-in-law, Captain Seward and his friend David Horndon, both, like the Pattison's themselves, 'Gospel believers'.

They advised her to consult Dr Thomas Simpson, M.D., physician to the County Asylum at York, by whose advice Mr Pattison was removed to Acomb House, York, a private madhouse licensed under the Act of 1828, and kept by H. B. Hodgson, for whom no medical qualification is listed. By an irony, The Retreat, York, offering humane and enlightened treatment, was close at hand, but this was a Quaker foundation, not considered suitable for a clergyman of the Church of England. Unfortunate in his illness, Mr Pattison was supremely unfortunate in its timing. He was confined just five years before the general movement to abolish 'mechanical restraints', chains, handcuffs, and strait-jackets for mental patients. 'Moral treatment', that is to say kind treatment, was in the near future, but for the present the fashionable remedies were still those of blistering, cold douches, dark rooms and circular swinging with the patient strapped into a revolving chair until vertigo and vomiting ensued. The conditions of confinement, in the absence of public inspection, were more often than not appalling. 'I went into the passage', reported a Commissioner visiting the York Asylum, 'and found four cells, I think of about eight feet square and a very horrid and filthy situation; the straw appeared to be almost saturated with urine and excrement . . . I turned up the straw in one of them and pointed out the chain and handcuff which were concealed beneath.'[14]

Mr Pattison later called his cell 'the most noisome den to which a clergyman of the Church of England and that clergyman a gentleman could have been consigned.' After three months his symptoms began to subside, except for one fixed fatal idea. 'On every subject but one', wrote Mrs Pattison to Mark at Oxford, 'your Father's mind is perfect and even vigorous – that one is home . . . I am *not* to see him'.[15] He was enraged that his family had allowed him to be confined and humiliated. His threats against his wife were so violent that the physicians advised her not to visit him, and it became one of his principal grievances that she had been 'too dainty' to enter his 'loathsome dungeon'. On 19th November 1834 he was discharged, but his outbursts of rage made it clear that it was not safe for him to come home. Mark Pattison left Oxford temporarily and looked after his father in lodgings in York during the Christmas vacation of his third year.[16] Mr Pattison continued to brood over his treatment which he now held responsible for the failure of his career. 'By this *fatal, fatal* step I have been deprived of every prospect in life however glittering that prospect was. I am satisfied that kind and soothing measures would have saved me much pain,' he wrote pathetically. He dwelt on 'the filth, meanness, noise and cant to which I was so long and so unnecessarily exposed. I never can forget the scenes I have gone through. No time can blot it from my memory, were I to live till the day of doom.'[17] In April 1835 he came home to Hauxwell Rectory, officially cured. His mind was clear, but his personality never recovered. Three-year-old Dorothy Pattison's first conscious memories of her father were of seeing him sit for two hours, scowling at an open book without turning a page, or pace angrily up and down under the tall beech trees of the avenue, shouting abuse at anyone who came near him. The children learnt to keep out of his way and indeed he showed no interest in any of them except Frank. 'I do not think', wrote Eleanor, 'that he feels anything but himself and his injuries.'[18]

Mr Pattison's mental condition seems to have followed a cyclic pattern, with violent episodes in 1834, 1842, 1853 and 1860. These outbreaks were always precipitated by some complaint against his family. Between them he remained morose, suspicious, resentful and depressed.

He was able to take the duty of his parish, to preach and to write competent business letters, but suspicion and hatred of his wife and children settled into a fixed, unalterable system of delusions, which very seldom lifted during the next thirty years. Mrs Pattison still adored him, though her love was mixed with fear. Her features began to set into the anxious, frightened expression her daughters were to know so well. Most of her time was devoted to soothing and placating her husband, trying to avert the rages which reduced the whole household to shuddering dread. Duty was her god and she never failed to do her duty by the children, but from sheer weariness she could bring little affection and no gaiety into their lives.

Sister Dora's first biographer, Margaret Lonsdale, writing without access to family documents, described her as the pet and darling of a large, happy, Rectory family. With a writer's natural wish to dramatize her heroine's self-sacrifice, she also invested the Pattisons with a 'high-bred' county background, not supported by the evidence. In reality Dorothy Pattison's was a sombre childhood, and in all her life she was never to know the happiness of an ordinary home. Her father's paranoia blackened and blighted the life of all his family. 'This misery', one of them wrote later, 'has been going on ever since we were children.'[19]

NOTES

1. Pattison, 68. Loose folio pasted in back cover.
2. Ibid., 144, ff. 33, 76, 95.
3. P.P.R., Exeter, 564. This was the source of the mistaken statement in Lonsdale, 1, that he 'belonged to a Devonshire family'.
4. P.P.R., Walpole, 203.
5. *Memoirs*, 24.
6. Ibid., 8.
7. Register of Baptisms, Hauxwell.
8. T. Whitaker, *History of Richmondshire*, I, 323.
9. *Memoirs*, 34-5.
10. Pattison, 61, f. 28.
11. Ibid., 61, f. 10.
12. Ibid., f. 34.
13. *Memoirs*, 24.
14. Hunter and Macalpine, *Three Hundred Years of Psychiatry*, 698.
15. Pattison, 61, f. 40.
16. *Memoirs*, 138.
17. Pattison, 61, ff. 49, 52.
18. Ibid., 43, f. 81.
19. Ibid., 45, f. 34.

CHAPTER TWO

The Children

1835–1844

For the next few years Dorothy disappears as an individual. With Elizabeth, Sarah and Rachel she was handed over to the care of sisters and servants in a group always spoken of collectively as 'the children'. Elizabeth and Sarah formed an inseparable couple of sensible, rather prosaic small girls. Rachel and Dorothy formed another, in which Dorothy was leader and gentle, affectionate Rachel was led. Among the elder sisters, Jane, Eleanor and Mary were forceful, domineering characters, resembling their father before his illness. Fanny, Grace and Anna, like their mother, were timid, introspective and inclined to depression. These three proved particularly vulnerable to the abnormal stresses of their home. All were pious, studious and intensely serious-minded; a sense of humour was a rarity in the Pattison family circle. Mark, the eldest, and Frank, the youngest, as brothers, were set apart and adored, though Mark, who remained at Oxford seeking a fellowship, was necessarily adored from afar. Girls could expect few personal rights, no freedom and only a limited share of notice.

In this large family there was no time to give individual attention to unimportant members, even when they were ill. When Dorothy was five the nursery was invaded by measles. 'I am surrounded by children crying, sneezing, sniffing, coughing, spluttering,' wrote Eleanor rather resentfully to Mark.[1] She was twenty, an intellectual girl who longed to read and study, but who was forced into the duties of nursemaid while her mother accompanied Mr Pattison on a visit to his doctor in York. Next winter all the children had mumps; only Frank who was already

established as his father's favourite and less confined to the
nursery escaped the infection. 'The children' all had swollen
faces, could not swallow and were miserable. 'The house has been
like a hospital for the last six weeks,' was their mother's somewhat
chilly report. However, illness had its compensations. 'We
finished that most entertaining book the Pilgrim's Progress last
night,' wrote twelve-year-old Anna.[2] Evidently the little Pattisons
had learnt to find their own amusements.

Indeed the courage and resource of these children was miraculous. Dorothy in particular showed spirit from the start. Indoors
her refuge was the kitchen, with its huge, perpetually glowing
fire-place; it remained her favourite room as long as she lived
under the Rectory roof. There she was sure of a welcome from
Bessy the housemaid, from Wright the parlourmaid, who gave
'affectionate service for nineteen years' and above all from Sally,
kind Mrs Sarah Watts the cook, with her blazing range and clean
white apron. The scrubbed stone flags, the vast oak dresser and
the glittering copper saucepans of an old-fashioned Yorkshire
country kitchen taught lessons of good housekeeping. There, too,
Dorothy learnt a further lesson, never forgotten throughout her
life's work; the warmth and goodness of simple people. Two of
these early affections, for Wright and Mrs Watt, lasted to her
life's end. At the New Year of her seventh birthday, the children,
with the help of their elder sisters, gave a supper party and
entertainment for the Rectory servants and thirty friends from
the cottage in Hauxwell village. They were thanked and cheered.[3]
Their treats were rare. Mark's visits home were longed for and
long remembered; he gathered the little ones round his favourite
seat in the garden and read aloud to them from Southey's tales
and ballads.[4] Sometimes Mrs Pattison took the girls with her in
the carriage to pay calls or over the straight, bleak moorland road
to shop in Richmond. On one day which threw the household
into a turmoil, the Dowager Duchess of Leeds, passing on a
journey, called at the Rectory. The children were more at ease
without their parents, when they were sent with the coachman in
'a very pretty Phaeton for two horses' up the green flank of
Wensleydale to see the waterfalls at Aysgarth. Their happiest
times were winter afternoons when their parents went out and
'games of chess, draughts, backgammon and riddles were carried

on with a tumult in the dining room'.[5] Silence fell abruptly and the games were quickly packed away when the sound of carriage wheels on the gravel announced their father's return.

These were occasional treats, but Dorothy's constant joy, from as far back as she could remember, was to escape out of doors. The Rectory garden sloped towards the south, with a wide view over Wensleydale before the great whaleback of Witton Fell closed the skyline. There was a tulip tree, a cedar behind the house, a tall Wellingtonia and Dorothy's favourite, a great rustling copper beech which overshadowed one corner of the lawn. Beyond lay the park of Hauxwell Hall, its avenue of lime trees peopled all the summer by her sister's bees. Behind the house lay still more exciting territory. The Rectory has gone now, but the glebe farmyard remains. A high wall of stone encloses the tithe barn still used for hay, the empty coach-house, the stables, the loose boxes with their long-disused racks and mangers cob-webbed over. In Dorothy's childhood the glebe was a busy working farm, with sheep and cattle. Children helped in the hay-fields all over the dales; sometimes at hay harvest a farmer and his family would work right through the night.[6] The barns were the domain of old Tommy Bowles, a dalesman from Hawes, full of strange superstitions and ghost stories, which Dorothy adored, and with a countryman's minute knowledge of the wild life of the moors. He taught her to observe the least sign of a coming change in the weather, the stillness of frost, the stirrings of a thaw, a darkness in the sky which heralded snow. Later she said this early training in minute factual observation was of the greatest help when she began to learn nursing.

In the stables were the horse that pulled the gig, and the handsome black mare on which Mark had gone hunting at six in the morning throughout the season. Rampaging through the bales of straw were a tribe of cats, while outside in the yard were hens, ducks, goslings and 'the bee house'. Here the children were allowed to build castles among the haycocks and visit the lambs in their hill fold. Dearest of pets was 'poor old Dido' the retriever, who died at last of old age; the children gave her a full scale funeral and buried her under a gravestone bearing a Latin epitaph, composed by Eleanor. As Dorothy grew older her territory began to extend to the village and the countryside around, where the trout beck ran, the winding dell overhung with oak trees, the green lanes and distant villages stretching before the Rectory and the expanse of wild moorland and heather behind. Her physical vitality was immense, and confinement unbearable to her. 'I liked tomboy games best,' she remembered. People often asked her had she thought of nursing as a child, and she replied rather doubtfully, 'Well, when I was a little thing, I used to like the idea of washing, tending and nursing dolls or people. But don't think from that I was one of those good, quiet children! I was a romp and used to riot about, just as wild, merry and noisy as a boy. When I grew older I was good at all boyish sports – riding, shooting, rowing, swimming, archery, skating – and climbing trees.'

In the winter of 1837–8 Rachel fell ill with rheumatic fever. Dr Bowes warned the family that she must be watched day and night. Dorothy demanded to help. 'I had a darling sister,' she wrote later, 'a little older than myself and as we were about the same age we loved each other specially. She fell ill; I begged and entreated to be allowed to sit up with her and was refused. But at last I got into the room and so, seeing I was there, they thought they might as well let me stay and I helped to nurse her till she was well again.'[7]

When Rachel was allowed up and they took up their lives together the two little girls aged nine and six had a conversation. 'We got talking, as girls will, about what we would do when we grew up. With me it always used to be "Oh, I'll be a nurse or a lady doctor and do everything for my patients." But my sister used to say "No. I'll not do that – I'll get married. The first one that loves me I'll take!" And do you know,' said Sister Dora relating this conversation forty years later, 'wasn't it singular? We both grew up and did exactly what we said!'[8]

At about seven Dorothy began regular lessons every morning in the dining-room.[9] There was no question of school, or a professional governess; her teachers were Jane, Eleanor and Frances. They seem to have been at boarding-school during the family's happier days and were still carrying on their own studies under the direction of Mark from Oxford. The process of improvement, as conducted by their brother, was of an abrasive thoroughness. 'I have fathomed the shallows of your scholarship

37

enough,' he wrote to Eleanor, 'to see that you will find sufficient novelties (i.e. difficulties) in much easier Latin than Tacitus.' Or again, 'Desultory reading will never do for you what persevering hard study will, if you avoid your old snare of thinking you have actually *done* much when you have read over a certain number of pages or chapters.'[10] His devoted sisters winced now and then under this continual correction, but patiently returned to their books, and attempted to apply the same high standards to teaching the little ones reading, writing and multiplication tables. They did not have to teach Frank more than his letters, for as soon as he was old enough he was summoned every day to his father's book-room to begin his Greek and Latin grammar. Mr Pattison would have given ready assent to the celebrated Oxford sermon, recommending the study of classical languages 'which not only elevate above the common herd, but lead not infrequently to positions of considerable emolument'. In some country rectories it was the custom for sisters to share their brothers' lessons. Many clergy daughters, among them Emily Davies, the future founder of Girton College, got an excellent education in this way. No one ever had the temerity to suggest such an arrangement at Hauxwell, or to propose that the younger girls should be sent to school.

By contrast, their religious education was the subject of their mother's anxious care and their father's sternest authority. Mr Pattison and his wife belonged to the older group of Evangelicals, the school of Wilberforce and Simeon, which called for 'regularity and sobriety' in worship. Mr Pattison was jealous of his authority as a minister of the Established Church. He had a gentlemanly contempt for itinerant lay preachers, 'ranters' or 'noisy professors'. Instead, the parishioners and the rectory children were summoned twice a Sunday to St Oswald's, an isolated church half buried among tall trees. There their father read the Prayer Book services, the clerk making the responses on behalf of the congregation. At sermon time the Rector put on a voluminous black Geneva gown and ascended the pulpit[11] for the 'Gospel preaching'. The gospel according to Mr Pattison consisted of election, reprobation, punishment, atonement, conversion and the absolute eternity of the torments of hell. 'To my home religion almost narrowed to two points,' Mark Pattison remembered. 'Fear of God's wrath and faith in the doctrine of atonement.'[12] Evangelicalism was above all the religion of the home, and the same doctrines were repeated daily in extempore family prayers, which every member of the family was compelled to attend.[13] Mr Pattison read the Scriptures, prayed, exhorted and castigated while his daughters and the maids knelt with their faces buried in a row of dining-room chairs. 'Lay open the universal sinfulness of nature' was the advice to a 'gospel preacher', 'the darkness of the mind, the frowardness of the tempers, the earthliness and sensuality of the affections . . . declare the evils of sin in all its effects . . . and Hell to receive all those that die in sin.' The discipline of Bible study was rigorous, with an intense, introspective, anxious application of texts to everyday situations. Dorothy loved singing hymns, but even those composed for children dwelt on the fear of death and the peril of damnation.

> *'Tis dangerous to provoke a God!*
> *His power and vengeance none can tell,*
> *One stroke of his almighty rod*
> *Can send young sinners quick to hell!*

Evangelical parents were warned to be careful lest the rod should be spared and the child spoiled. In Wesley's famous words, 'Whatever pains it costs, break the will if you would not damn the child. Let a child from a year old be taught to fear the rod . . . from that age teach him to do as he is bid, if you whip him ten times running to effect it.'

This upbringing implanted in sensitive natures a haunting sense of sin and a dread of judgment, which remained as childhood faded. 'Today I am fourteen,' wrote Agnes Jones, another future pioneer of nursing, in her diary. 'When I look back at the past year I see nothing but sin, depravity and unhappiness.' 'I keep trying to do right,' wrote Charlotte Brontë to her schoolfriend, Ellen Nussey, 'I abhor myself, I despise myself.'[14]

Nothing could alter Dorothy's passionate and self-willed nature, as child or woman, but her upbringing left her with a profound sense of her own failings. 'Oh don't talk about my life!' she once cried to the amazement of a friend who praised her self-sacrifice, 'If you really knew it you would be down on your knees, crying for mercy for me, a sinner!'[15] Meanwhile she continued to be the most wilful child in the Hauxwell nursery. For instance there was the episode of the hated bonnet, which she told to some young friends forty years later, with evident enjoyment of its absurdity. Dorothy and Rachel were given what they considered extremely ugly velvet bonnets for Sunday church-going wear. Dorothy had innate feminine vanity and a fastidious taste in clothes, which she never lost. To wear anything ugly was hateful to her, and she complained loudly about the bonnet. Complaints were useless; to waste a hat simply because one did not look well in it would be both worldly and extravagant. Rachel, always docile, submitted, but Dorothy had no intention of giving up so easily. One very rainy day Mr and Mrs Pattison set out for an engagement which involved a long drive. Dorothy ran to her elder sister and said, 'Be quick; now's our chance for spoiling our bonnets, so we can't ever wear them again!' She dragged out the hat-box and put on the bonnet, urging Rachel to do the same. Then she ran, not to their own bedroom window, but to the forbidden holy of holies, their father's study, flung open the window and stuck her head well out in the rain, until the velvet was soaked right through. Rachel timidly copied her. 'Now we'll put them back in the box,' said Dorothy. 'Not to hide them, just to finish them off.' Sunday morning came: where were the bonnets? 'Quite spoilt,' said Dorothy firmly. 'We can never wear them any more.' Mrs Pattison, who always insisted on strict, unquestioning obedience, was outraged. As a punishment she forced the two children to wear the ruined bonnets publicly to church every Sunday for months.[16] It was essential, the parents agreed, to break Dorothy's sinful will and to mortify her vanity would bring repentance, though in reality a religion of threats and prohibitions could do very little to form the character of such a child.

There was, of course, another side to the Evangelical faith, which trained up men and women of all beliefs or of none to dedicated lives. This was a deep devotion to spiritual values, an ardent longing for a deeper spirituality, which expressed itself in work to relieve earthly hardship and suffering, but never felt that 'works' alone were enough to transform the world. Dorothy Pattison's early Evangelical training in practical charity prepared her to take part in a great Tractarian experiment, the revival of the religious orders in the Anglican church. Within the household, good housekeeping was the rule. The nineteenth century convention that a lady existed to be waited on never found acceptance in the Yorkshire dales, where all hands were needed to provision a large household. Women of all social classes were active and skilful housewives, and girls were brought up to practical work. The sisters were trained in self-discipline, hard work and method. All was kept in perfect order, 'the kitchen managed', the kitchen-garden harvest, fruits and vegetables, preserved. They were taught to sew neatly, turning and re-making their own frocks, so that their small dress-allowance might be used for charity. A sampler worked by Sarah in 1839 now hangs in the vestry of Hauxwell Church, its faded verse expressing perfectly the spirit of an Evangelical home.

> *Jesus permit thy gracious name to stand*
> *As the first effort of an infant hand*
> *And as her fingers on this sampler move*
> *Oh teach her infant heart thy name to love*
> *With thy dear children may she have a part*
> *And write thy name thyself upon her heart.*

The parish of Hauxwell was large in extent and its small population scattered between the hamlets of Hauxwell East and West, Barton and Garriston. The only other educated family in the parish were the Misses Catherine and Anne Gale, patrons of the living, at Hauxwell Hall, half a mile away. They were descended from a family which included a Dean of York and Roger Gale the famous Yorkshire antiquary of the eighteenth century. They seem to have been conscientious landowners, but Mr Pattison had quarrelled with them and attacked them from the pulpit with a rancour which made his daughters blush for shame. Although the Rectory stood at the entrance to the avenue of lime trees leading to the Hall, the two households did not exchange visits for fourteen years.[17] The Pattison daughters had no social life whatever. Instead they spent their time in good works.

The sisters went far into the parish to help where they were needed. They had no money to give away, but were allowed to eat bread and cheese and give away their own dinners. They went two together, an older with a younger, visiting the hungry, with cans of food which they re-heated over the peat fires of cottage kitchens. They ran with quiet efficiency a clothing club for the Hauxwell women, arranging every November to measure, count and order cloth for the sewing party which met each week and sewed children's clothes, a service much appreciated by mothers in the village.[18] They opened a voluntary school in the village and gave an annual Christmas party for their children with presents made by themselves.[19] In the single schoolroom half-way up the village street, the Rector's daughters, under the direction of Jane gave daily lessons to some thirty Hauxwell children in the three Rs and whatever else their invention could devise. They drove out with pony and trap to fetch children from outlying hamlets and farms, and people in Hauxwell can still remember their grandparents speaking of this early school bus service. The summers of 1843 and 1844 brought them a new field of work, when epidemics of scarlet fever swept through the village. 'Young and old are going one after another, without any Christian rite,' wrote Fanny to Mark, about 'minding the sick people in the village. They have with them a good many hands, so we have a good deal to manage, but we do not dislike it, as it puts us in the way of doing a good many things we had no idea of before.'[20]

The younger girls were not supposed to share in the dangerous work of visiting the scarlet fever patients. In fact they were forbidden to enter the damp, airless cottages while the epidemic lasted, but Dorothy was deeply interested in her sisters' accounts of nursing, and anything forbidden was an irresistible challenge to her. She told the story of what followed to a young friend, who wrote it down as she heard it.[21]

Fever was very bad in our village and an old woman we knew well took it. I was going past her house one day and I thought I would ask how she was, when I found the poor old soul was left to suffer alone, with no one to do a hand's turn for her. My mind was made up in a moment. I hung up my hat and jacket behind the door and told her I had come to stay with her; never once thinking what a state they would be in at home at my absence. I stayed on until evening and then sent a message home to say where I was, and that I was going to stay all night.

The Children

The answer returned was 'You went without permission, now stay where you are until you are sent for.' So there I was, really and truly a nurse. Well, I washed and nursed her and read to her; but she grew worse and worse, and on the next night she died. There was a kind neighbour, who had looked in several times to see how we were getting on, and who came in and helped me to lay her out. She stayed with me a little while. Then she had to go home, and I was left alone with a dead person who had died under my care, in a fever-stricken house, myself having run away from home and not daring to return without permission. Then the reaction of all my excitement came on and I felt tired and frightened.

As soon as possible in the morning, I sent a very humble message to the Rectory. 'The poor woman has died. Please might I come home?' Back came the answer as before. 'Stay where you are until you are sent for.' Imagine how I felt, cast off by my own parents, as I supposed and all through my own terrible wilfulness. I was full of the wildest terror, thinking whatever should I do if I was never allowed to go home again.

In a little while, however, a carriage drew up at the door and our old nurse stepped out.[22] 'Put on your hat immediately, Miss Dorothy, and get into the carriage,' she said as sternly as possible.

It appeared that she was to take me to the seaside for a month, to get a good airing before I went among my sisters and brothers again. Then I began to dance for joy, chattering as fast as I could and pestering her with all sorts of questions, which she sternly tried to repress by saying, 'How, for shame, can you go on so? Don't you know you are sent away for a punishment?'

And all the time we were at the seaside, if ever I wanted any of the little boys and girls I played with on the sands to come and take tea with me, she always refused. 'No, no, Miss Dorothy, little girls as is sent to the seaside for a punishment ought to know better than to ask for favours.'

As the time grew near when I must go home, the old dread and misgiving came back; and I used often to ask Nurse if they were dreadfully angry.

Dorothy really believed she might be cast off for ever for her wickedness. She was genuinely bewildered to be welcomed home with kisses. 'I didn't know what to make of it all,' she said remembering the scene. They did not know what to make of it either; they might well have reflected that this was no ordinary child, but no one had very much time to give thought to the matter. They were struggling to preserve their own sanity in a renewed attack of their father's madness. The cause of this disaster was a desperate quarrel with his eldest son Mark.

NOTES

1. Pattison, 43, f. 159.
2. Ibid., 43, f. 204.
3. Ibid., 43, f. 253.
4. Ibid., 45, f. 141.
5. Ibid., 44, f. 255.
6. M. Hartley and J. Ingilby, *Life and Tradition in the Yorkshire Dales*, 76.
7. Ridsdale, 7.
8. Ibid., 13.
9. Lonsdale, 2–32, says she was too delicate for lessons 'like other children', but there is nothing in the correspondence at this date to support this.
10. F. C. Montague, *Some Early Letters of Mark Pattison*, 3–4.
11. Horton Davies, *Worship and Theology in England*, iii, 213.
12. *Memoirs*, 326.
13. Ibid., 172.
14. W. Gérïn, *Charlotte Brontë*, 33–4.
15. Lonsdale, 152.
16. Ibid., 4–5.
17. Pattison, 62, ff. 3 and 10.
18. Ibid., 46, f. 208.
19. Ibid., 44, f. 138.
20. Ibid., 46, f. 100.
21. Mark Pattison's opinion was that 'Dorothy had a far more vivid imagination than her father; she spent a faculty of invention which would have placed her in the first rank as a novelist in embellishing the everyday occurrences of her own life'. Clearly two points in the narrative are misleading, for it is implied that Dorothy Pattison,

44

like other middle-class children of her time, had a nurse and went to school, neither of which is true: but the main point of the narrative has never been challenged.

22. Sarah Watts, the Rectory cook, who stayed with Sister Dora to her death.

CHAPTER THREE

Dark Springs
1837–1845

When Dorothy Pattison was five years old, the pattern of her next twenty-five years was already being laid down by her brother Mark's experiences two hundred miles away. It was not possible for an intelligent and serious young man to live in Oxford during the late 1830s and early 1840s, without being drawn into what Mark called 'the whirlpool of Tractarianism'. Bitter controversy was beginning about all that concerned man's relationship with God. Evangelicals still believed in the literal truth of the whole Bible and the sinister machinations of all Roman Catholics. Church-going to them was a moral and social duty; a parson was primarily a preacher. Middle-class society since the Industrial Revolution had settled into a comfortable materialism, which individual religion did little to disturb. Now, for the first time, Mark Pattison, and many of his generation, met a challenge to these beliefs.

Dr Pusey, the Regius Professor of Hebrew, John Keble, Professor of Poetry and author of a greatly loved collection of poems, *The Christian Year*, above all J. H. Newman, the brilliant and profound vicar of St Mary's, Oxford, confronted him with a radically different statement of faith. Their series of *Tracts for the Times*, begun by Newman in 1833, presented the Church of England as a divine institution, created by God to embody unseen spiritual realities. Its clergy, far from being mere preachers, stood in direct succession from the apostles, as priestly mediators between God and Man; its prayer book was a divinely appointed rule of faith. These doctrines were conservative; essentially they restated the High Church ideals of the seventeenth century,

46

but they struck Mark Pattison with the force of total revolution.

The very intensity of evangelical piety in which he had been brought up, the blind beliefs to which he was devoted, his hunger for assurance of salvation all led him irresistibly into the great Oxford Movement to recapture the teaching, practice and spirit of the Early Church.[1] Respect for Dr Pusey's learning and the spellbinding charm which Newman wove around the young men of his circle completed the conquest of the stiff and shy young B.A. from Yorkshire. It was not in Mark Pattison's nature to change fundamental opinions without much anxious introspection. His brief journal entries for 1839 reveal his mental distress, 'unwell and idle, though not so wretched as last week', 'wasted time shamefully', 'walked alone'.[2] Each afternoon he walked alone, to Cumnor thicket, to the Wytham hills, on the Banbury Road, or along the Binsey tow-path, brooding over a dilemma in which reason seemed useless. Country associations still had power to charm him; he walked round Oxford market to view the Christmas beef, and when the Isis froze, promptly bought a pair of skates and skated to Iffley. Yet after each brief distraction his mind swung back to the obsessive problem. What would become of him if he died before accepting the doctrines of the true Church? All his upbringing combined to surround this question with terrors. With Newman's approval in the winter of 1838–9 he began to prepare for Holy Orders, which he interpreted both then and later in a manner totally incomprehensible to both his parents. They do not seem to have been present when he was ordained deacon in 1841. He lived and attended retreats at Littlemore with the young men who formed Newman's disciples, he translated passages from St Thomas Aquinas for Dr Pusey, he fasted, he recited the offices, he joined in waspish Oxford jokes at the expense of 'our stepmother the Church of England', and watched with anxious suspense for every smile or frown which might show his place in Newman's estimation. It was a period in his life on which he was later to look back with intense distaste, when 'reason seemed entirely in abeyance' and time which should have been devoted to scholarship was wasted on 'degrading superstition',[3] although he compelled himself to record his high church fanaticism with total honesty. From about 1838 to

47

1845 it dominated his career. When he gradually moved on into the reasoned scepticism of his maturity, he left his sisters with their always precarious home life in ruins for ever.

For the effect of the Oxford movement at Hauxwell was overwhelming. Mark Pattison complained in his memoirs of 'a vague consciousness of being wronged'⁴ because he loved his sisters more than they loved him. In this he was surely mistaken, for every letter shows the girls accepting the opinions of 'our Oxford oracle' with uncritical adoration. By 1838 these opinions were beginning to cause his mother some alarm. 'I pray you will be preserved from the errors of your Oxford friend,'⁵ she wrote, for to her rigidly Evangelical way of thinking 'the charge that the Pusey school are almost Papists does not appear ill-founded'.⁶ Hostilities were suspended during the anxious year of 1839 while Mark competed unsuccessfully for fellowships in four different colleges. When at last, almost resigned to the boredom of a country parsonage, he was elected on November 9th into a Yorkshire fellowship at Lincoln College, Mr Pattison wept with joy at the fulfilment of his life's ambition. The girls, of course, were proud and delighted; they talked of nothing else for weeks, and planned a visit to Oxford the following summer, but their mother's disquiet remained. She taxed her son with, surely understandable, reserve and constraint in his letters, adding, 'there does seem to be a decided leaning towards that Church from which we have always considered it a blessing to be separated.'⁷ It was widely believed by Evangelicals that the Tractarians were 'concealed Romanists', intent on perverting others.

By contrast Mark's sisters were swept away on a flood of Tractarian enthusiasm. Older and younger trooped down the single narrow lane which connected Hauxwell with the coach road from Bedale to Leyburn and the outside world. At the coach stop by the iron gates of Constable Burton Hall, copies of *The British Critic* sent by Mark were handed to them from the mail coach. Every evening the sisters read this Tractarian journal aloud. 'My favourite article in the B.C. was Rites and Ceremonies,'⁸ confessed Eleanor rather naïvely. As the sister nearest to Mark's thoughts and studies she took the lead. In their monotonous and lonely lives a new excitement had dawned; moreover, they were intelligent enough to read the works of Keble, Pusey and Newman and try to understand the Tractarian theology. They felt, without knowing why, that they had been starved of something essential. This now revealed itself as an ardent longing for a deeper spirituality than the teaching of their childhood could provide. They flung themselves, without considering the conflict this must arouse, into all the approved practices of Tractarian piety. It seems clear, in the perspective of a hundred years, that their hunger for fasts and festivals, for a humble place in the fellowship of the Church, was simply another expression of their mother's longing for salvation. She had taught them that they could only be saved by lonely submission to the iron will of providence. Now they began, with what joy and gratitude, to hope for a place as members of the Church created by God. The Church of England, the Book of Common Prayer, the sacraments took on a new meaning and beauty in the light of Newman's teaching 'that material phenomena are both the types and the instruments of real things unseen'. How could they fit themselves to be humble members of the Communion of Saints?

On 20th June 1841, Mark returned to Hauxwell to preach in his father's church. The text was I John iii v. 3, 'Every man that hath this hope in him purifieth himself even as he is pure.' Dorothy, aged nine, took her place with her elder sisters in the high Rectory box pew to hear the conclusions her brother drew from this verse. 'When a person confesses that he does evil, that he lives in perpetual sin, confesses that he does not even make any efforts to resist sin, to purify himself and at the same time rests in comfort upon the hope of heaven, that man is neither consistent nor reasonable in his prospects. . . . It is often said that youth is the natural season of enjoyment. The very plain answer to this sort of arguing in defence of sin is that our lives are so uncertain, we cannot calculate upon age and leisure in which to reform. . . . *Never* allow yourself any indulgence that you know to be wrong.'

Mark's sisters did their best to follow this austere call to spiritual perfection. As a first step they adopted his daily programme of prayer and spiritual reading, with all the ardour of total revolution. Mark believed, like Newman, that 'Antiquity was the true exponent of the doctrines of Christianity and the basis of The Church of England.' He therefore urged his sisters to return to the practice of the early Church. To the younger children the change was bewildering but enthralling. They listened fascinated as their sisters, in imitation of Mark, recited the monastic hours, beginning with Prime at seven each morning, and crept out of bed to hear Compline at half past ten every night. They sewed linen surplices for their adored brother to wear in church, instead of the customary gown and bands, they illuminated texts, they learnt early examples of F. W. Faber's saccharine hymns by heart. Dorothy could recite these to her dying day. Each one of them felt faint glimpses of beauty and harmony, never suspected in all their years of compulsory religious instruction.

They still attended, of course, their father's Church, almost unchanged since the fourteenth century, with long, narrow, rather dark nave, low chancel arch, rank grass in the churchyard and great beech trees overtopping the embattled tower. Dutifully they filed into the dining-room for family prayers, but now even this custom was called in question. The most intelligent, certainly the most headstrong, of Mark Pattison's converts to 'the Oxford theology' was his cousin Philippa Meadows, daughter of Mr Pattison's widowed sister Mary at Ainderby Steeple. Philippa, who dominated the household of her adoring mother and her grandmother, old Mrs Pattison, dismissed any hesitation on the part of her cousins with brusque impatience. She was an oddity, a woman of about thirty with a total absence of feminine softness or charm, and a driving, speculative masculine intellect, which Mark considered could match in power the ablest brains he knew at Oxford. Once she had accepted Mark's Tractarian arguments, all her resources of knowledge, her prodigious memory for history, Latin, Greek and logic, directed themselves against the weaknesses in the Anglican claim to be 'a portion of Christ's one Holy Catholic Church'. She was early critical of family prayers, as a source of 'the greatest irreverence in this country'. From family prayers it was logical step to the family itself, 'the exaltation of the family is contrary to the genius of true religion'.[9] Her cousins, who had been brought up to instant uncritical submission listened breathlessly when Philippa criticized their mother with all the force of her character and conviction saying, 'my aunt's doctrine of filial obedience seems to me *extreme*'.[10]

None of these discussions could remain unheard by their

father. Loneliness and cold closed in on Hauxwell in the winter of 1841, isolating the household. During the long, dark evenings with nothing to occupy him, Mr Pattison's increasing resentment of Philippa and her mother, of Mark's opinions and his influence upon his sisters, grew steadily, with the menace of a gathering storm. Two of his most powerful obsessions, pride in Mark and horror of Roman Catholicism, clashed, and the shock was too much for his sanity. At last the paranoid suspicions and resentments, which had been dormant since his breakdown, found a focus. As God's gospel minister was he to condone Popery in his own house? The storm was ready to rage over the heads of his children. One evening in mid-winter, about a month before Dorothy's tenth birthday, it suddenly broke. The day had been quiet; the first snows had already begun to fill up Hauxwell's narrow lane, the streams were freezing into silence, while their father dozed in his chair beside the grate. Stealthily Fanny drew out a forbidden book from Oxford, probably Pusey on Baptism, and began to read. Her father's eyes opened, and fastened upon her. His face slowly suffused with rage. Suddenly he began to bellow with a violence that held them rigid in their places.[11] 'You are all a pack of infidel schoolgirls with a Romish priest at your head,' he shouted. 'I am not the only one to detest him and his Popery.'[12] It was useless to try to hurry the younger children out of the room, away from the terrifying scene, since his chief complaint was that his elder daughters were plotting 'a crusade against Christianity, and an attempt to convert the children'. For four nightmare years, from now on, Sarah, Rachel, Dora and small Frank were to be in the centre of the battle. They were fought and re-fought over, like some devastated village in the wars of religion. The confrontation in the Pattison family during the early 1840s reflected in miniature the troubles of the Church of England, which indeed was almost in a state of civil war. The effect of Oxford Movement intransigence was to drive the Evangelicals into opposition and to confirm Low Church prejudice.[13] No possibility of reasoned discussion, compromise, or even of civilized agreement to differ was considered by the High and Low Church factions. Locked in what was largely a sham battle, since many of their essential beliefs were the same, the warring Anglicans failed to notice the advance of their real challenger, reasoned scepticism, which increasingly attracted some of the finest minds of the age.

Meanwhile Hauxwell Rectory resembled one of those scenes in a Charlotte M. Yonge novel portraying a large clergy family; but here the pious cast of characters was reflected in a hideous distorting-glass of hate. Philippa, of course, urged her cousins to defy their father for conscience's sake. 'I certainly should not submit an enlightened conscience to one whose *sanity* is doubtful and whose *moral defects* are manifest,'[14] she wrote, from the safe distance of Ainderby. She and her mother were both forbidden the house. So, which was much worse for his sisters, was Mark, contemptuously described by his father as 'the Father Confessor'. His name was never spoken in public,[15] though the elder sisters wrote regularly begging him for letters and demanded to know every detail of his life in Oxford.

Although their home was so remote and their daily lives so narrow, they acquired a detailed knowledge of University politics and Tractarian controversy. One of Newman's most ardent followers, W. G. Ward, a Fellow of Balliol, was censured for heresy by Convocation of the University and stripped of his degrees. Within a few days, Mark's sisters in snow-bound Hauxwell, knew every detail of the meeting at Oxford.

Nothing to be seen but snow drifting through the streets. Yet through all this 1000 MAs had found their way – Mr. Clayton from Newcastle, Elder from Durham – with many more who could ill afford it to Oxford by 1 o'clock and before that time the streets leading to the theatre[16] were well trodden by the stream of gowns of all colours and shades, which the lumber closets of tailors and scouts had turned out for the occasion.

When Ward left the Sheldonian, having been degraded by the assembled MAs to the status of an undergraduate, some students staged a demonstration in his favour.

He was received with cheers by the crowd of undergraduates who had collected round the exterior gate, while the V.C.[17] was decorously but unmistakably hissed – one impudent dog even going so far as to hurl a snowball at his red sleeves.[18]

To read such letters gave the elder sisters the sensation of living, even vicariously, and of occupying at least a corner in Mark's Oxford life.

To the younger children, university affairs mattered less than the loss of an elder brother, who might have taken a father's place in their lives. Rachel and Dorothy hoarded every memory of walks and stories with Mark on his last visit; Dorothy was not to see him again for seven years.

From the darkness of this period at Hauxwell changing scenes emerge. Their father's loathing of Mass was so obsessional that the very name of Christmas met with Mr Pattison's particular resentment, 'the termination of it being so dreadfully Papistical'. In 1842 he refused to mention the word when giving out Church notices.[19] The children's Christmas Day was much like a normal Sunday. At seven in the morning the three little girls, with Bessy the kindly housemaid, crept into their sisters' bedroom to sing a Christmas hymn to them. They spent the morning at church, took an afternoon walk, went to church again and were allowed to sing carols quietly round the fire after their father had finally retired to his study.[20] They had no Christmas tree, presents, decorations or games.

The New Year of 1843 promised worse things. Ten days before Dorothy's birthday it froze hard, and the children's spirits lifted with the promise of a skating party at Newfound England, a farm reclaimed from the moors above Hauxwell. They were gathering in the hall with their skates, when the door of their father's little book-room at the front of the house was flung open and he burst out, shouting violent abuse. He spat in Eleanor's face and cursed her so loudly that not only the servants but the villagers heard him.[21] The Papists were to be banished upstairs, not the skirt of their dresses nor the sound of their feet to be heard in a good Protestant household. For several months after that the elder sisters lived in their bedroom, where they were allowed the luxury of a small fire against the iron winter of the North Riding. Sarah, Rachel and Dorothy waited on them with devoted kindness, carrying trays of tea and toast, smuggling up Pusey on Baptism, to be hidden in the box of Tractarian volumes, which their father had threatened to burn, under the bed. 'We literally never move into the garden or even from room to room without having ascertained in what corner of his dominions he is.'[22] Dorothy, boldest and most agile of the children, was particularly adroit at spying out the movements of the enemy.

Hauxwell Rectory was a small house. It has now been pulled down, but it was hard to believe it could ever have sheltered a family of fourteen with its servants.[23] The lack of privacy, the impossibility of escape anywhere indoors, increased the strain on health and nerves. The nights were exhausting to all, for Mr Pattison hardly slept. When he did he complained of frightful nightmares and woke, sometimes weeping, more often shouting abuse at his wife and family for two hours on end. Sometimes his threats of violence turned them all out of bed, and the children, huddled in their nightgowns on the landing listening to the ugly sounds. 'Papa and Mamma at it again,' they said with matter-of-fact acceptance.[24] Mrs Pattison submitted meekly, even when her husband packed his clothes and threatened to leave her, taking Frank with him. Jane, the eldest daughter, now about thirty, had to interpose to prevent her father from striking her mother. No one could prevent him throwing a dish at her during an attack of rage at the dinner table. 'Mama felt it,' wrote Eleanor, 'but she was afraid to show her resentment. No Spring ever felt so hopelessly dark.'[25]

The one remaining outside interest of the prisoners in the Rectory was their small day-school, which they knew was valued in the village. Now even this was taken from them. One morning, the elder sisters found a crowd of children waiting for them on the doorstep of the little stone-built schoolroom. 'Why are you not in your places?' 'No more school! Master has locked school and taken t'key.' Jane had been founder and headmistress of the school from its beginning; with the courage of desperation she faced her father and pleaded for its reopening, arguing that it did nothing but good in the parish. The Rector's reply was an angry tirade on his duty to prevent 'the propagation of error'. The village would have been left without a school, had not the Misses Gale of Hauxwell Hall, anxious for their unfortunate tenants, engaged a schoolmaster and reopened it under their own management. Jane and her sisters tried not to feel jealous at the happy shouts in the playground, from which they were now excluded.[26] Their father was incensed and raved night and day against them.

At other times Mr Pattison's mood swung from rage to black

depression. Then he would refuse to speak to anyone 'above Sarah'. He refused to enter 'the Papist rooms' and sat slumped for hours in his chair beside the book-room fire, to which the younger children carried his meals on trays. A chance caller at the Rectory was dumbfounded to be met by the Rector with the question, 'Will you take your dinner with the Papists in the dining-room or the poor persecuted Protestant here?' He was cunning enough to seize the chance of exploiting Low Church prejudice against his undutiful children, especially from the pulpit. They belonged, he said, to the Almanac[27] party, while he was faithful to the Bible. In the course of at least one sermon he wept and in exaggeratedly broken voice informed the puzzled villagers of Hauxwell that 'he has thought right to rise up and leave the ungodly people who surrounded him and should advise them to do the same even though they should prove their nearest and dearest relations.'

The girls, listening, shrank into themselves with shame and prayed that the high Rectory box-pew would hide their burning cheeks.[28] Church services were conducted 'at a scrambling gallop'. Morning and evening prayer at home were given up. Easter was a time of special dread. Mr Pattison refused to allow his younger daughters to be confirmed and threatened each year to deprive the elder of their Easter Communion.[29] The pious young women never doubted the validity of the Sacrament, but felt revulsion from receiving it at their father's hands. Mr Pattison was by no means alone in his peculiarities among the clergy of remote Yorkshire villages. Their Archbishop was senile when he died at 90 in 1847. Robert Wilberforce, when appointed Archdeacon of the East Riding, wrote of the scandal caused by several mad or drunken clergymen. In his present condition at least, Mr Pattison was clearly unfitted for the office of priest, yet, as Eleanor lamented, 'all the doctors in the land would not pronounce him mad, seeing him only at a visit – no Bishop can lay hold on him – nobody will believe us'.[30] The feeling that no one knew what they suffered was desolating.

Why did Mrs Pattison take no steps to protect her children from a father who was clearly not of sound mind? The answer requires a considerable effort of theological and historical imagination. One undoubted reason was her belief in Evangelical dogma, as bigoted, if less violent than her husband's. She sincerely believed that her daughters might fall into the clutches of Rome, the scarlet woman, the beast of the Apocalypse. To save their souls she must prevent this, even if health and happiness were sacrificed in the process. The second was the fantastic, almost unbelievable, obedience which Evangelical parents, as of right, exacted from their children. 'I know nothing like the petty, grinding tyranny of a good Evangelical family,' said Florence Nightingale in a moment of bitterness, and Charles Simeon the Cambridge Evangelical advised a young man with a strong and sincere vocation to holy orders to give up the whole idea and read for the bar as his father wished. 'You are *certain*,' he wrote, 'that you are acting according to your duty in obeying the wishes of your father.'[31] In this implacable court no appeals of conscience or pleas for mercy could expect a hearing. Mrs Pattison met any complaints by her children with a pious rebuke. 'Let us pray it may please God to bring us *all* to better feelings and lead us all into the path of duty from which we have *all* deviated. The Divine blessing cannot be upon a family so sadly divided.' Mrs Meadows offered to give a home to one or more of her nieces, pointing out that they were in physical danger, but their mother refused. 'She seems to view any interference with his will as a breach of duty by her children,' wrote Philippa to Mark.[32] Mrs Meadows wrote to Mark urging a separation, and recalling her brother's violent rages for upwards of thirty years. She pointed out that the entire household lived on the watch against a blow or a missile. 'The minds of all will be sacrificed if something is *not done*.'[33] Of course, nothing was done. When Mark wrote pleading with his mother on behalf of his sisters, her reply was an icy rebuke. The coldness this caused between them lasted for years. The fact was that Mrs Pattison, worn out by incessant child-bearing, frightened, exhausted, still loved her husband and continued to love him almost to the end. Belief in his divine election was an article in her creed; nothing would induce her to accept that he was, as she put it, 'unfitted to be God's minister'. One kind word from him would make her forget past injuries, and hope again for the future. Gradually her daughters came to see that in any contest with their father they could never win. The most they could do was to persuade their mother that Mr Pattison was not well, although his physical health remained extraordinarily good. Dr Bowes when consulted, could only recommend soothing him. Dr Simpson, to whom Mrs Pattison wrote secretly for advice during 1843, suggested antimony and 'leeches to the temples'. She dared not call in another doctor for fear that resentment would make her husband worse. The girls were forced to realize that there was no hope. 'Look forward to the future I cannot,' wrote Jane, 'there is no hope for us of deliverance.'[34]

The cold winter, which set in early in 1843, confined the girls to the house. 'Our life, which is never various at any time, becomes deadly monotonous in winter,' wrote Fanny. 'If this winter is to be worse than the last I know not how it can be got through,' and again, 'Nothing will ever be done; it will never be better, but gradually get worse and worse. Do you not see that we are almost prisoners for life, with no prospect of escape?'[35] To their credit, miserable as they were, the elder sisters at least realized that the young ones were even more to be pitied than themselves. 'The little helpless, young ones,' as Jane called them, grew up in dread of their father. 'It really is pitiable,' wrote Eleanor to Mark, 'to see them so utterly trodden down and neglected by those who should bring them out and in fact educate them.'[36] During the hubbub of these years regular daily lessons were an impossibility, and the young ones never wholly recovered what they lost at this time. Compared with their older sisters, Elizabeth, Sarah and Rachel remained poorly educated, though Dorothy later made up some of the gaps in her education by sheer effort of will. Eleanor was a natural writer; her description gives a convincing picture of what the children daily faced. 'His look is dreadful, his eyes glare round the room, his colour is changed and altogether he is fearful to look at. Ever since he threw that dish we have all become so frightened of him; we never hear a strange sound in the house but what our hearts beat, and if we meet anyone unexpectedly, we give a start thinking it may be him.'[37]

As so often when a family is vulnerable, disasters fell upon this stricken household. The weakest were the first to suffer. In January 1844, Grace, a gentle, domesticated girl of twenty-two caught pneumonia. In spite of all Dr Bowes's prescriptions it was impossible to relieve the congestion in her lungs; by mid-February he warned the family that she was suffering from consumption and there was no hope. The sisters did all they could to give comfort. Dorothy was allowed to fetch and carry, to help to change the bedclothes after Grace's deathly sweats and to warm milk which was all that the patient could swallow. They took turns to sit by Grace's bed and read to her, but as she lay with eyes closed, saying nothing, it was impossible to tell whether she listened or not. Once she whispered that from the beginning of her illness she had felt quite sure she would not recover, for she felt so worn and wearied out.[38] On Ash Wednesday the sisters began their usual Lenten practice of the Hour Services, which threw the house into an uproar, as Mr Pattison rushed from room to room to break up the 'Popish meetings'.[39] Grace was seen to tremble at the angry shouting, and to twist the sheets in panic when she heard her father's step near the door. She died on 27th March at two in the morning, with all her sisters, who had been woken to say farewell to her, gathered round her bed. She was fully conscious and her bitter cries long echoed in the ears of the younger girls.[40]

Mrs Pattison dutifully accepted this further visitation of a mysterious providence. 'Let me bless the God who has sent it and pray that it may have its due influence, for we sorely need chastisement,' she wrote. The same summer Anna, who was still in her teens and the best classical scholar in the family after Eleanor, collapsed with a depressive illness from which she was never to recover, although she lived on into middle age. One hand became paralysed, and she complained pathetically, 'My whole body feels so weak and shakes terribly.'[41] She was taken to Tynemouth to consult a specialist in paralysis, but already she had slid into that passivity which provided a retreat only less secure than death. She settled into the life of a chronic nervous invalid, unable to do anything for herself. Once again Dorothy's willing hands were pressed into service; she brushed Anna's hair, dressed her and fed her. When Anna went away to the seaside for treatment Dorothy missed her patient; the outbreak of scarlet fever in Hauxwell provided a substitute and her escapade in the cottage of the dying woman dates from this summer of 1844. She was twelve, full of brains and character, though no one so far had observed them. She was searching for an outlet for her energies, some work with more meaning than the futile, unhappy daily round at home. The events of 1844 confirmed that her chosen work should be nursing.

In 1845 Mr Pattison was persuaded to take a 'composing draught' prescribed by Dr Simpson. Its effect was to depress him; he buried his face in his hands if anyone tried to speak to him, but he became calmer and, to the inexpressible relief of his family, began to sleep through the nights.[42] Gradually comparative quiet was restored. It became possible to communicate with the outside world and to take up the girls' neglected education again; but young people's growing up will not wait upon circumstances, and in 1845 another serious illness, this time her own, brought Dorothy Pattison's childhood to an end. Nothing could restore the years which had vanished in conflict and fear, and this ravaged childhood was to set her apart.

It was not until many years of nursing had sharpened her insight that Dorothy saw the tragedy of her father's wasted life. Mr Pattison was not fully responsible for his own words and actions, but his daughters were hardly equipped to understand their father's condition. They could only see that his formal intelligence was unimpaired, and so were his manners when he chose. He received a lawyer on business 'with the greatest urbanity' and conducted Frank's education just as he had Mark's. He could preach and take services, although he increasingly neglected his ill-fated parish. After 1847 he seldom took duty, he never entered one of the cottages. All his energies went into persecuting his daughters, while their mother preached submission to the loathed tyrant as a religious duty. Mrs Pattison did indeed love her children, as her later actions were to show beyond all doubt. Yet tragically, from a sense of duty, she maintained an attitude which wounded them far more deeply than their father's naked and paranoid hatred. To an appeal for an affectionate meeting by Mark she replied, 'May we meet where sorrow and sighing are no more,' a postponement which chilled him to the marrow, as well as leaving immediate problems unsolved. There is no doubt that he and the elder Pattison daughters were embittered against their mother, and influenced the younger ones to feel the same. They pointed to the tranquil, cheerful affection of other families. 'It is so painful to contrast our situation, hated by one parent, not loved by the other.'[43] The sense of injury was

Dorothy Pattison

ineradicable. The household was secretive, furtive, divided. The girls were driven to petty deceptions to carry out the most harmless plans, and the more thoughtful of them worried about the effect this must have on the younger children. Anna wrote to Mark, just before illness overtook her. 'I am afraid you will say as so often before that the ordering of our individual conduct is the thing we each ought to attend to. I trust your warnings have not been thrown away, though the task is *very, very* difficult where right and wrong is not fixed save by tyrannical will.'[44] Mrs Pattison felt that her daughters did not confide in her, and suffered because of it. 'It is one of the chief sorrows of our sad family,' she said, 'that we cannot be united in anything.'[45] Yet the chief sufferers from lack of trust and affection were always the children. Years later, when they were both eminent in public careers, Fanny exclaimed to Mark, 'If she had only cared for us, independent of what he thought, *how* we should have loved her!' The Pattison girls suffered agonies of social embarrassment in public and fear and humiliation at home. Their troubles have a certain topical interest now that the mentally disturbed, after a century of rigid seclusion, are again being advised to live in their own homes. By his wife's devotion Mr Pattison was maintained in home and profession, but the cost to his family was appallingly high. The conflict in their minds between duty and rebellion was perpetual. They were sensitive and intelligent, but the atmosphere of bitterness and alienation, in which they grew up, undermined their confidence in human relations. Moreover, they carried the burden of a dark inheritance. Suspicion and resentment, unbalanced excitement and dragging depression were woven into the fabric of their lives.

NOTES

1. *Memoirs*, 208.
2. Pattison, 7 *passim*.
3. *Memoirs*, 185–9.
4. Ibid., 36.
5. Pattison, 43, f. 205.
6. Ibid., 43, f. 200.

60

7. Ibid., 43, f. 211.
8. Ibid., 44, f. 32.
9. Ibid., 63, f. 3.
10. Ibid., 63, f. 142.
11. Ibid., 44, f. 210.
12. Ibid., 46, f. 110.
13. L. E. Elliott-Binns, *Religion in the Victorian Era*, 111.
14. Pattison, 53, f. 142.
15. Ibid., 46, f. 110.
16. The Sheldonian Theatre.
17. The Vice-Chancellor of the University.
18. F. C. Montague, *Some Early Letters of Mark Pattison*, 12–14.
19. Pattison, 46, f. 234.
20. Ibid., 44, f. 241.
21. Ibid., 45, f. 5–6.
22. Ibid., 45, f. 203.
23. J. Sparrow, *Mark Pattison and the Idea of a University*, 33.
24. Pattison, 45, ff. 69, 167.
25. Ibid., 45, f. 64.
26. Ibid., 48, f. 231.
27. That is the calendar of church festivals and saints' days.
28. Pattison, 45, f. 26.
29. Ibid., 45, f. 54.
30. Ibid., 62, f. 149.
31. D. Newsome, *The Parting of Friends*, 120. The receiver of this advice, John Sargent, fortunately disregarded it and became the beloved, saintly rector of Woolavington, Sussex.
32. Pattison, 63, ff. 142, 148.
33. Ibid., 62, f. 91.
34. Ibid., 45, f. 272.
35. Ibid., 45, ff. 128, 154.
36. Ibid., 46, f. 228.
37. Ibid., 62, f. 18.
38. Ibid., 46, f. 11.
39. Ibid., 46, f. 15.
40. Ibid., 46, f. 22.
41. Ibid., 46, f. 104.
42. Ibid., 46, f. 82.
43. Ibid., 62, f. 42.
44. Ibid., 48, f. 276.
45. Ibid., 61, f. 72.

CHAPTER FOUR

Brother and Sister
1846–1853

❉

It is characteristic of the troubled Pattison correspondence that Dorothy, who for fourteen years had never been mentioned by name in letters from Hauxwell, makes her first appearance as an invalid. On 8th August 1846 Mrs Pattison wrote to Mark, 'dear Dorothy has been almost taken from us and restored again – at least I think so.'[1] The proviso was not merely a pious formula, for Dorothy's illness was pleurisy, which, after the death of Grace, filled the whole family with alarm. Grace had surrendered without a struggle, but Dorothy fought her illness. In the painful struggle to breathe she remained almost gay, and this spirit sustained her during a long and wearisome convalescence. 'She is much better and we hope sea air will strengthen her for the winter,' wrote her mother.

Dr Bowes's first proposal was that Dorothy should spend the whole winter in the South, but Mr Pattison was unwilling to allow a daughter out of his sight for so long. 'As to the South winter scheme it is fast dying away, nothing has come or is likely to come of the thousand plans that have been whispered here,'[2] reported Fanny wearily in October. Continual whispering behind closed doors suggests the whole claustrophobic world of the Rectory. Dorothy escaped, for she was sent for some weeks to Redcar, still a small fishing village on the north Yorkshire coast. There were fishing boats, old shrimp-women, sailing ships passing on their way to Newcastle, a rocky coast and miles of clean, firm sand. The St Luke's summer of 1846 was long and fine. Dorothy adored the seaside and spent whole days on the shore.

She returned in November to a situation which confirmed her

determination to nurse. A boy in the village, a former pupil of the little school, had been ill for weeks with rheumatic fever and was now dying. Day after day he asked for Dorothy, and on the day she was expected home from Redcar he lay listening intently for the gig to come up the lane.[3] 'There she is! There's Miss Dorothy,' he cried, long before anyone else could hear the sound of wheels, and he was right. As soon as she knew the sick child was asking for her, Dorothy flung on bonnet and cloak and ran to his parents' cottage. She did not ask permission; since her illness she had grown from a child to a young girl, and appeared already certain that anyone ill had first claim upon her. She spent every day with him until he died. For some months she was considered too delicate for school work, but in the winter of her fifteenth birthday regular morning lessons with Fanny began. After so many years of irregular teaching, this discipline was very unwelcome. She preferred the ghost stories and old wives' tales of the kitchen, where she had spent so much time. 'I didn't like lessons,' she admitted frankly. 'German I specially hated, I thought it had such an uncouth sound and besides, I argued, what could be the use to me of learning music or languages.' She protested vehemently to Fanny, 'I don't want to be a fine drawing-room lady – I want to be a nurse. I shan't want them in this world or the next!' Timid, gentle Fanny was later to find her life's vocation in caring for orphan children; Dorothy remembered her patience, though, with a characteristic distortion she described her, not as a sister, but as a professional schoolmistress. 'My teacher was very patient and discerning in her management of me,' she said. 'Instead of setting me down as the ignorant girl I was, she tried to make me understand a nurse should learn *everything* she has time to learn; cooking, nursing and surgery would come later. How could I be certain I should never have French and German patients and all people would like music. After that I took an interest in every subject I studied.'[4]

As well as their morning lessons, Rachel and Dorothy took turns to read aloud each afternoon, while their sisters stitched at church needlework or hand-made shirts for Mark. Sometimes Fanny decreed 'parler Français' days, and read a French text while the young girls knitted Mark's Christmas presents, a kettle-holder for his Oxford fire-side or woollen wristlets to keep out treacherous collegiate draughts. To vary the monotony of these endless days, every one the same, the amateur governesses tried to devise new schemes of work. Eleanor wrote 'a pair, i.e. an elder and a younger one to choose some country in Europe and get it up completely, geography, manners, customs, history and give an account of imaginary travels there. We think it will do the children good.'[5] It comes as something of a shock to realize that the youngest 'child' was fourteen and the older partakers in this schoolroom pastime already young women in their late twenties, with no prospect of more adult occupation. Their only reward was the gratitude of their younger sisters. 'Their attachment and love to us is very great,' wrote Fanny to Mark, who could no longer picture the little girls he had last seen in 1841. 'They cannot do too much for us or feel too affectionately.' In 1847 Rachel was allowed to visit Mark at Oxford, an experience of mingled pleasure and dread for the shy young girl, overwhelmingly aware of her own ignorance. 'It puzzled me so,' she remembered years later, 'you don't know what a country life begets in a mind . . . oh, how I wished I was different, fit to be there – I did detest myself.'[6] Mr Pattison was calmer and more rational; he even told his wife that she might invite Mark for a visit in the Spring. Frank, an astonishingly cheerful and normal schoolboy, considering his upbringing, was sent to Rugby, apparently on his elder brother's advice. 'Such an increase of regard and good feelings,' wrote the poor mother, 'could all recollection of the past and anticipation of the future be removed, the present might be very comfortable.'[7]

Religion, however, could still provoke skirmishes in the no-man's-land between the High and Low Church parties of the household. Dorothy listened to Eleanor preparing Sarah for confirmation that summer, and longed to be confirmed herself at the Bishop's visitation in June 1847. She asked her father, pointing out that she and Rachel, at fifteen and eighteen, were both of full age to renew their vows. Mr Pattison, impregnable in his double authority as parent and priest, refused permission. The two girls felt that 'a great blessing had been neglected'. They were so bitterly disappointed that they could not even speak of the matter to their sisters; secretly they comforted one another as best they could.[8] Dorothy felt a longing to receive the sacraments, and as

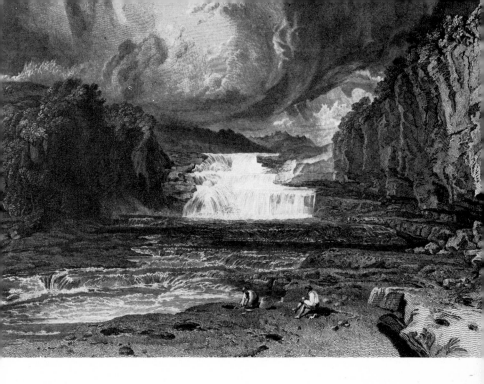

5a & 5b. Aysgarth Force and Semerwater: two scenes in Wensleydale
visited by the Pattison sisters

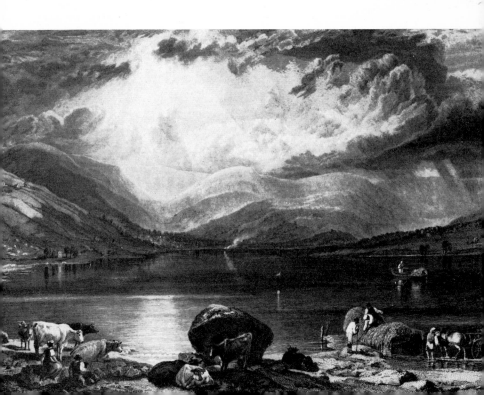

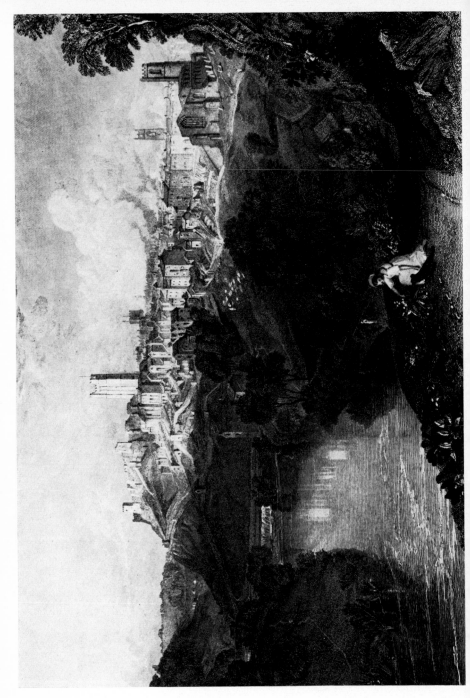

6a. Richmond, Yorkshire, from an engraving after J. M. W. Turner she had already shown, did not easily give up when she had set her heart upon something. That Christmas, for the first time in years, Mr Pattison felt well enough to go and visit his brother-in-law Captain Seward, who lived since his retirement at Cheltenham. Could she not take advantage of his absence to make her first Communion on Christmas Day? The duty was to be taken by a neighbouring clergyman, Edward Wyvill, squire and rector of Spennithorne, a village on the coach road from Bedale to Leyburn. With Mrs Pattison's permission and the Rector safely out of the way, Mr Wyvill was asked to call. 'We told him how it was she had not been confirmed, how much she wished this in her frail state of health, and that we had Mama's sanction though my father knew nothing about it.' Edward Wyvill, from his letters, was a kind as well as a courteous man, whose position as a member of one of the oldest county families in Yorkshire assured his independence. 'He said if we were quite sure she wished it herself it would be a mistaken sense of duty to keep her back – that he should be very glad to see her on Christmas Day.'[9]

Eighteen forty-seven ended with the happiest Christmas for years. At Easter 1848 Mark, convalescent after one of the many illnesses which plagued him at Oxford, was invited to visit his family home for the first time since 1841. He had contrived to meet some of his sisters during a stay at Tynemouth in 1844, and Rachel had visited him at Oxford, but Dorothy he remembered only as one of the anonymous band of 'the children' haunting house and garden. He found her at sixteen a young girl of startling beauty.[10] She had grown tall during her illness; her slender figure was supple, her features clean-cut, her cheeks youthfully rounded, almost to the last. Her dark auburn hair was brushed back to expose small, shapely ears, but no brushing now or starched caps later could ever subdue it. Her eyes were a clear, brilliant hazel, which, when the pupils were dilated, shone almost black under strongly marked brows. Her skin was fine-grained and delicate, faintly flushed over the cheekbones where the colour ebbed and flowed with a continual play of changing expressions. In later life people would turn to look after her as she passed in the street. Her voice and her laugh were fresh, unaffected, gay.[11] She adored being amused and amusing other people with her lively wit; the dreariness of life at home which so depressed Fanny or poor Anna gave an edge to her smallest pleasures. She was unquestionably, as Mark found, a natural charmer. She was also appallingly ignorant.

On her side Dorothy was fascinated by the scholarly stranger, who was also her brother. It was not easy in the crowded Rectory, where everybody wanted a share of Mark's attention, to have any private conversation with him, but she soon discovered a way to get him to herself. She remembered it years later. 'It was long ago,' she wrote, 'when you ceased to ignore my existence. How very bright life looked then, when there seemed so much to attain to. . . . You used to set out at five o'clock and walk along the Hunton lane as far as the water, and I used to put on my cloak and slip out through the garden when I thought you would be coming back, to get a walk with you alone. How you used to enjoy the song of the birds, and as we passed the dining-room window we had our joke every evening about the party sitting in silence round the tea-kettle!'[12] They crossed the grass together, the reclusive scholar, and the lively, pretty schoolgirl hugging her cloak around her against the cold of the Yorkshire evening. Feminine charm always had the power to rouse Mark from his habitual, sardonic depression. Instinctively Dorothy felt her way with him. 'You are a deep well,' she said later, 'and wells take a great deal of diving into.'[13]

To the elder sisters Mark seemed in some ways so changed as to be incomprehensible, and his fondness of 'the society of Rachel and Dorothy', caused them some heartburning after their years of earnest devotion to opinions they believed he shared.[14] The truth was that Mark was changing, if not in character then in ideas. Just as a strong emotional need had led him into Tractarianism, now secular rational interests began to lead him away from it. Eventually, though the process was only just beginning, they were to lead him away from belief altogether. At the time of Newman's conversion to Catholicism, when he left Oxford for Oscott, gossip said that only the accident of missing the coach to Birmingham prevented Mark Pattison from following him.[15] In fact the loss of his beloved leader was a profound shock, to be followed by another nearer home, the conversion to Roman Catholicism of his cousin Philippa. After the death of their grandmother Pattison, Philippa had gone south with her mother, to live in Keble's parish at Hursley. The high Anglican position could not long satisfy her ruthless logic; 'Keble himself,' wrote Mark, 'far from being a saint was discovered to be an addle-headed old hypocrite.' By 1847 both women were living in lodgings near the Holly Place Church in Hampstead, and receiving instruction before their reception into the Roman Catholic faith.[16] They drifted into the lonely rootless life, at English watering-places and foreign spas, which was so often the fate of converts. At Hauxwell all visits or letters to them were forbidden; their names were not to be mentioned. Mark must have felt some unease at the part he had played in their history.

For himself, though he maintained to the last a conventional observance of his duties as a clergyman of the Church of England, he was increasingly absorbed by his work as tutor and Sub-Rector of Lincoln College. The proper end of study began to reveal itself, he wrote, not as the maintenance of faith, but as the search for truth. He was a skilled, devoted and, by 1848, highly experienced teacher. His sister Dorothy, clever though ill-educated, had fallen into good hands. For the next twelve years Mark directed her reading; her freedom and her future work owed everything to his tutorship. The many letters she wrote him during these years have remained unpublished. In their pages a figure approaches the reader out of the unknown, a figure more complex and much more human than the plaster saint of the Sister Dora legend, a young girl of fighting spirit, self-will, humour and a deepening vocation. Mark's state of mind at this time was critical for Rachel and Dorothy. He was turning away from the religious preoccupations he later described bitterly as 'the nightmare which had oppressed Oxford for fifteen years'. The time was 1848, the year of revolution; liberty was in the air. Political and social questions all over Europe forced themselves upon his attention.[17] He was determined that his young sisters should not grow up with minds blinkered and fettered, as he believed his own to have been. He pointed out to them how much the Brontës had been able to achieve in an isolation comparable to their own. They must accept *'the Plan'*, a formal scheme of reading and writing under his direction. Rachel and Dorothy, responding with passionate gratitude to his love, were willing to accept the most caustic criticism as evidence of his care for them; Dorothy welcomed his letters as 'the greatest treasure for me'. Sitting alone in the dining-room with a bright fire, they struggled every morning through Tacitus, Pascal's *Pensées*, and a stiff course of political economy.[18] This last subject bewildered Rachel. 'My head feels bursting,' she confessed after a session with Adam Smith's *Wealth of Nations*. Dorothy's chief failing was lack of patience. 'My spur towards reading has partly died away,' she wrote in 1849. 'You warned me of that. Still the Plan forces me to it, which is good for me . . . I know I try to arrive at perfection without going through the drudgery and am therefore disappointed.'[19]

The only form of entertainment during the long, lonely winters at Hauxwell was reading. Mrs Pattison was a lover of books, as may be seen from her commonplace volumes of this period. Mr Pattison, though usually morose and withdrawn, would on his good evenings summon his family to the book-room to hear him read from Macaulay's *History of England*. He still read magnificently. Mrs Pattison later copied long passages into the commonplace books for reference and discussion, alongside extracts from Bishop Burnet's *History of his own Times*. On the evidence of the commonplace books there were, as one might expect, a good many pious volumes in the house, but there were also accounts of travels to Palestine, to Tartary, to Japan, Stewart's *Elements of Philosophy*, Montalembert on *The Political Future of England*, Chall on *The Natural History of Mankind* and Hugh Miller, the great Scottish quarryman-geologist on *The Testimony of the Rocks*.[10] Mrs Pattison's principles did not permit fiction, but the girls, once she had gone to bed, read novels aloud every evening and formed a society, inspired perhaps by the Brontës, to impersonate their favourite characters. Some of their reading was among classics they found in the house, *Northanger Abbey* and *Persuasion*, but they were also hungry for new novels. Rachel and Dorothy, as the youngest, undertook to walk over the bleak moorland road eight miles to Richmond and eight back, to borrow books from the circulating library in the Market Square. One new novel which they enjoyed reading in 1850 must surely have been smuggled into the Rectory, '*The Scarlet Letter*, a book one could not read without holding one's breath'.[21] More important, one could not read it without learning something about men and women.

As well as being anxious about his sisters' neglected education, Mark was concerned over Dorothy's health. In fact he need not have been. Old Dr Bowes, sorely tried by the various invalids of Hauxwell Rectory, was at his best in her case; he seems indeed to have been ahead of current medical opinion. 'Let the girl be a great deal in the open air,' he said. By this piece of inspired commonsense he secured for Dorothy health both of body and mind. She and Anna, as the most delicate members of the family, were sent again to spend the summer of 1848 at Redcar under Mary's care. By the autumn she was strong and well. Returning to Hauxwell she took up the freedom which Dr Bowes's prescription had secured for her. That winter she was well enough to follow the hounds on foot, the following spring she was the first visitor to Newfound England to hear the early cuckoo;[22] by her eighteenth summer she was often out gardening at six in the morning and still walking on the lawn by moonlight. She learnt to ride, first a donkey, then the Rectory horse. The younger girls went 'an exploring expedition' to the top of Swaledale, another to the Aysgarth falls and the lake at Semmerwater in Wensleydale, a third to the top of Sandbeck by the light of a summer moon. It was impossible, wrote Mark in old age, to live in the Yorkshire dales without feeling the poetry of landscape.[23] Under his sympathetic direction Dorothy, at a most formative age, grew sensitive to the freedoms and solitudes of the countryside. No one had cared so much before for her inner thoughts and feelings and she responded with touching gratitude. 'Never a day passes,' she wrote at seventeen, 'but some of your words recur to my mind and comfort me. . . . To you I owe the banishing of all desires which make me discontented with my lot. You showed me that I might be happy and find plenty to do. It is indeed the case and this place which I used to think so dull has many charms. I go over some of our walks again and love to consider what we talked about at each step; I only wish we had visited my spot on the moor; Wordsworth has become my companion; I have found someone else much interested and that is Fanny. We walked out reading it aloud to each other . . . I am a great deal in the open air and have found many flowers which were unknown to me.'[24] Mark, who prided himself on being an excellent amateur naturalist, urged her not to be satisfied with vague enjoyment of country things, but to use reference books to identify plants or insects and to record her observations. The days out of doors, which seemed idle, laid the foundations of an interest in natural science, essential to her medical work. Her character was moulded by these natural surroundings, as well as by harsh experience. Where Mark found only beauty in hills and rocks, waterfalls and moorland, Dorothy felt a sense of the power of nature. The wild, harsh landscape of the moors challenged her to fighting self-reliance, and the desires which made her discontented were to return with ever-increasing force in the years ahead. Between the heather and the sky, she felt an intense freedom.

Yet always when evening came she had to leave the dale, drowsy in the summer haze or glittering, smooth and level, under the snow, and return to the stifling neuroses of the Rectory. From these early experiences of delight and terror she learnt that dramatic instinct for the light and shade of life, which was later to fascinate every chance acquaintance.

Dorothy was not shy. The Misses Gale, with great kindness in spite of the Rector's hostility, invited different Pattison girls from time to time to their dinner-parties. For the first time in their lives the Rectory daughters wore evening dress, the best frocks from their late grandmother's wardrobe carefully 'made over'.[25] It was difficult, however, to find one subject of conversation in common in the drawing-room after dinner. Dorothy was happier visiting the relation of Edward Wyvill at Constable Burton Hall down the lane.[26] The colonnaded Hall and landscape gardens, both by John Carr of York, were minor masterpieces of eighteenth-century design. Edward Wyvill's father, Christopher Wyvill, had devoted his whole career to championing radical causes, an extension of the parliamentary franchise, Roman Catholic Emancipation and complete religious toleration. 'In him,' said his monument, 'the Love of Liberty was the natural glow of Christian Benevolence.'[27] The atmosphere in his family's home was tolerant and reasonable, in contrast with the bigotry of the Rectory. 'There certainly is an air of happiness about that house,' wrote Dorothy wistfully, 'they all appear on such affectionate terms with one another that it is quite enviable.'[28] In this sympathetic atmosphere her interests expanded and her spirits rose.

Dorothy took every opportunity of going on housekeeping

errands to the county town. She walked the old road over open moor, past the Tollgate at Halfpenny House, past Hart Leap Well, to the sharp turn and the unexpected view over the river. Richmond must be one of the most beautiful towns in England; George IV declared it 'the noblest prospect he ever beheld'. The great square keep of the Castle towers on its crag, high above the winding valley of the Swale. Far below, the river, overhung with trees, roars past the bridge and over the weir on its way to the meadows of Easby Abbey. Around the ruined castle clings a network of medieval streets and squares, into which the ingenuity of the eighteenth century has fitted terraces of handsome stone houses. From their windows the gardens fall suddenly and steeply down Richmond Hill. Richmond people, and Dorothy on her mother's side was Richmond-bred, are proud of their long history. 'There remain of its ancient glories,' wrote the historian of Richmondshire, 'besides the castle ruins, two very ancient churches, monasteries, chapels, chantries, guilds, crosses, a fine stone bridge and a famous Grammar School.'[29]

Of these the Grammar School interested Dorothy and her sisters most. Early in the nineteenth century it had become one of the great schools of the north, under the headmastership of James Tate. He was a Canon of St Paul's, a Fellow of Sidney Sussex College, Cambridge, and an admirable classical scholar, described by Sidney Smith as 'dripping Greek'. The school owed everything to him, and after his death it was rebuilt in his honour. In September 1850, the new building 'in the Gothic style' was formally opened with great festivities. In these the Pattison sisters helped. They painted heraldic banners with the arms of school and college, they commandeered greenery from the Hall gardener to make wreaths and garlands, and they served at the festival supper for the schoolboys who, in return, drank their healths with three cheers. It was 'such a gala day as we are not likely soon to forget'[30] in their monotonous lives. The charm and intelligence of Dorothy made a deep impression on the new headmaster, son and namesake of the great James Tate. The whole Tate family was renowned, said a Yorkshire writer, for 'cheerfulness, courtesy and charity'. The family was large and well-educated. The new headmaster had been a Scholar of Trinity College, Cambridge; three of his brothers and two of his sons were Cambridge men. His youngest son, James, was the same age as Frank Pattison, his schoolmate at Rugby. His wife was warm-hearted and kind; the whole large, cheerful, interesting household made Dorothy welcome like a member of the family. She met their guests, among them a son of the Rector of Croft near Darlington, 'young Mr L. Dodgson who is going to Christ Church after Christmas',[31] the future author of *Alice in Wonderland*. The change from the gloom of Hauxwell Rectory was exhilarating.

Dorothy and Rachel were at last confirmed in 1850. Perhaps the Rector finally gave permission in a fit of indifference; his eyes were beginning to trouble him and he took less and less interest in his parish. After 1850 his signature does not appear in the Hauxwell registers; Edward Wyvill took the duty for him and the registers are also sometimes signed M. Yates, who seems to have been licensed as curate.[32] His parishioners charitably accepted Mr Pattison as 'not always himself', a phrase still used round Hauxwell in speaking of him today. No proceedings were ever taken to question his fitness for his duties in any ecclesiastical court. Her father's withdrawal, and the coming of the kind and civilized Edward Wyvill brought one great happiness into Dorothy's life. For the first time since childhood she could enjoy the church services, so long dreaded by the entire family. With Mr Wyvill's encouragement in 1851 she took lessons in singing and playing from the organist at Richmond, and began the training of the village choir and singing lessons for the schoolchildren. She worked hard at her music and it became a lifelong source of happiness. Such was her power to create and share enjoyment that many beside the pupils collected in the schoolroom to hear the lessons.[33]

It seemed that nothing would ever happen to vary home life, until in October 1851 the news that the old Rector of Lincoln College, Oxford, was seriously ill threw Hauxwell into a turmoil. There was every possibility that when he died Mark, as sub-Rector, would be elected into his office. Letters from home showered upon Oxford, showing that Mark's family knew the minutest details of college politics concerning what they called '*the all-important subject*'. Probable votes among the Fellows were canvassed, cast and counted as his sisters sat over their mending. 'Though I cannot help detesting the intrigue, I should so like to see you head of Lincoln,' wrote Fanny. Eleanor voted her brother 'immeasurably superior and the Maker of Lincoln College', while Rachel was convinced that 'every right-thinking person in the University must see that *you ought* to be Rector'.[34] By early November Mr Pattison, past quarrels temporarily forgotten, talked of nothing else as he sat over the fire. Even Mrs Pattison, ever fearful of the snares of worldly ambition, offered her son 'my most earnest prayers that you may be guided in all your doings (especially at this eventful period of your life), by That Spirit which cannot err'.[35] To Dorothy the election seemed like the blowing of the wind from a world of decision and action which she could imagine only in daydreams. The village, led by the family, confidently expected Mark's success; in fact the schoolmaster asked him to send the result 'by Electric Telegraph to Richmond that I may convey the joyful tiding to the young ladies at the Rectory'.[36] Nothing so joyous, so exciting, had happened in their lives before.

From this peak of expectation they suffered a sickening plunge into disappointment and misery. On 14th November 1851 came the news that the Fellows of Lincoln, meeting the day before, had elected as their new Rector James Thompson, described as 'a grotesque divine', more suitable as master of a workhouse than an Oxford college.[37] Indeed sporting undergraduates were known to make bets on whether their jovial billiard-playing Rector could read or write. It was some time before the Pattisons or the outside world in general could unravel the tangle of Common Room intrigue which had led to this ludicrous fiasco.[38] The affair became one of the great, classical scandals of Victorian Oxford. All Mark's sisters knew as the days dragged on towards Christmas was that their dreams of triumph were dashed. 'Among all the disappointments and annoyance of life let us look on High and endeavour to improve these sad events,' urged Mrs Pattison, but her children were too heartsick to listen to her pious advice.[39] The result, wrote Mark bitterly, was 'a just punishment for having fixed my hopes on an immediate name and position for a member of our family'. The loss to his sisters was lasting; it cost them their brother as they had known him. For the Rectorial election of 1851 was the turning-point in Mark Pattison's life. For a time he was plunged in a stupor of misery. 'The fiasco was so terrible,' he wrote, 'that I did not feel it worth while trying to keep up appearances.' As his father had never got over the tragedy of 1834, so, to a minor degree, the son never forgave or forgot the events of those days in 1851. Years later he could write 'the killing sense of disappointment comes to me in gusts as keen as ever'.[40] He was to grow morose, suspicious, increasingly self-absorbed, but for the moment all he could feel was a blank, dumb despair, which paralysed his mind and filled his whole being. He woke to it every morning, though indeed it never left him even in sleep. 'You must estimate the crash sufficiently,' he wrote to his sisters, 'which, as far as my academical career is concerned is utter, complete and hopeless.' His very looks changed; his long hooked nose, sparse beard and withered skin reminded one observer of a bird of prey. He grew wizened and wintry, his silences more prolonged, his sarcasm more biting, even towards his sisters who loved him so blindly. Yet the sisters shared generously in his distress; they were all 'excessively, miserably, disappointed' on his behalf. Dorothy and Rachel were too young and too unworldly to see how closely it concerned themselves. As Mark's favourite sisters they could have hoped for help, hospitality, perhaps even a home in Oxford if he became Head of a House. By his defeat, Dorothy was condemned to ten more long years at Hauxwell. Already at twenty she was beating her wings against the bars of home; she would be thirty before the battle for personal freedom was won.

This independence had not been in any way Mark's intention when he began to educate her four years before. He always regarded culture as an end in itself. 'All my energy was directed upon one end,' he wrote, 'to improve myself, to form my own mind.' Continually, and to his sisters rather inconsiderately, he pointed out how lucky they were to enjoy rural solitude for reading and thought.[41] Fatally for his own happiness he expected to mould the people he loved, especially if they happened to be young women, to his own ideal. He had no conception of the growing independence and strength of Dorothy's character. As she read, wrote and studied under his direction, thought appeared to her in a very different light, as the prelude to useful action. This point of view began to show itself in the earliest letters she wrote him, while she was still a schoolgirl. 'Sometimes I feel so *useless*,' she wrote during her prolonged convalescence, 'as if I had nothing to do but please myself and though I try to argue and prove the contrary, I am not convinced. At other times I see I have plenty of duties and am only sad to think how few I perform. I long to be able to look at my own actions with a less partial eye.'[42] She had never been a spoilt child, and she was not thinking of pleasing herself when she felt the first stirrings of a profound disquiet. 'Do you think Emulation is wrong?' she asked anxiously at seventeen. 'This question has been very much in my thoughts. . . . There are times when books and walks which one day pleased me seem insipid the next and then how I long to converse with you, for I am perplexed to know what is right.'[43] The sisters had all been taught to feel what Eleanor called 'a keen sense of their own inferiority in mind, education and sex,' and they could not help contrasting this with the care lavished on the education of Frank who was now cheerfully passing through Rugby with the minimum of work. As his anxious sisters reported, 'he does not care to get forward, he has no ambition, no industry and no desire to go to college'.[44] The rest of them accepted this contrast as one of the facts of nature, but Dorothy, by the time she reached her twentieth birthday, could no longer do so.

More seriously for her immediate peace of mind, she could no longer accept the tyranny of her father's absolute rule with the same weary resignation the other women of the family had learnt over the years. Her ineradicable generosity was already roused by the wrongs of others more than by her own. She saw her sisters promised a trip to London, for which they prepared with great excitement, and which was then cancelled without warning, when their trunks were already packed and the carriage at the door. 'We are not too disappointed,' said Fanny, 'for we never expect to go anywhere until we are actually on the railroad.'[45] Dorothy raged on their behalf. On another occasion she saw their silent misery when the whole village was invited to a party for the school which they had founded, and from which their father had shut them out. 'You can have no idea', Dorothy wrote to Mark, 'what a deep interest they took in the school, how all their thoughts were centred on it and what a blow it has been to them. It really was melancholy to go up the village and see it deserted and we the only people cut out. I cannot mind as I had nothing to do with the former school, but I *longed* that I could give them some comfort.'[46]

Few things roused her to such open anger as the treatment of her childhood friend, the farm-hand Tommy Bowles. In a fit of temper Mr Pattison dismissed the old servant who had been twenty-five years with the family and was now too old to find another post. He was only saved from the workhouse by the kindness of a daughter-in-law who took him in. To part with his young ladies was a terrible grief. 'I think if anyone with any heart at all had seen the tears running down that old man's face it must have moved them,' wrote Dorothy, choking with indignation. 'I do not know that I have ever felt so powerless, so tied, not able to do anything to show the anger I was feeling.'[47] There was also the spectacle of their mother, broken by a marriage, in which twenty years of continuous childbearing had been followed by twenty years of domestic strife. 'Mama looks quite haggard, so worn and worried it makes me miserable to look at her.' Mr Pattison was now engaged in a quarrel with his sister over the trusteeship of their own mother's will, and suspected his wife of complicity. 'I do not know that I ever saw him treat Mother so ill, he treats her with such contempt that we cannot bear to witness it, and she feels it most acutely.'[48] In fact by 1852 he was moving towards another of his periodic outbreaks, but this, as always, his wife refused to recognize. As Eleanor and Fanny reported in a metaphor of undisguised bitterness, she 'licked his hand whenever it was raised to strike her' and ordered her daughters to do the same.[49] When Mark wrote to urge her to protect his sisters from their father's rages, she regarded this criticism of 'God's Minister' as 'another bitter drop in the cup which it has pleased My Heavenly Father to give me'.[50] An acrimonious correspondence followed, and in the summer after Dorothy's twentieth birthday, Mark went for his usual fishing trip to Scotland without calling at Hauxwell as he had promised, to his sisters' great distress. For a long time Dorothy refused to give up hope of seeing him; lying awake at night she imagined every sound of a gig in the lane, or every quick step on the gravel might be his. When she realized he would not come, the disappointment was cruel. She was left with 'that craving I feel in my heart for something further than this'.

Mrs Pattison began to look ill and lost weight; her daughters said she had 'gone to nothing'. She suffered several sharp attacks of bronchitis through which Sarah and Dorothy nursed her. She got up from them exhausted and increasingly crippled with rheumatism.[51] During the winter of 1852–3 she could hardly stir outside the house. She was sad and querulous; it wrung Dorothy's heart to see her. The year drew in. The dark evenings with nothing to do made Mr Pattison restless and irritable; he would walk aimlessly up and down the sitting-room for half an hour at a time. Ominously, he began to be wakeful and noisy at night. The thought of long lonely winters imprisoned at Hauxwell in the shadow of this self-torturing pair, who destroyed their own children, oppressed Dorothy and Rachel like a physical weight.

What was to become of them? This was the question they discussed at night, when the servants had gone to bed and they could at last find privacy beside the dying kitchen fire.[52] They had been reading an Anglican sermon by the future Cardinal Manning on 'Our Appointed Work in Life', and it had left them both saddened, for it was so clearly addressed only to men. 'People say women's work is in her home, to learn home duties,' said Rachel; but Dorothy, always bolder, objected. 'What if she feels she could do more, could read, and that the more she does, the more she could do, and that everyday occupations tie her down and hinder her, what should she do?'[53] Rachel applied timidly to Mark for guidance 'it is not that I wish to avoid these things but I want to know how far I may refrain from them and how far it is lawful to indulge oneself in one's own way?' In the same year, thirty-two-year-old Florence Nightingale wrote, 'Why have women passion, intellect, moral activity – these three – and a place in society where no one of the three can be exercised?'[54] Many less articulate wives and daughters felt the same longing to serve, though the Pattison sisters in snow-bound isolation had no idea they were not alone.[55] Dorothy longed for an active life. Her intelligence, her imagination, her strong will, all clamoured to be put to work, and belief, for her, demanded action. The only hope of escape seemed to be marriage; but in January 1853, the month of Dorothy's twenty-first birthday, a renewed crisis showed how hazardous marriage might be for a member of their family.

NOTES

1. Pattison, 61, f. 48.
2. Ibid., 61, f. 59.
3. Lonsdale, 7, says Dorothy had been 'travelling abroad'.
4. Ridsdale, 18.
5. Pattison, 62, f. 10–11.
6. Ibid., 62, f. 199.
7. Ibid., 62, f. 190.
8. Ibid., 48, f. 181.
9. Ibid., 62, f. 202–3.
10. No photograph exists of Dorothy Pattison before the age of twenty-seven and no portrait in colour before the last year of her life. All accounts however agree that her earlier beauty lay in colouring and expression.
11. Lonsdale, 11–12.
12. Pattison, 53, ff. 133–5, 179–81.
13. Ibid., 53, f. 134.
14. Ibid., 47, f. 202.
15. Sparrow, *Mark Pattison and the Idea of a University*, 76.
16. *Memoirs*, 227. Mark Pattison remembered their 'perversion' preceding that of Newman, but Pattison, 62, f. 64, establishes it as 1847.
17. *Memoirs*, 236.
18. Pattison, 47, ff. 322, 485.
19. Ibid., 47, f. 511–2.
20. Ibid., 68 and 69.
21. Ibid., 50, f. 166.
22. Ibid., 47, f. 485.
23. *Memoirs*, 123.
24. Pattison, 47, f. 322.
25. Ibid., 47, f. 284 and 62, f. 162.
26. Lonsdale, 42, does not identify by name the family friend and neighbour to whom Dorothy turned for advice as long as she lived at Hauxwell, but Edward Wyvill seems the only available neighbour to fit the part.
27. V. H. H. Green, *Church of St. Andrew, Fingall*, 8.
28. Pattison, 48, f. 362.
29. T. D. Whitaker, *History of Richmondshire*.
30. Pattison, 48, ff. 158–9, 178, 350.
31. Ibid., 49, f. 191.

32. V. H. H. Green, *Hauxwell Church*, 20 and personal information.
33. Pattison, 49, f. 219.
34. Ibid., 49, f. 273.
35. Ibid., 49, f. 266.
36. Ibid., 49, f. 282.
37. J. Sparrow, *Mark Pattison and the Idea of a University*, 100.
38. They are described in *Memoirs*, 272–87, and analysed in V. H. H. Green, *Oxford Common Room*, 150–62.
39. Pattison, 49, f. 294.
40. V. H. H. Green, *Oxford Common Room*, 169.
41. Pattison, 48, f. 276.
42. Ibid., 47, f. 511–2.
43. Ibid., 47, f. 322.
44. Ibid., 48, ff. 348 and 352.
45. Ibid., 49, f. 122.
46. Ibid., 48, f. 231.
47. Ibid.
48. Ibid., 48, ff. 296 and 301.
49. Ibid., 45, ff. 35 and 70.
50. Ibid., 45, f. 267.
51. Ibid., 50, f. 234.
52. Ibid., 50, f. 166.
53. Ibid., 48, f. 10–11.
54. F. Nightingale, *Cassandra*, printed as Appendix A in R. Strachey, *The Cause*.
55. J. Manton, *Elizabeth Garrett Anderson*, 40–50.

CHAPTER FIVE

Affairs of the Heart
1853–1857

At Hauxwell there seemed no room for affairs of the heart. The sisters had very little social life of any description. The theatre, card playing or dancing were considered too worldly; even the simplest gaieties, visits from friends, croquet-playing or musical evenings such as their contemporaries enjoyed, seem to have been denied them. It was therefore a total surprise when Eleanor, who at thirty-six seemed to her young sisters a middle-aged woman, announced her engagement to Frederick Mann, curate at the village of Patrick Brompton, near Bedale, the son of a Colonel. Their surprise was as nothing to their father's fury. The old scenes and paroxysms of rage were renewed, with the old manic force, but this time in public. In January 1853 Mr Pattison stormed out of the Rectory 'shouting that Mr Mann was master of the house and not himself' and that he would not return 'till he could call his front door his own'. He took the gig and drove to the King's Head, the fine coaching inn which stands in the market square at Richmond. Mrs Pattison, appalled by the scandal in a town where her family had been respected for generations, set out in a hired fly to fetch him back, but her husband would not even see her and she was forced to take shelter with Dr and Mrs Bowes. The Rector remained at the King's Head, publicly 'raving and threatening to knock Mr M. down'[1] for his presumption as a poor and obscure country curate in offering marriage to a member of the Pattison family. He shouted, for all to hear, that the couple could starve and disgrace themselves, he would not give them sixpence, 'and I do not believe he ever will' reported Mary.

Mr Mann appeared to his fiancée's sisters as a far from romantic figure, but even Dorothy admitted he behaved well. Mr Pattison, beside himself with rage, was prepared to use even his own madness, as a weapon in the fight. 'I am not pretending to be passionately in love,' wrote Eleanor to Mark, 'I am only deeply grateful to Providence for having given me a refuge and a home at last, but he is going to tell Col. Mann there is insanity in the family to influence his son to give up the affair. Tell me what I must do.'[2] Frederick stood by his promise of marriage, even in the face of this threat, but the sisters were deeply angered by it. They remembered how, at their mother's command, they had always kept their father's condition a secret from the world outside the village; 'we have always kept his affliction to ourselves when we might often have cleared ourselves by mentioning it'.[3] Now all this sacrifice was in vain. They assured Eleanor of their love and support in the most practical way by sewing her trousseau, and a neighbour gave her meals and a bed, when her father was at last persuaded to return home. Eleanor had one encounter with her father however. He ordered her to fetch a bucket and scrubbing brush from the back kitchen. When she brought them, he pointed and said, '*There* is your dowry; *there* is your future.'[4]

Mrs Pattison's chief concern, as always, was for her husband. She consulted Dr Bowes, who advised holding the wedding as quickly as possible, so that the offending couple could be hurried away to Frederick's new parish at Wyham in Lincolnshire. Meanwhile the Rector should be kept as quiet as possible. 'I could hardly wish him to be present on the occasion, as the excitement of it would quite overcome him,'[5] wrote his anxious wife. The sisters only felt a longing for it all to be over, 'to carry through the whole affair with as much decency as we can.' On 25th January 1853, Edward Wyvill performed the marriage ceremony at Hauxwell, while the Rector, in a paroxysm of thwarted fury, locked himself into the hay-loft behind the house. 'O God,' exclaimed Mark when he heard of it, 'for what cause is this curse inflicted upon us!'[36]

Mark felt bitterly the humiliation his sisters endured at this time, but perhaps even he did not realize its full effect upon Dorothy. At twenty-one she endured an experience which marked

her for life. From this time began her passionate desire for independence, her inner reserve, her iron will to work. The kindness
of local families, though she acknowledged it, grated upon her.
She could accept with real gratitude only the sympathy of the
servants and the villagers whom she loved.[7] The one exception
to this rule, because of his tact and understanding, was Edward
Wyvill, 'the only person we know who, while he is very civil to
Father, really seems to take an interest in our well-being'. She
kept in touch with Mark, but since his failure to achieve the
Rectorship he had withdrawn from personal relationships and
spent much time on solitary fishing-trips or travels abroad. In
college he was beginning to acquire his lasting reputation for
boundless learning and icy unsociability, 'the inscrutable sage in
the rooms under the clock'.[8] Dorothy still loved him, and longed
for his support, yet like all his sisters she learnt to fear his freezing
manner of sitting in judgment upon them. There was no hope of
seeing Mark while their father's present state of mind lasted, but
from sheer force of character she persisted in the reading he
recommended, philosophy, history, politics, music and languages,
botany, and current affairs from newspapers which she never saw
unless Mark sent them.[9] Only, as 1853 and 1854 dragged wearily
along, she sometimes wondered: for what?

Eleanor's defection introduced a new obsession, which became
as much of an *idée fixe* with the Rector in the next decade as
Popery had been in the 1840s. None of his daughters must marry;
they must all stay at home to keep the family and the family
fortune intact. 'Since Eleanor's marriage,' reported Fanny, 'he
vows we shall go nowhere and see no one. Now in a free age like
the present, how is this to be borne?'[10] Such behaviour, not
unknown in other Victorian fathers, is usually explained by
unconscious sexual jealousy. This may have played a part here,
but it seems more likely that Mr Pattison's fundamental hunger
was for power, since he was equally determined to keep his
favourite son Frank under his control. The way to assert power
over his children was through money and threats about money;
allowances, settlements, wills and codicils form a recurrent theme
for the rest of his life. Frank had left Rugby, a pleasant, healthy,
active young man, with no intellectual interests, but a liking for
horses and open-air life. His great wish was to enter the army,

the profession of his grandfather and his cousins the Sewards. Mr Pattison refused either to buy Frank a commission in the cavalry or to set him up in business. He was kept at home in idle boredom, escaping when he could to hang round the famous racing stables at Middleham in Wensleydale.[11] The daughters were to be brought to heel by refusing them money for any purpose whatever. 'The Jailor has taken a new phase of tormenting us,' wrote Dorothy in open revolt. 'He will not pay for anything, not even necessary articles of clothing.'[12] The sisters were ashamed to go into the shops at Richmond, where their mother's father had been Mayor, knowing that their bills were unpaid. For the next few years they were forced to make their own clothes from the cheapest materials, which quickly wore out and did not keep them warm in the northern winters. Dorothy, attempting to write to Mark from her bedroom, had to break off the letter because her numbed fingers could no longer hold the pen. Her sisters suffered so much from cold that their cousin Captain Elliot Seward actually sent Fanny a warm cloak to wear after an illness, and Mark lent his mother ten pounds to distribute pocket money to these young women in their twenties and thirties.[13] She herself was continually worried by lack of petty cash; as her daughters reported, 'her purse is in a miserable condition; he gives her nothing'. She was especially distressed to be unable to help Eleanor, now facing her first confinement at the age of thirty-seven in extreme clerical poverty. Even to this repressed and inhibited woman a first grandchild was a moving event. The daughters determined to help their sister; by re-using old linen they made every stitch of the baby's clothing, and smuggled it out of the house to post to Lincolnshire.

Why did they endure it? For Mrs Pattison the subjection of women was a matter of religious belief, since it was directly due to the Fall as narrated in the Book of Genesis. Her daughters, taught by their brother, took a less fundamentalist view. They were able bodied and intelligent women. Why did they not leave home? The answer involves the whole legal and economic position of women before the pioneers of the feminist movement had done their work. These latter were not, as was sometimes said at the time, unchristian and undutiful, nor, as is sometimes said now, neurotically ill-adapted to their feminine role. Like other

Victorian reformers their first concern was to remove unnecessary human suffering. It was still true, when J. S. Mill wrote fifteen years later in 1869, that 'The sufferings, immoralities, evils of all sorts, produced in innumerable cases by the subjection of individual women to individual men are far too terrible to be overlooked'.[14] A deserted wife had no right to maintenance until 1886, a separated wife, even in cases of cruelty and assault, until an amendment of 1895. A wife's property, unless withdrawn by legal settlement, remained in the absolute control of her husband until 1870; the guardianship of children rested entirely with the father until an act of 1886.[15] Mill's essay dealt mainly with the legal position of wives, but all these disabilities applied equally to daughters, as Mr Pattison's daughters were soon to discover. In 1854, goaded beyond endurance, they asked Mark whether if they left home they would have any legal claim upon their father for support. Mark, at what cost to his pride one can only imagine, consulted a lawyer. The answer was, 'No, not a penny.'

Their only other resources would be to run away from home and find work. 'Surely,' urged Fanny, 'there is no disgrace in working for oneself rather than submit to this?'[16] But, apart from the fact that they had no ready money even for their fares, what were they trained to do? The only occupation open to educated women was that of governess. In 1851 it was estimated that there were 24,770 governesses in Britain; for one post, at a salary of fifteen pounds a year, 810 applications were received. Nursing, which Dorothy longed to do, was the work of a domestic servant, unimaginable for a clergy daughter. Mark's advice to his sisters was 'they had no alternative but to stay at home and stick it out to the end'.[17] The misery of Hauxwell was exceptional, but Mill ends his essay with a haunting picture of a wilderness of suffering concealed beneath the surface of respectable family life. 'How many,' he wrote, 'are the forms of animalism and selfishness, often under an outward varnish of civilization, living at peace with the law, maintaining a creditable appearance to all who are not under their power, yet sufficient to make the lives of all who are so a torment and a burthen to them?'[18]

A woman in such a situation needed great courage to make her escape. This Dorothy Pattison possessed, but for the present she could not bring herself to use it. She was held prisoner by the very instinct which made her long to work as a nurse, compassion for suffering. While Mrs Pattison dragged out her weary invalid's existence, her daughter could never leave home. It was not even that she loved her mother greatly; the compulsion to serve was stronger than ordinary affection. 'She suffers a great deal of pain', reported Dorothy to Mark, 'and scarcely ever finds a comfortable position. Her helplessness is pityable and it grieves me to fulfil all the little offices of kindness to her from duty not from love, but oh she is so unlovable! You may pity her weakness, but that is the tenderest feeling you can imagine.'[19] Nevertheless she did not, apart from one attempt, consider leaving her mother to be nursed by anyone else. Just so, twenty years later, Florence Nightingale, after years of fame and independence, returned to care for the blind and senile mother with whom she had been in conflict since girlhood. To such women helplessness and suffering presented an overpowering claim. The duties of nursing were shared between Dorothy and Sarah, a quiet dependable girl, whose great kindness now showed itself. Dorothy's instinct was to surround a sick person with a cheerful atmosphere, not easily achieved in the Pattison family circle. Mr Pattison seemed to be beyond help; he looked wretchedly ill, seldom got up before eleven and hardly left his chair in the book-room all day.[20] Dorothy found an ally in Frank, still at home with no occupation. The pony-cart stood idle in the coach-house because Tom, the horse which pulled the dog-cart, was too powerful for its harness. Frank ordered and trained a pony from the famous Middleham horse fair, and after months of persuading Mr Pattison to pay the bill and Mrs Pattison to enter the carriage, Dorothy was able to drive her mother out for a change of air in good weather.[21] The autumn of 1854 was fine; hopefully, Dorothy tried to please the invalid with the beauties of the great sweeping valley around them. 'I wish you could see some of the tints we have here,' she wrote to Mark at Oxford, 'browns, reds and greens – it is rich.'[22]

At the same time, she made her last open attempt to leave home, inspired by a desire to serve which she felt her parents must recognize. The occasion was the war in the Crimea, which penetrated even the remote world of the Yorkshire dales. The mill at Aysgarth in Wensleydale spun yarn, from which women at their cottage doors knitted the first Balaclava helmets. November and December of 1854 brought the first news of Florence Nightingale's work in the Barrack Hospital at Scutari. Everything in Dorothy's everyday life was reduced to insignificance by the comparison. 'I feel ashamed to be weighing petty trifles here', she wrote, 'while Miss Nightingale is acting so heroically abroad.'[23] She made up her mind to beard her father, sitting sullen and silent in his chair beside the fire, and begged to be allowed to volunteer as a nurse. His reply was, 'You would be worse than useless and you have plenty to employ you at home.'[24]

Considering Dorothy's age, not yet twenty-three, and her total lack of training, this was probably true. Yet, unlike hundreds of girls who dreamt of volunteering for the Crimea, she had the ability and the will to learn. Her father's objection was in reality deeper-rooted than the reason he gave. It involved one of the more curious paradoxes of Victorian social history, the contrasted attitudes of High and Low Churchmanship towards women's work. By the middle of the nineteenth-century many people were disturbed that the Church of England, with its middle-class clergy and institutions, was unable to reach the working classes in the cities of the industrial revolution. High Church clergy, sometimes banished for their unpopular opinions to poor parishes, discovered overwhelming squalor, often neglected since the 1760s. Parish priests tried to organize work among the sick poor and children, paupers and prostitutes, but were limited by lack of reliable workers for district visiting, night refuges, fever nursing, orphanages or ragged schools. Who would be willing to do this hard, thankless work, and show in practical terms that the Church of England was at last concerning itself with social justice? The question answered itself. Groups of pioneers, members of the new Anglican religious communities for women, were waiting to be used. There were never enough of them and they had to improvise their own training, but from the first they proved their worth. 'The sisters who work in my parish', wrote an Anglican clergyman, 'are not creations of fancy or romance. On the contrary they are willing to do what others will not do.'[25] The sisters lived among the people for whom they worked. They formed strong ties of personal affection among the poorest classes, and by devoted service they were able to cut across class barriers in a way the clergy very seldom could. Their freedom from social convention made pioneer work possible, especially that favourite of Victorian good causes, the reclamation of prostitutes. Fourteen of the most experienced nurses with Florence Nightingale in the Crimea were Anglican nuns. By the middle 1860s Anglican sisterhoods offered a young woman wishing to do teaching, welfare work or nursing opportunities she could never hope to find as an individual.[26] The Oxford Movement, so traditional in its theology and doctrine, found itself strangely allied with the revolutionary struggle for the emancipation of women.

This fact was quickly seized upon by the Low Church party as a threat to the sanctity of family and domestic life, one of the fundamental dogmas of Evangelicalism. Serious teaching or nursing work was attacked, less as bad in itself than as a rival to the infallibility of the husband and paterfamilias. 'I believe no blessing will ever come', wrote A. C. Tait, while Bishop of London, 'on work however self-denying which is undertaken to the neglect of those higher duties which belong to *home life* and which are imposed by God himself.'[27] Samuel Wilberforce, Bishop of Oxford, in what he clearly regarded as the ultimate condemnation, complained of the 'un-English tone' of religious communities. This prejudice of the British public could be aroused to violence, as in the churchyard riots which took place at Lewes in 1851 during the burial of a young nursing Sister from the East Grinstead community. Florence Nightingale regarded *'Family'* as the idol, the fetish of the Evangelical party, jealously reserving women for its own uses. It was unthinkable that an Evangelical clergyman, who was also father of a family, would be willing to surrender his daughter to a conflicting authority. Moreover the calling of nurse, 'earning her guinea a week' in private families by the most menial duties, could never be reconciled with Mr Pattison's idea of his own family's social position.

Dorothy could hardly have expected her father to let her leave home for a nursing training; but she was still young, philosophy did not come easily to her, and she cried bitterly before she accepted his decision as irrevocable. Her desire for vigorous action brought one result; at some time in 1854 or 1855, she was allowed to go with Frank to the Meets of the two local hunts.[28] One was the Bedale subscription pack, the other, the pride of the

district, the Wensleydale hounds. 'Our vale possesses a pack of
hounds,' said a local writer, 'which will follow any animal from
a jack weasel to an elephant.'²⁹ Their cry, and the sound of the
hunt servants' horn, meant freedom and action to Dorothy.
Hunting became a passion. Hounds met at six o'clock in the
morning at inns and country houses scattered all over the dale.
The freshness of these autumn mornings, the light wreaths of
mist, the diamonded grass, were unforgettable. Tom, released
from the shafts of the Rectory dog-cart, pulled hard on the bridle
and kept his young rider up with the field. The country of the
Yorkshire dales provides rough riding, with steep fells, river-
crossings and sharp stone walls to jump, but it had no terrors for
Dorothy. 'It was a fine day, a very large field, and we had a
splendid run,' she wrote to Mark. 'Tom was in first-rate condition, he took Witton Fell with the best hunters, though the
descent was the most difficult part to me, for I could not hold
him in. We ran to near Masham and I kept up the whole way,
though Tom pulled hard on the bridle as usual. There is nothing
like a run after foxhounds for getting to know the countryside;
I will make you laugh one day with an account of my hunting
days.'³⁰ In a season's hunting Dorothy's sisters noted how fast
she developed independence, quick judgment and physical cour-
age.³¹ Other riders noticed the daring young horsewoman, so
slender and supple in her close-fitting, side-saddle habit, her
cheeks flushed by cantering against the wind. She was allowed so
few pleasures that a day's hunting had all the charm of a magical
adventure. Rachel, who sometimes accompanied her, was gentler,
more timid and too delicate for hunting over rough country. The
affection of the two sisters, and perhaps some remembered gossip
about their unhappy home life, added an element of mystery to
their charm.

What followed remained a mystery to their family, and could
only have happened in a home where total repression had produced a habit of almost total concealment.³² Meets of the local
farmers' hunts were easy-going, sociable affairs. Among those
who gathered at inns and village greens were two young dalesmen
who had ridden by the old bridle road along the slope of Penhill,
still a short-cut from Aysgarth to lower Wensleydale. They are
called in Rachel's letters by the initials R.S. and P.S., but it

becomes clear that they were Robert and Purchas, two of the
four surviving sons of a farmer, John Stirk, and his wife Abigail
of Thoralby.[33] The village of Thoralby is scattered among
wooded ravines in the wild and rugged Bishopsdale, set below a
waterfall called the Silver Chain. Its weather-beaten farm houses
are built of stone, with huge, cavernous fireplaces. A hundred
years ago, it was exceedingly remote. Its people had spoken the
old Norse language until the reign of Queen Elizabeth I, and
still spoke a dialect of Norse derivation. Their staple food, oat-
cake, was called havercake from the old Norse 'hafri' for oats.
Thoralby means Thorold's Farm and Stirk 'a young bull'.[34] The
Stirks were working farmers. John, father of the boys, had only
become a farmer on his marriage into the Tennant family, farmers
at Burton Rust. Previously, like his own father before him, he
had been a 'badger', that is a licensed hawker selling foodstuffs
from place to place. Badgers were mentioned in a statute of 1552,
but the term survived only in dialect. Among the Stirk relatives
were a miller and a series of farm labourers. Robert and Purchas
cannot have had very much schooling, for the only secondary
school in the dale was the old Grammar School founded in 1601
at Yore Bridge. In 1845, when they were aged fourteen and
twelve, Yore Bridge was said to have no pupils, and a headmaster
who spent his days fishing in the River Ure.[35] Whatever their
lack of education, they were attractive young men, handsome and
good riders. Robert was nearly of an age with Rachel, and
Purchas with Dorothy. The two couples fell in love. For Rachel,
Robert and Purchas the passion was lasting, for Dorothy merely
a stage in her restless search for an ideal.[36] Even Rachel, so fond
of her sister and so gentle in her judgments, considered that
'Dorothy used P.S. ill'. She continued to meet him intermittently
until 1861, without ever speaking a word about it at home. Mark,
whose intuition was sometimes almost feminine, guessed that she
was concealing something from him and in 1858 pressed Rachel
for information. 'You say I was obscure,' replied Rachel with a
sharpness very rare for her. 'You would be yourself did you ever
see and know D. as I do. It is impossible for the present to be
otherwise. She is a riddle to me.'[37]

For already by the summer vacation of 1855 a rival to Purchas
Stirk had presented himself and Dorothy was to spend the next

five years driven by cross currents of feeling between the two men. The new suitor was young James Tate, son of the head-master of Richmond, whom she had known since his years at Rugby with her brother Frank. In August 1855 James drove over to Hauxwell to spend the day with his school friend and renewed his acquaintance with Frank's sisters.[38] He was twenty-three, a year younger than Dorothy and perhaps rather young for his age. He may have been somewhat overpowered by the weight of learning among his brothers, uncles, father and grandfather, for he had failed twice to gain admission to Oxford. 'I am afraid we cannot bring scholarship enough into the field,' wrote James Tate senior from Richmond Grammar School to Mark, fatherly anxiety struggling with headmasterly disapproval. 'At University College the matter was decided by the *Mathematical Paper*, and here again, alas, we are not strong.'[39] On Mark's advice the young man made a third attempt and gained admission to Corpus Christi College in 1854.[40] The girls at the Rectory found him much improved by his first year at Oxford, a rather double-edged compliment. Dorothy said, 'Mrs Tate has always been so kind to us.' Like many girls from unhappy homes, she was drawn to the young man by the charm of his parents' family life. On his side James seems to have fallen hopelessly in love with the beautiful and vivacious young woman, so much more forceful in character than himself. He was a helpful, biddable suitor, who haunted the Rectory, gathering letters, small presents and messages from the Pattison sisters for Mark at Oxford.[41] Mark, who loathed ladies' fancy work, received these offerings rather grimly, putting them away in a drawer he reserved for the purpose. He may have been equally grim towards James, for Dorothy wrote to her brother, 'you must promise me to be merciful in your bearing – you know what I mean, dear Mark'.[42] It says much for James's devotion that he was willing to face the bitter and taciturn figure of Dorothy's elder brother. James Tate possessed at least one clear advantage as a suitor. He could present himself openly at the Rectory, unlike Purchas Stirk, who had to rely on hasty, stolen meetings.

By all the standards of the day Dorothy's conduct in encouraging the attentions of two young men at once was totally disgraceful. Yet one can hardly condemn her. Kind Aunt Mary

Meadows wrote to Mark that she feared 'your poor sisters suffer want of judicious and friendly counsel and loving authority'.[43] Dorothy suffered more than any of them from this lack, for her looks always attracted attention and her natural instincts were strong. She longed to be in love and dedicate her life to marriage, as to a great cause. A marriage of convention or convenience repelled her, but a man whom she could love with the full force of her nature was hard to find. The pity, humanly speaking, was that her choice was so limited in these early years. One sees her, in her letters, struggling, willing herself to be in love, but in the end always too honest to deceive herself. Her handwriting, which had been graceful, grew angular and jagged with nervous tension. She appeared gay, even brilliant, but Rachel realized that she was secretly unhappy.[44]

One romantic satisfaction Dorothy had; she could recognize true love when she saw it. She was the first to hear, in the spring of 1856, of Rachel's secret engagement to Robert Stirk. She welcomed 'dearest Robert' as a brother, and remained fond of him until the last year of her life. In June Rachel told her sisters of the engagement, but made them promise not to reveal it to their parents or to Mark,[45] who she knew only too well would consider the match unworthy of her. In one way at least Mark resembled his father; he was painfully conscious of etiquette and social nuances. He was once heard to say of a distinguished self-made man, 'Could anything turn him into a gentleman?' Particularly, therefore, Rachel extracted a vow of secrecy from Fanny, who was due to visit Mark at Oxford during the long vacation. In a fatal hour for her peace of mind, poor Fanny gave the promise and kept it. Mark, when he finally found out the truth, never forgave her for this deception. With the streak of cruelty which existed in his sensitive nature, he deliberately withdrew his love and confidence, though Fanny pursued him down the years in letters of humiliating, grovelling self-abasement. 'Once again for the last time,' she wrote, 'I appeal to your better feelings, if for *one* wrong done to you you will cast me away as unworthy of your love.'[46]

Mark, in this respect his father's son, felt Rachel's engagement as a personal affront. The elder sisters too were not sympathetic. 'Rachel can never be happy,' wrote one of them, 'with her refined

mind in the society into which she must be thrown.'[47] Dorothy
defended the engagement stoutly, without any of the fear of
Mark's sarcasm which her sisters showed. 'R. thinks that watching
her own corn grow and making her own cheeses would be better
than spending her days here and I say it would too,' she wrote.
'I would be a nurse sooner than be governed by one who cannot
govern himself.'[48]

It did not in fact matter what any of them thought. Rachel,
usually so docile and so anxious for approval, was on this point
quite immovable. Her engagement continued as a perilous secret,
adding to the tensions of the household. Mark was not the only
member of the family to show signs of their troubled inheritance.
The family was rent with dissension. Eleanor, in a series of
voluble, near-hysterical, letters from Wyham, accused her sisters of
failing to help her in her poverty. Dorothy longed to experience
life in London or some big city,[49] but pitied her mother too much
to leave, and, staying, felt that she carried a burden of deceit about
her own love affairs. Fanny was jealous of Rachel and Dorothy,
and lachrymose over her loss of Mark. Jane and Mary were prim
and censorious to their younger sisters. Slowly the family affections, so long woven together by dread of the common tyrant,
loosened and frayed, while from January 1857 a deep cover of
snow kept them all indoors for three nightmare months. 'Ours
is a case past help,' wrote Fanny, 'it grows more galling every
year. I have now lost all hope. Father is our bitterest enemy and
Mother does not care one jot for us.' She was too inhibited to act
on her knowledge, but her comments show real insight into their
situation. 'I believe that as a family we make our own troubles,'
she said. 'It seems a sort of fate that comes over us and we cannot
help ourselves. It is not strangers or the world which makes our
miseries – it is ourselves.'[50]

Dorothy had been sincerely glad of Rachel's engagement. She
tried to be equally unselfish towards Frank's plans for escape,
although she knew how much she would miss his cheerful company. At twenty-three he was still hanging about at Hauxwell
with no job and no prospects for the future. After the railway was
extended to Leyburn in 1856 he threatened to go as a guard on
the new line, unless his father gave him enough money to look
for a post in London.[51] The threat of social disgrace worked as

he had hoped with Mr Pattison. He received an allowance, on which he went to London and eventually found a permanent appointment in the accounts department of H.M. Customs House. Later he married, and settled in London. He remained a kindly but distant brother. Among the family, he, Elizabeth and Sarah seem to have inherited from some Yorkshire ancestry a sturdy, taciturn, common sense. All three eventually found ways to leave home, and none was forgiven by their father for this act of defiance.

Family affairs were so critical that in July 1857 Mark felt he must pay one of his rare visits to Hauxwell. Self-pity had absorbed him during the years since his great disappointment over the Rectorship; yet he was forced to realize the helplessness of his mother and sisters. He came and stayed with the family for five weeks.[52] There is no written record of the discussions on this visit, but various decisions seem to have been taken. Rachel, despite all arguments, steadfastly refused to give up her engagement. Reluctantly, Mark promised to return and perform her marriage in the New Year. 'That you have played a kindly part,' wrote Aunt Meadows, 'is a satisfaction to me. I think there will be two honest hearts knit to you to their lives end. Your value to your sisters has been expressed in every letter, and we all know this act of kindness has cost you much self-denial.'[53] It was hard for Mark to resign a favourite sister, on whose teaching he had taken such pains, to a life of housekeeping and farm work which he never ceased to feel was unworthy of her. Everyone tacitly agreed that Mr Pattison, slumped like an abdicated Lear in his study chair, should be told nothing until the last possible moment, when Rachel insisted she would interview him herself.

Mrs Pattison prepared to make her will, a decision fateful for herself and her daughters. Normally, of course, her entire property would have been in the control of her husband; but, as she explained to Mark, by the will of her mother, Jane Winn of Prior House, Richmond, who had died in 1813, 'a very trifling sum and the rent of two fields' had been settled upon her,[54] to be controlled by two trustees. Both trustees had died; Mrs Pattison had appointed Mark and Richard Bowes junior in their place. The latter who was to play an increasing part in Hauxwell life, was the son of old Dr Bowes, had qualified at St Bartholomews in the

1830s and had served as a medical officer in Malaya before returning to practise with his father and his brother John at Richmond.
Mrs Pattison's capital was only £1161, but apart from a small
bequest to Frank, she bequeathed it 'equally amongst my nine
daughters, share and share alike to and for their respective sole
and separate use'.[55] This will, witnessed by the doctor and the
village schoolmaster, could only be altered by the joint act of both
parents. If it stood, each daughter would receive a sum of money,
however small, outside her father's control. This plain fact was to
produce the last, most disastrous crisis in the Rector's relations
with his wife and family.

Dorothy was able to talk freely to her brother for the first time
in years. She said nothing about her love affairs, but much about
her ideas. At twenty-five she was fully aware of 'a craving for
work in the world, in a corner of which she seemed condemned to
sit apart from the busy crowd'.[56] She poured out her passionate
regrets for 'the feeling of powers unused which might have
achieved something. Alas my dearest brother, what fruit have
they borne? . . . Is it not true that says "Hell is paved with
regrets"?'[57] Mark was embarrassed by the violence of these emotions. Though he prided himself on freedom from intellectual
prejudice he was socially an intensely conventional man. Perhaps
as a general reply to the discontents of his sisters, he preached a
sermon at Hauxwell church on 12th July 1857 on the text 'The
Kingdom of God is within you'.

'Most of us,' it concluded, 'have felt or still feel at times
uncomfortable and discontented in the place where we are. . . .
If we are disposed to think in this way, let us correct our thoughts
by dwelling on this verse "The Kingdom of God is within you".
. . . We may have entered into the Kingdom of God, without
quitting Earth, without moving from our places.'[58]

After Mark had returned to Oxford and the affairs of the world,
Dorothy did her best to follow this advice, to convince herself
that, as he repeated, 'place and circumstance do *not* make our
happiness.' It was uphill work. She wrote to him constantly,
though he was clearly a highly critical correspondent. 'How can
you say,' she wrote for his forty-fourth birthday on 9th October
1857, ' "my details were all on the outside"? Why, they were
intended to give you an idea of what was occupying and interest-

ing me, so that you might be able to picture me. . . . You must
not think that I do not enter into your feelings, for believe me I
do, but a steel pen and paper will not convey to you what I
want to say. I do so long for a good conversation with you. . . .
You may be sure I shall be thinking of you tomorrow. Have you
missed me since we parted?'[59]

Mark Pattison's pupils and old friends noticed sadly that 'he
could not be brought to believe how many loved and regarded
him'.[60] To this lonely, suspicious middle-ageing recluse the exchange of affection was an unaccustomed and dangerous luxury.
Yet even his chilly heart was warmed by Dorothy's devotion. For
the next three years she was perhaps as close to him as he ever
permitted anyone to be in his life. On her side, Dorothy clearly
loved her brother intensely; her letters leave no doubt of that.
She learnt feminine tact and skill by constantly teasing him into
good humour and coaxing him into generosity. He had an
authority over her mind which her two suitors could not rival,
neither the correct, rather colourless Oxford undergraduate, nor
the rough-riding young farmer on the fells. Yet he lived a life,
at Oxford, travelling abroad, among his books, in which she
could never fill more than a corner. Soon Rachel, her companion since childhood, would be married and gone. What could
the future hold for her, imprisoned at Hauxwell, alone? 'Oh the
fight,' she wrote, 'not to waste my time in useless regrets. God
grant my yearning for good may be carried into *action*.'[61]

NOTES

1. Pattison, 50, f. 112–16.
2. Ibid., 50, f. 157–9.
3. Ibid., 50, f. 163.
4. Personal information: the Rev. Dr. V. H. H. Green.
5. Pattison, 50, f. 124.
6. V. H. H. Green, *Oxford Common Room*, 170.
7. Pattison, 50, f. 205.
8. John Morley, quoted J. Sparrow, *Mark Pattison and the Idea of a University*, 109.
9. Pattison, 50, f. 389.

10. Ibid., 51, f. 297.
11. Ibid., 51, f. 291
12. Ibid., 51, f. 94.
13. Ibid., 52, f. 143.
14. J. S. Mill, *On the Subjection of Women* (2nd edn.), 107.
15. Ibid., Notes 20–22.
16. Pattison, 51, f. 297–8.
17. J. Sparrow, *Mark Pattison and the Idea of a University*, 38.
18. J. S. Mill, *On the Subjection of Women* (2nd edn.), 69.
19. Pattison, 53, f. 133–5.
20. Ibid., 50, f. 282.
21. Ibid., 50, f. 416.
22. Ibid., 50, f. 290.
23. Ibid., f. 412.
24. Lonsdale, 14, says 'he wisely refused'. It is never clear how much Miss Lonsdale knew about the Pattison family, or how much she suppressed in deference to their feelings.
25. A. M. Allchin, *The Silent Rebellion*, 147.
26. Ibid., 120.
27. P. Anson, *The Call of the Cloister*, 303.
28. Pattison, 54, f. 281. Rachel, recounting this six years later, could not remember the exact date.
29. M. Hartley and J. Ingilby, *Life and Tradition in the Yorkshire Dales*, 113.
30. Pattison, 53, f. 181.
31. Lonsdale, 8.
32. Pattison, 52, f. 9.
33. *Aysgarth Parish Registers*. Their name was later spelt Stirke.
34. P. H. Reaney, *The Origin of English Surnames*, 263. Old English 'styrc'; the k spelling suggests Scandinavian origin.
35. Correspondence in *The Wensleydale Advertiser*.
36. Pattison, 54, f. 281. Dorothy's love affair was not revealed to Mark until 1861, and the name and parentage of Purchas Stirk have been untraced until now.
37. Pattison, 52, f. 214.
38. Ibid., 50, f. 224.
39. Ibid., 50, f. 224.
40. *Alumni Oxoniensis*.
41. Pattison, 51, f. 98.
42. Ibid., 52, f. 437.
43. Ibid., 52, f. 9.
44. Ibid., 54, f. 27.

45. Ibid., 51, f. 266.
46. Ibid., 51, f. 349.
47. Ibid., 51, f. 282.
48. Ibid., 51, f. 282.
49. Ibid., 51, f. 363.
50. Ibid., 51, ff. 211 and 349.
51. Ibid., 51, f. 318.
52. Ibid., 136, f. 67.
53. Ibid., 52, f. 9.
54. Ibid., 62, f. 209.
55. P.P.R., 1861, f. 546.
56. Lonsdale, 15.
57. Pattison, 53, f. 179–81.
58. Ibid., 71, f. 72–81.
59. Ibid., 51, ff. 393–5.
60. J. Sparrow, *Mark Pattison and the Idea of a University*, 56.
61. Pattison, 53, ff. 188–91.

CHAPTER SIX

A Chain of Iron
1858–1859

On 5th January 1858 Mark married Rachel to Robert Stirk. He remembered it as 'the most melancholy wedding I ever attended'. Mr Pattison was made ill by the shock, but rallied enough to forbid Rachel to enter the Rectory again, or her sisters to visit her. The sisters were present to give the disgraced bride 'countenance, support and sympathy', while Mrs Pattison resigned herself yet again to the mysterious dealings of Providence. Only Aunt Meadows, writing from abroad, seems to have spared a thought for the other family involved. 'It cannot have been a joyful day for old Mr. and Mrs. S.,' she wrote, 'their first-born married like a *culprit* and I shd. take it Mrs. S. will not relish patronizing. How the familiarity grew up between the parties baffles every feeling I have.'[1] Whatever their feelings, Rachel's new family were very kind to her. She went to stay with them at Thoralby, until her new home was ready. In the spring she and Robert moved into the Manor at Bellerby, a long grey farm-house, standing back from the one street of stone cottages which forms the village. A row of pine trees leans away from the north wind. Behind the house moorland and heather stretch into the heart of the Pennines.

It was only a few miles, but a world away from the Rectory at Hauxwell, where Dorothy remained. Rachel felt the freedom to speak and act naturally and the absence of deception like the lightening of a physical load. Dorothy, for the first time, had to carry the burden of home life without her. Mr Pattison, at seventy-one, had begun to look old and frail, 'his sight greatly diminished',[2] he needed continual attendance by his daughters, because he could no longer read or write for himself. He talked of going to London to consult an ophthalmic surgeon, but could never bring himself, in spite of Dorothy's urging, to set out on the journey. Instead he groped about the house, increasingly helpless and irritable. His wife, Dorothy reported, 'is still his devoted slave',[3] but she could no longer wait on him hand and foot as she had done in the past. She was now crippled by arthritis, unable to dress herself or lift the slightest weight, barely able to cross the room with Dorothy and Sarah supporting her, complaining constantly of pain. 'She seems to care about nothing,' reported Dorothy. 'A little attention from her husband is the only thing that pleases her and as this is very rare she is generally insensible to everything except her own ailments, which, I fear, are very great.'[4] Dorothy's instinct as a nurse was to create an atmosphere of hope and cheerfulness; she went out in search of the first spring flowers and brought a bunch into the house, to encourage her mother to go out in a wheel-chair. Love of nature was one of the very few pleasures Mrs Pattison allowed herself. Now even this failed her. There seemed nothing for either parent to look forward to but increasing helplessness and death. Dorothy had maintained her gaiety and fighting spirit through years of confinement at home, but the care, night and day, of these two querulous and helpless invalids began to wear her down. 'Oh, *how* I miss Rachel,' she wrote. 'My room feels very lonely at nights without her.' Her sisters, preoccupied each with her own disappointments and grievances, dragged still further on her spirits. Home life, wrote one of them, 'lays upon us all like a chain of iron'.[5]

In April Dorothy could bear absence from Rachel no longer. As soon as the footpaths were passable she set out, in open defiance of her father's orders, for Bellerby. By taking every possible short cut across stiles and stepping stones, she managed the walk in a couple of hours. She was overjoyed to find Rachel, 'charming mistress of the house', and readily admired farmhouse, garden, dairy and the great sweep of land and cloudscape, seen from the moorland road. She had never seen Rachel so lively and bright before.[6] 'Now the Hauxwell atmosphere is gone,' explained Rachel, 'a weight within me is relieved. I feel an individual at last, not ruled by fear or circumstances, but able to rule them.' 'I feel,' replied Dorothy sombrely, 'that I am growing old without having lived.' Rachel was alarmed by the change in her. 'It grieves me to see dear Dorothy,' she wrote to Mark, 'she looks so ill and her spirits almost broken.'[7] Mark wrote urging Fanny to comfort her younger sister, to which Fanny, goaded beyond endurance, replied sharply, 'Remember you have other sisters in the world besides Dorothy.'[8]

Every spring Mark set off with rod and tackle, or box of books and a large store of tobacco for a fishing holiday. This year he remembered a rod he had left at Hauxwell and announced that he would call to fetch it. This news raised Dorothy's spirits and she wrote at once. 'We will do our best to make you comfortable, though I know our best is not what it ought to be. I had a hearty laugh at your directions for packing up the fishing rod as if it were of such great importance. You could not have given more directions for packing up a baby! Is fishing the only temptation to come – no, I know you better.' She added, however, 'As for your doing "any good" here, I can hold out no hope, for our affairs seem hopeless.'[9]

The sight of Dorothy was enough to convince Mark that her health was in danger. On this excuse he persuaded their parents that she must have a holiday, and that he would take charge of it. In August 1858 they set off together on a tour, Dorothy quivering with mingled excitement and apprehension. It was the first time she had been further than Redcar, and she felt Mark's critical eye upon her. Most of the Pattisons suffered acutely from isolation and shyness. Mary, in company, was rigid as a statue, Fanny frankly terrified, Rachel, in her own words, 'so bewildered'. Mark himself had experienced tortures of embarrassment when he went up to Oxford as an undergraduate; he had even cut the Provost of his own college in the street because he was too shy to greet him.[10] His silences as a don unnerved generations of undergraduates. A favourite Oxford story told of Pattison's walk with a freshman to Iffley. Not a word was spoken until the freshman plucked up courage. 'The irony of Sophocles is greater than the irony of Euripides,' he nervously remarked. Pattison merely gave him a stony glare and kept silently on to Iffley, where they turned. Then Pattison broke the silence. 'Quote,' he snarled.[11] At the same time he was severe on the manners of others. 'If a youth on being presented to his superior in age or station, or to a lady, offers to shake hands,' he observed sourly, 'I have little hope of him.'[12] He noted in his diary, as French idioms which particularly appealed to him, 'tout l'aplomb des convenances' and 'on peut y déployer du savoir faire'. It was difficult for his sisters, fresh from the country, to keep their self-possession in his company, and Mary, visiting him the previous summer, had lost her courage and fled home. 'From Mary's account,' explained Dorothy, 'the reason she left was not anything in your conduct to her, but that she believed she was in your way. If she had only been more *natural* it certainly would have been pleasanter, but it was truly her eager desire to please you made her otherwise.'[13] Now she herself must meet the same exacting test.

They spent the first half of August in lodgings at Abbot's Bromley, in a house with a view over distant Cannock Chase. Then they moved on to Shrewsbury with expeditions, which delighted Dorothy, to Leominster, Kineton and Ludlow. From 11th–16th September they stayed at 'Jane's', near Builth, for Mark to fish the superb upper reaches of the Wye. 'Jane' was the parlourmaid Wright, who had married James Bowe and left saying 'she hoped we would never go into South Wales without going to see her'.[14] It was a happy meeting for both women, who were really fond of one another, and seems to have stayed in Dorothy's mind for the rest of her life, since she left Jane Bowe in her will the only personal bequest outside her own family.[15]

Indeed the whole holiday was a success. Dorothy, in her own words, made herself agreeable, so that landladies and travelling companions 'took to me especially'. She diverted Mark with conversation and soothed him in the evenings with playing and singing. When he criticized her letters, saying, 'You cannot take trouble,' she defended herself cheerfully. 'Don't read them with critical eyes, but picture the writer. Why my very going and *enjoying* my visit to you so much, shows I am not Hauxwell-bound and your time has not been spent in vain.'[16] With amazing vitality she threw off the weariness and depression of months. Everyone found her fresher, prettier, transformed in manner and conversation. She knew that she was charming Mark, and delighted in the fact.

The climax of her holiday was the journey home. At the age of twenty-six she had apparently never travelled alone by railway, had an independent meal in a restaurant, or visited a large city. Now, by an innocent stratagem, she was able to achieve all these ambitions at once, and moreover to see the first art exhibition of her life.

In a breathless, very human letter to Mark she revealed how she achieved this; for all her inexperience in worldly affairs, she fulfilled her intentions first and left the explanations until afterwards. They had parted at Shrewsbury station, where Mark gave her the first-class fare and warned her she must change at Manchester and Leeds. To have money actually in her purse gave her an undreamt-of freedom of action.

'as you said June 13th was very *sensible* and very much to the *point*, this shall be the same . . .' she wrote.

'Well, when I arrived at Manchester we were half an hour behind time . . . I found I had to take a fly to the Leeds Stn. Then the next train would depart in a $\frac{1}{4}$ of an hour but if I went by it I should not be able to proceed further than Thirsk that night. Well now, it struck me I had far better stay in Manchester, get a peep at the Exhibition and a great deal of pleasure out of an accident. I had not much time to make up my mind for the train was starting, but it grieved me to give up the sight of the Exhibition.'[17]

The Exhibition, which attracted Dorothy's attention, opened on 10th September, at the Royal Manchester Institution. It was one of their annual Art Exhibitions, forerunners of the City Art Gallery.[18] Part of the letter is missing here, but it appears that she had difficulty in finding lodgings.

'. . . it seemed hopeless, but as we were coming down a nice street I saw Apartments in the window and found a very nice room. . . . After this I sallied forth and was delighted with the streets, then returned to the refreshment room and got my tea, then a kind friend saw me home to my lodgings which I found very comfortable. I rose early and sallied forth, a lovely fresh morning; at 9 I went to my friend in the refreshment room and got my breakfast, then took an omnibus to the Exhibition. . . . I staid till 2 then took the train and arrived here last night . . . I felt sure you would like me to see the Exhibition and as you had said I could come first class from Leeds I thought I might spend that money on seeing the Exhibition and so the expenses would be equal. I am so sorry for the way in which we parted, you never wished me good-bye and I never thanked you half enough for the great treat you had given me.'

Dorothy returned as autumn, or as the servants called it in dialect 'the back end' was closing in on Hauxwell. Somehow she must keep a grip on her new-found freedom, somehow keep in touch with the outside world. She feared neither cold nor rain; in black frost or the first feathery flakes of a snow-shower she would saddle Tom and ride out, or if need be walk. She was drawn, first one way, then the other, in two directions, up the moorland paths to Bellerby, or over the old pack-horse road to Richmond. At Bellerby there was the harsh landscape, the perpetually-blowing wind, the realities of farming and the love of Rachel and Robert. There was also the chance of meeting Purchas Stirk, who sometimes rode over to help with the heavy seasonal work. At Richmond, in dignified Georgian Frenchgate, was the home of her girlhood's friends, the Tate family. The lofty stone houses looked over St Mary's churchyard and the Grammar School buildings to the winding valley of the Swale. Here Dorothy was welcomed into an atmosphere of affection. Mr Tate was at work upon a new edition of a Latin text-book;[19] his wife was kind and hospitable as ever. James had taken his degree in the previous summer. Characteristically, no one asked him what career he wanted to follow. It seems to have been taken for granted by everyone that he would follow his father into holy orders and teach at the Grammar School.[20] Equally, it was assumed that he would become, as Mrs Pattison put it, Dorothy's 'accepted lover'; she was tempted to marry him to escape from home. Mr Pattison summoned the young man over for 'a book-room conference, much more quiet and amicable than was anticipated'.[21] The women, listening anxiously from another room, heard none of the expected shouts and threats. James, diffident and well brought up, was no match for the Rector. He asked for an engagement and was told, 'At present it is most imprudent.' There was some truth in this, as the maximum salary for a curate was a hundred and fifty pounds, and some existed with a family on as little as fifty pounds a year.[22] In any case, James was too polite to argue; he merely asked, in the classic phrase of the Victorian suitor, 'May I hope for the future?' Mr Pattison replied, 'By then I shall be gone,' and forbade him to enter the house. James meekly submitted and the interview was at an end.[23]

Dorothy was deeply chagrined. Her romantic dreams had been of a St George who would fight the dragon and carry her off to freedom. It was galling that James had cut a less courageous figure than her commonplace brother-in-law, Fred Mann. She had a quick temper. There was a furious quarrel, 'a lovers' quarrel' Mrs Pattison called it, between Dorothy and James, and within a fortnight she broke off the unofficial engagement between them.[24] Mrs Pattison, Mary, Jane and even Mark, all sincerely concerned for her happiness, pointed out that James was 'an excellent young man', 'likely to make her very happy', and most suitable as to family background. Rachel, who knew much more about Dorothy than she was prepared to tell, wrote to Mark 'That James loved her I have known for a long time and so have you, but I *never* believed that Dorothy returned it. She is uncertain and decidedly miserable about the whole thing'.[25] She would not say more for fear of betraying Dorothy's secret interest in her own brother-in-law, Purchas Stirk.

The two sisters were much together this winter. In November Dorothy went to Bellerby to stay with Rachel until her first confinement. She was anxious, because the childhood attack of rheumatic fever had weakened Rachel's heart, yet she could not help being happy, because they were together. The moorland farm-house was like a fortress, shutting out the world. 'Nothing like a bright red fire on a frosty night, shutters up and no candles. Then one can defy wind, cold and snow.'[26] The two women talked by firelight, just as they had by the Hauxwell kitchen fire, in younger days. Purchas Stirk came several times to Bellerby during the month Dorothy stayed there; he was as much in love as ever. Rachel could not make out whether her sister returned this love or not; secretly Dorothy was deeply disturbed. Away from Purchas she could dismiss him, but his physical presence affected her as James's never had. Months later she confessed as much to Rachel. Her austere and rigid upbringing had never admitted the possibility of sexual feeling; it was quite outside the understanding or control of her conscious mind. No wonder she seemed to Rachel 'a complete riddle'. For the present she put love out of her thoughts; a sudden emergency demanded all her energies. 'Thank God,' she wrote to Mark on 4th December, 'Rachel is safe and doing well. She gave birth to twin girls this morning, but alas neither of them lived. They both breathed, they were perfect in form and feature and perfectly beautiful. . . . Oh, Mark if you had heard her piteous entreaties to be told even one was living, it was heart-rending. Forgive this hasty scrawl but I have the whole house to look after and she does not like me to leave her long.'[27]

This poignant shared experience drew the two sisters even closer together. In all the family correspondence, so full of quarrels and misunderstandings, there is never a hint of deception or jealousy between them. Rachel accepted Mark's growing affection for Dorothy with fine generosity. 'I had often thought', she wrote, 'that you did not appreciate her as she deserves. Of course she is ignorant, we are all frightfully so, considering our opportunities, but I consider her more original, a more active and intellectual mind, more capable to follow and enjoy you than me.'[28] Secretly Rachel was deeply troubled by her sister's passionate and wayward nature. For the next six months Dorothy turned restlessly this way and that, like an animal in a trap, struggling to escape. Finally, she took the nearest way out. Marriage promised freedom; in June 1859, she renewed her engagement to James Tate. The Rector was infuriated. 'Father and I are on the worst of terms,'[29] reported Dorothy coolly. The Tate family were delighted and carried Dorothy off to stay with them. Since James was forbidden to enter the Rectory, they insisted Dorothy must visit them as often as possible. This she seemed only too happy to do. Yet Rachel had a nagging feeling of unease at the whole affair. 'I cannot understand what broke it off before,' she wrote, 'I can only hope D. is certain *now* of her own mind. She is my own peculiar favourite and I long to see her happy, but above all I should like to see her sure of herself.'[30] Mr Pattison was determined to prolong the engagement indefinitely, but Rachel thought the only safety for Dorothy lay in marrying at once. Dorothy herself put off making any final decision by declaring that she could not think of marrying while her invalid mother still needed her. She was torn by conflicting feelings. She really loved the

D*

Tate family and was grateful to them. 'The Tates are very, very good to me and I am very happy here,' she wrote, and added, echoing Rachel, 'I am beginning to feel an *individual* at last, living and acting for myself.'[31] Yet anyone could have seen that she was not in love with James from the joy with which she accepted an invitation to visit Mark at Oxford that summer. 'How can I ever thank you,' she wrote. 'My dear, what greater joy can you offer than being with you; only think what a long time it is since we met, and how I shall have you all to myself. You talk of my granting you "this favour" when the favour is all on your side. I am delighted with the idea of seeing new places – such a treat for one who scarcely ever passes beyond the bounds of Hauxwell – and besides, I *do* so enjoy railway travelling! I shall grudge every hour you are without me, but I am staying with the Tates and cannot get away before Monday, as they have made engagements for me every day.'[32]

Mark called for Dorothy at the Tates' house, on his way south from a fishing trip in Scotland. She was uneasy at the sight of her brother and her fiancé together; once again she begged 'be merciful in your bearing – you know what I mean, dear Mark'. As they travelled together, she let slip the revealing remark, 'Oh, *how* you have spoilt me for dull conversation!'[33] She forgot the past and the future in the charm of his company. Mark Pattison suffered, as much as he made his sisters and friends suffer, from the morbid suspicion deep-rooted in his character. It was perhaps a strain of paranoia, inherited from his father. When it was lulled, his feminine sensitivity made him a most sympathetic and perceptive companion, especially to women. His fondness for young girls was later a subject of ribald comment in Oxford, and Walter Pater described him as 'romping with great girls among the gooseberry bushes'; but his kindness to his sister Dorothy was generous and disinterested. Their two months together from 22nd July to 25th September 1859 were among the happiest in both their lives.

Their first visit was to Rugby, where Dorothy was able to visit the scenes of *Tom Brown's Schooldays*, which Mark had given her to read. Then they settled in country lodgings at St Ippolyts, a pretty village near Hitchin in Hertfordshire. There they enjoyed long, leisurely days of forced intimacy, with 'a long ramble, poetry during breakfast and music at night till the embers darken'.[34] Mark had fastidious taste; he did much to cultivate Dorothy's charm of manner and form her for the public part of her future life. Free from the eternal constraint of home she fell into the liveliness, the quicksilver changes of mood, and un-affected friendliness to all comers which were to be hers for life. From St Ippolyts they moved on to Fen Drayton, where a former Fellow of Lincoln College held the living, and they were guests at the Rectory. From here they drove to visit Cambridge, where Dorothy stood enchanted on a bridge, staring like a child at the beauty of the Backs. They went to a service in King's College Chapel. 'It is still ringing in my ears,' she said later, 'I would it might in my life.'[35] From Cambridge they went for the visit to London, on which Dorothy had so often and so vainly begged her father to take her. From London they travelled, early in September, to Oxford at last. For Dorothy it was like a dream to pass under the gateway of Lincoln College, cross the Quad, climb the scrubbed oak stairs and enter at last the rooms so minutely drawn and described by Rachel twelve years before. She sat on the sofa by the window gazing out at the battlemented stone walls, the velvet grass. She was seeing Mark in his rightful home at last. On his side too, it must have been a strange experience. He had always dreaded the loneliness, the heavy langour of Oxford during the Long Vacation, and fled from it whenever he could. Now, in the company of this ardent creature, so inexperienced in the most ordinary pleasures of life and so responsive to his every look and word, Oxford was transformed to the golden city of his youthful ambitions. She could not of course stay in College, walk un-chaperoned in the streets or sit alone under the great plane tree in the inner quad called The Grove. With thoughtful care for her comfort he found her lodgings nearby, arranged for her to have daily papers, sent her laundry to his own washerwoman, and had dinner sent up for them both to his own 'Garret'. Mark Pattison was extremely careful about spending money; indeed, his mean-ness formed part of his legendary personality. His accounts included 'This account book 6d.' Yet, as these accounts show, he spared no trouble or expense to make Dorothy happy on this first, and as it turned out last, visit to Oxford.[36] He bought her a new straw bonnet, which was much admired and which, she said, 'I shall prize highly, remembering the loving way it was given.'[37]

Thanks to Mark's careful accountancy, we know it was bought from Elliston and Cavell, at a cost of 8s. 6d. 'I am ashamed of how much money has disappeared to treat me to such luxury,' she protested, but half-heartedly. An innate feminine vanity lay very deep in her character; no austerities would ever destroy it and for many people it formed part of her charm. 'She was essentially feminine in all her instincts,' said an acquaintance, 'a woman who was loved not in spite of her faults, but was loved faults and all.'[38] She could be devious too. Among all the affectionate confidences of these weeks she said nothing to Mark about her doubts over her engagement to James, or her feelings for Purchas Stirk.

She settled into his life, graceful and contented as the cats, whose company soothed his irritable nerves. A corner of his room became 'my corner', where she cut the pages of books fresh from Parker's bookshop, copied references and wrote to his dictation.[39] Whenever the sun shone, she coaxed him out of doors, to sit in a sheltered corner in the Parks, or walk up and down in the shade of the great elms in Christ Church Meadow. She made him promise not to give up this exercise when the time came for her to leave him.[40] She even persuaded him to give a breakfast party, at which she seems to have made a conquest of 'your nice friend Mr. Ward'. On 9th September Mark took Dorothy, apparently for the first time in her life, to the theatre. That week the Theatre Royal company presented *The School for Scandal*, with Mr N. Ray and Miss Eburne as Sir Peter and Lady Teazle. 'A genteel and numerous audience' attended, and the screen scene in particular drew rounds of applause.[41] Mark could not have chosen better; Sheridan appealed both to Dorothy's love of comedy and her instinctive feeling for elegance. Her pleasure, in turn, drew him out of his habitual, morose dissatisfaction with the human condition and especially the condition of Oxford.

It is clear that there was also a more serious side to their relationship. In the leisurely walks and talks of their shared holidays in 1858 and 1859, the conversation of Mark and Dorothy Pattison turned inevitably to questions of religion. Having already experienced two of the great religious movements of the nineteenth century, Evangelicanism and Tractarianism, in her own home, Dorothy was now to meet a third, the Liberal reaction. The second half of the nineteenth century has been called 'the age of honest doubt' in religious history.[42] Believers who had been brought up, like the Pattison children, to accept every word of the Scriptures as equally and divinely inspired, received in the mid-century a series of shattering shocks from the scientific revolution, from advanced historical studies and from textual criticism. The first tremors of the earthquake date from the publication in 1831 of Lyell's *Principles of Geology*, which upset the traditional dating of the Creation. The full blast was felt in 1859 with the publication of the *Origin of Species*. At the same time Buckle's *History of Civilization* applied the historical method to the records of Christianity, to the discomfiture of readers who found natural cause and effect taking the place of a minutely-supervising Providence. Textual criticism of the Old Testament revealed a variety of literary forms, chronicle, poetry, myth and legend. How could the New Testament or Christian dogma be insulated from these disturbing studies? F. D. Maurice went so far as to question the doctrine of eternal punishment, the ultimate deterrent of every Evangelical nursery for three generations, because it rested on a possible mistranslation. Meanwhile J. S. Mill's *On Liberty*, published in 1858, prepared the way for the toleration of differing religious opinions, and a concern with the social implications of Christ's teaching.

These new ideas, so strange to a daughter of Hauxwell Rectory, were all familiar to Mark Pattison, for he was a contributor to the famous volume which first set them clearly before the public, the *Essays and Reviews* of 1860. This 'liberal theological tract for the times'[43] roused orthodox churchmen to fury. It was received, wrote Mark, 'with blatant and ignorant howling'.[44] Bishop Thirlwall, speaking in the Upper House of Convocation said, 'this was a question between infidelity and Christianity and we ought to prosecute'.[45] Dorothy read *Essays and Reviews*, and later said that she had both copied her brother's manuscripts and written to his dictation during the two years when he was at work on it. She was ignorant, but intelligent enough to understand his main arguments.

Mark Pattison's contribution to *Essays and Reviews* was *Tendencies of Religious Thought 1688–1750*,[46] a dispassionate examination of eighteenth-century theories of belief and their rival claims. A very few quotations are enough to demonstrate its tone. 'We have not yet learnt, in this country, to write our ecclesiastical history on any better footing than that of praising up the party, in or out of the Church, to which we happen to belong.' He allows himself a certain sardonic amusement at the spectacle of nineteenth-century churchmen allotting blame for the manners and morals of the eighteenth century. High churchmen blame the Toleration Acts, latitudinarians blame free-thinkers and non-jurors in equal shares, Nonconformists blame 'unscriptural worship', 'while the Catholics rejoice to see the Protestant Reformation at last bearing its natural fruit'. For himself, he sees much to praise in the commonsense eighteenth-century doctrines 'which have been long the butt of the Evangelical Pulpit. To abstain from vice, to culti-vate virtue, to fill our station in life with propriety, to bear the ills of life with resignation and to use its pleasures moderately – these are indeed not a little.' He is scrupulous to point out the limitations of this theology, but still contrasts it favourably with that of his own day, when 'nothing is allowed in the Church of England but the formulae of past thinkings, which have long lost all sense of any kind'. The serious and thoughtful Christian, according to Pattison, should feel it his duty to make a fresh examination of the grounds on which his faith stands 'whether on Authority, on the Inward Light, on reason, on self-evidencing Scripture'. 'Whoever undertakes this,' Pattison somewhat bleakly concludes, 'would probably find that he had undertaken a per-plexing but not altogether profitless inquiry.' To this inquiry, within her limited resources, Dorothy Pattison now addressed herself, with disturbing results.

While drafting this essay, Mark Pattison was already exploring a subject he handled in a paper published three years later, *Learning in the Church of England.*[47] One point in particular emerged, which was to concern Dorothy Pattison increasingly for the whole of her working life. Pattison posed the problem, which he did not pretend to answer, of 'how the Church may be brought home to the classes which have never yet been at home within it'. At present, he rather dourly observed, 'remedial measures of social relief originate outside the clerical body and often find in it their most uncompromising opponents'. Dorothy had been brought up to regard the solid material comfort of Hauxwell Rectory as an unquestioned right. Now her brother confronted her with a new, profoundly disturbing fact of life, 'the clash of interest, unsoftened by any bond of union, between labour and the employer of labour. . . . The great social difficulty of our time is the gulf between the rich and the poor'.

The great Victorians responded to the religious crisis of the 1860s according to individual temperament and character. Some sought God in the soul of man, carrying on Christian charitable work without Christian dogma, trying, like William Hale White, 'to gain admittance into the house of the poor and do some practical good.' Some, of whom George Eliot is perhaps the most famous, created a system of ethics endowed with all the authority of the discarded religion, a new morality 'whose music is the gladness of the world'. For many Arthur Hugh Clough expressed their bewilderment as they prepared

> *To spend uncounted years of pain*
> *Again, again and yet again*
> *In working out in heart and brain*
> *The problem of our being here.*

The most sensitive shared the desolation of Matthew Arnold upon Dover Beach.

> *The sea of faith*
> *Was once, too, at the full and round earth's shore*
> *Lay like the folds of a bright girdle furl'd*
> *But now I only hear*
> *Its melancholy long, withdrawing roar,*
> *Retreating to the breath*
> *Of the night-wind down the vast edges drear*
> *And naked shingles of the world.*

Mark Pattison claimed that he personally felt only a great relief, a liberation in the shedding of his orthodoxy: 'Anglicanism fell off from me like an old garment, as Puritanism had done before.' Where in this range of opinion was his sister? Ardent, undisciplined, ignorant yet intelligent, she was possessed, as she confessed, by 'yearnings not tangible enough to have formed themselves into wishes. There is no standing still, yet what have I been doing all these years?'[48] Religious authority had kept her prisoner at home, on the grounds that the Bible ordained it. What if the scriptures were unauthentic, or even misunderstood? For a time she said 'the very foundations of faith' seemed to crumble. The experience was desolating, as even Mark was forced to admit. 'Agnosticism', he wrote in later years, 'has taken away Providence as death takes away the mother from the child, and leaves it forlorn of protection and love'.[49] The poignancy of this simile is revealing, and Dorothy shared the suffering it expresses. Yet she never lost her deep desire for personal dedication. Gradually in the future as she passed out of Mark's intellectual domination, faith would return; but it could never again be the old, unquestioned faith. She continually sought instruction and her beliefs never hardened into a fixed, unalterable system, like those of many of her contemporaries. There is no going backwards in questions of belief and a thought cannot be unthought. The reading, the discussions, the searching of these years, left Dorothy with a new depth of judgment and a new view of the Christian's duty in society. When she became famous, both Evangelicals and Tractarians claimed her as their own. Both perhaps were right; but she was also a product of the mid-Victorian crisis of faith.

Walks and talks came to an end on 24th September, when Dorothy was due to return to Hauxwell. It had been hard to return after the summer holiday of 1858. It was much harder to leave Mark now after two months of loving companionship, and the parting grieved them both. 'My dearest Mark,' wrote Dorothy from Hauxwell next day, 'I have arrived here safe luggage and all – oh how I wish I knew how you were this morning. Did it hurt you coming down to the station with me? You said the journey would make me forget our parting, but oh, my dearest brother, no such thing. I thought of you each hour, what you would be doing and then I thought of all the love and care you had bestowed on me and it made me weep afresh. Oh Mark I never knew how much you cared for me till we parted; I had no idea until then that I could be anything to you, a being so superior in every way.'[50] Pattison was famous wherever Oxford men gathered for his freezing irony. In justice to him it should also be remembered that he was capable of giving and inspiring affection such as this. Dorothy had parted from him with tears, but gradually cheered up. Every railway journey was an adventure to her, and this time she found an interesting companion. 'I travelled with a gentleman engaged in the work of *The Times* who kindly endeavoured to explain the items and advertisements to me.' Mark's deepest suspicions were roused by this gentleman; he evidently wrote pressing Dorothy for details, for he received the disarming reply, 'He was quite ordinary looking, but young.'[51]

Hauxwell was at its gloomiest, cut off from the world by curtains of pouring rain, which continued for days. It was more than a week before Dorothy could set off at eight o'clock one morning on the five-mile climb to Bellerby, to tell Rachel all her Oxford experiences. She found her sister cooking; the two women spent the morning together in the farm kitchen making Christmas puddings, and, said Dorothy, 'You may imagine how we did talk!'[52] Rachel was struck afresh by Dorothy's charm, and the new polish of her manner and conversation; she seemed like a being from a wider world. The walk home from Bellerby, through the rain and the gathering dark, was rough. 'I got lost coming home in the evening,' wrote Dorothy to Mark. 'It poured down and when I came to the stream I could not find the stepping stones, so I had to wade through it. I found my Father had spent the whole afternoon storming at Mama for my going to Bellerby. I should not mind if it came upon my own head, for I should not care, but I cannot bear to bring more trouble into her miserable existence.'[53] Old, frail and half-blind, the Rector had lost the power to frighten his daughters now. Increasingly he concentrated his persecution on his invalid wife, while their children watched in helpless horror. To come back to this situation after experiencing life outside was like stepping from waking sanity into a world of nightmares. The inhabitants were aroused for a moment by news of Mark, but quickly fell back into their old apathy. 'Your mother was pleased', reported Dorothy, 'that you had sent her a particular message, and it would have done your heart good to see Fanny when I gave her your love and a kiss. But the state of affairs here is deplorable. I was very much struck with the *careworn* expression in every one of them. Oh Mark, when I contrast my summer with my sisters' here, I feel what you have done for me.'[54] Almost ashamed of so much freedom, she took up the burden of another winter; endless winters, like a dark tunnel, stretched into the future, as far as she could see.

NOTES

1. Pattison, 52, f. 9. This reflected the gap in their social positions.
2. Ibid., 52, f. 384.
3. Ibid., 52, f. 381.
4. Ibid., 52, f. 651.
5. Ibid., 52, f. 506.
6. Ibid., 51, f. 153. (Among 1855–57 letters in collection, but must refer to 1858.)
7. Ibid., 51, f. 36.
8. Ibid., 51, f. 162.
9. Ibid., 51, ff. 52–3, 153.
10. *Memoirs*, 57.
11. V. H. H. Green, *Oxford Common Room*, 265, n. 2.
12. *Memoirs*, 59.
13. Pattison, 51, ff. 393–5.
14. Ibid., 40, ff. 23, 52, f. 271.
15. Will of Sister Dora (Dorothy Pattison), PPR, 1879, f. 38.
16. Pattison, 51, f. 95.
17. Ibid., 51, f. 269 (Among 1855–57 letters in collection, but is clearly the letter which continues in Pattison, 51, f. 394–5 and Pattison, 52, ff. 154–8).
18. Manchester Public Libraries, Archives Department.
19. *Richmond Rules to form the Ovidian Distich*, 1861.
20. Pattison, 53, ff. 94–102.
21. Ibid., 51, ff. 162 and 151 (the same letter, the sheets of which have become separated).
22. *The Times*, 9th September and 15th September 1858, Correspondence.
23. Pattison, 51, ff. 162 and 151.
24. Ibid., 51, f. 150.
25. Ibid., 51, f. 161.
26. Ibid., 51, f. 236.
27. Ibid., 51, f. 237.
28. Ibid., 52, f. 633.
29. Ibid., 52, f. 419.
30. Ibid., 52, ff. 377–9.
31. Ibid., 53, ff. 94–102.
32. Ibid., 52, ff. 436–7.
33. Ibid., 52, f. 507.
34. Ibid., 52, f. 469.

35. Ibid., 52, f. 506.
36. Ibid., 40, ff. 32–3, 39.
37. Ibid., 40, ff. 502–3; see photograph on p. 129.
38. *The Standard*, 11th October, 1886.
39. Pattison, 52, ff. 502–3.
40. Ibid., 52, f. 506.
41. *The Oxford Chronicle*, 3rd and 10th September 1859.
42. Horton Davies, *Worship and Theology in England*, IV, 173.
43. Ibid., IV, 182.
44. *Memoirs*, 315.
45. V. H. H. Green, *Oxford Common Room*, 221.
46. M. Pattison, *Essays* II, 42–118.
47. Ibid., 263–308.
48. Pattison, 53, ff. 179–81.
49. V. H. H. Green, *Oxford Common Room*, 318.
50. Pattison, 52, ff. 620–1.
51. Ibid., 52, ff. 502–3, 506.
52. Ibid., 52, f. 511.
53. Ibid., 52, f. 512.
54. Ibid., 52, f. 621.

CHAPTER SEVEN

The Labour of the Day
1860–1861

Mr Pattison had already made his will. By it, his capital, of between thirteen and fourteen thousand pounds, was invested to provide an income for his wife, and after her 'for my daughters who shall be living and unmarried at the time of my decease'. He disinherited his two sons, apart from a small holding of land and some scattered leases in various North Riding villages. His married daughters he disinherited completely.[1] The punishment, however, would not be complete unless the disobedient daughters were also cut out of their mother's will. By the spring of 1860 she was clearly failing. 'Poor Mother is much worse and much weaker,'[2] reported Dorothy, who was again sharing nursing duties with Sarah. The Rector wasted no time, but ordered his wife at once to revoke her small bequests to Eleanor and Rachel. Mrs Pattison had never refused her husband anything in her life, but she had been brought up as a banker's daughter. Total financial probity was bred in the marrow of her Puritan bones. Her daughters believed her weak, but her years of stoic endurance prove she must have been strong. Now she showed the force of her character; steadfastly she refused to alter her will, or discriminate unjustly between her married and unmarried daughters. All should 'share and share alike' in the proceeds of her marriage settlement.[3] Her husband was infuriated, but for once powerless in law. He browbeat her night and day, while his warped mind searched restlessly for some weapon of revenge.

Mrs Pattison went slowly but inexorably downhill; she was crippled by arthritis and suffered frequent chest infections. Dr Bowes noted a decline every time he visited her. She grew ever more feeble and helpless. Although she was only sixty-seven she had not a single tooth left in her head; her sunken eyes and wasted cheeks reminded her daughters of a skull. 'She does lead such a sad existence,' wrote Dorothy hopelessly, 'no one can ever interest her in anything.'[4] Three months later she was worse again. 'Poor Mama is very poorly. She is shrunk and looks so very ill and sad; in no way can we alleviate her sufferings. I persuade her sometimes to sit out, but she will not even bear being wheeled out in her Bath chair. Nothing interests her and she can do nothing.'[5] It is doubtful whether medical science could have relieved Mrs Pattison; chronic rheumatic arthritis was only defined in 1857 and its treatment remained empirical.[6] She might have been spared some pain by the use of slings to move her in bed; Dorothy was angry that nothing was even attempted to help her mother. Nor was she the only patient. Anna was deteriorating though she had still seven years to live. 'I am troubled by Anna,' reported Dorothy. 'She grows weaker in mind and does not see it: her walk and bearing is that of a silly person.'[7] The care of these two helpless, hopeless cases caused grave anxiety to Sarah and Dorothy, who were quite untrained for the work. Dorothy suffered ever after from the memory of it. Even when she was a highly skilled and experienced surgical nurse, she confessed that she could not enjoy medical nursing, or the care of women patients.

Yet in these depressing months her vitality, her instinct for health and happiness showed at its strongest. She had 'a little joke' with her mother every evening, while preparing the helpless woman for bed. The Rector, in his moods of black despair, turned to her as 'the sunshine' in his gloomy house. To Mark she wrote cheerfully, knowing how he detested the complaining letters of her elder sisters. 'The labour of the day being over,' she said, 'I can enjoy a quiet chat with you.'[8] She asked his opinions about dress material and fashions 'for you must remember you stand in the place of *Robes et Modes* to me.'[9] No pleasure was too small to dwell upon and enjoy. In the autumn she cherished the smoky gold of the trees round Hauxwell Hall, and a mushroom hunt on a fine morning. For Christmas she made him a cake and gifts 'useful ones which will not have to go into *the drawer*'. Her Christmas letter, according to Mark's diary, was the only greeting he received. In spring she sent him 'crocuses which you must plant in a pot and cover with moss and stand in your window, and when they come up bright and gay, give them a look now and then and fancy it is me looking at you. Now don't laugh at me but try it!'[10] With instinctive skill, she played on Mark's love of wild nature and the dales. The cry of the hounds, meeting at Hauxwell Hall, was enough to send her running to the window. She told him the details of every meet she attended, the wild gallops over Witton Fell, the wading on horseback through the river near Jervaulx Abbey. 'I cannot resist even the sight of a red coat,' she confessed.[11] She was first with the news of a freak storm, which swept up the valley late in May, with a bitter whirl of wind and snow showers. 'It blew down the horse chestnut tree behind the beehouse and in its fall injured the top of the Purple Beech, which grieved me, for I am fond of that tree.'[12] Nothing gave her more happiness than a visit from Eleanor's small daughter, Nora. Eleanor longed to visit her mother, but the Rector still refused to let her enter the house,[13] so Dorothy took charge of 'this most engaging child', inventing games for her and reading aloud *The Ballad of John Gilpin*, by request, over and over again, till Nora knew it by heart.[14] Even Mrs Pattison, from her invalid couch, raised a wan smile at the sight of them playing together. These minor country pleasures seem ordinary enough, but to enjoy them through the dreariness of Hauxwell Rectory showed heroic self-command. Slowly Dorothy's character was being forged into a steely strength.

In the New Year of 1860 the Rectory cook left, and Dorothy volunteered to act as cook to the household until a new one could be found. She enjoyed the new work and especially the right to occupy the kitchen. There she sat alone before the huge, glowing range, writing to Mark and watching her home-made bread rise, while the wind howled in the chimney and snow lay knee-deep at the door. 'I flatter myself,' she wrote proudly, 'that I could now get up a dinner which even you who are spoilt by your college cooking would not object to sit down to. Bread I can manage very easily. . . . If ever I have to earn my livelihood, I could do it now by seeking a cook's situation.'[15] Whenever she could get out she visited the sick in cottages all over the parish. Her letters were full of news of patients whom Mark would know by name.

'What with filling the cook's vacancy and tending the sick, my days seem fully occupied,' she concluded.[16]

Yet below the purposeful activity and the resolute cheerfulness lay an aching sense of time passing with nothing achieved. One evening in March 1860, glancing out of the window, the slanting light through the garden trees reminded her of the spring evenings in 1848, when as a girl of sixteen she used to meet Mark returning from his walk. 'How very bright life looked then,' she thought. As she set the tea table, she remembered their laughter, companionable and gay in the garden, 'about the party sitting in silence around the large tea kettle. I was lost in these thoughts, wondering how the individuals still gathered there had altered. I wish I could say *improved*, but if I spoke the truth I should use the word *deteriorated*. Always the same gloom and silence, and with this thought I stood sick at heart. Where have all my hopes gone that things would be better? There we were, not the same but worse, and so much of one's life gone.'[17]

Was the only hope of escape for her to be a marriage without real love? Increasingly it began to seem so. Throughout 1860 Dorothy was welcomed as a daughter, whenever she cared to visit the Tates at Richmond. She stayed with them briefly after Christmas and again at midsummer. James was away from home first preparing for ordination, later seeking a living. He had been easily persuaded to agree to an indefinite engagement;[18] he was too considerate to force the issue when Mrs Pattison was so ill, the Rector so hostile and his own prospects still uncertain. In May, however, he was presented to the living of Marske-next-the-Sea, near Redcar, and both families began to demand more definite plans. 'I had expected matters to be settled this summer as to when they were to be married,' wrote Fanny to Mark. He had pressed Dorothy for news of 'her affairs', and had been put off several times with the reply that 'they are standing still for the present'.[19] Now he wrote again and received one of her evasive letters, with details, as he suspiciously complained, 'all on the outside'. Dorothy liked Marske; the stipend was small but the parsonage house good. She liked the farmers and fishermen of the village and hoped it would never become a watering-place; the sea was delightful. She said nothing about love or happiness, nothing about her inner thoughts, though the change in her

religious beliefs was serious for the future wife of a clergyman.
'When James will take possession,' she ended vaguely, 'I have not
heard. I will let you know. But oh my dear Brother, do not think
it will be any hindrance to your kind offer of *our* meeting again
this summer.'[20] Mark was not really much more enthusiastic
about his sisters marrying than their father was; he was sometimes heard in college 'expressing the most extraordinary opinions
as to the relations of the ordinary man with young women'.[21]
He seemed to accept the lion's share of Dorothy's affection and
her undivided attention on his summer holiday as his due. As
to where they should go, 'All is new to me,' said Dorothy, 'so I
shall enjoy anywhere, but it must be new to you, too. It is such
fun to explore it together!'

She delayed her holiday until the end of July, not for any
reason connected with her engagement, but because of Rachel's
second confinement. For weeks beforehand, she confessed,
she could hardly keep away from Bellerby.[22] She was with
Rachel and shared her joy at the birth of her first surviving
daughter, Mary; 'she is so happy it does my heart good to see
her'. Once again she was drawn into the life of the Stirk family,
including Purchas, sharing their company and the duties of a
working farmhouse. They kept a stable of horses, and Robert
had equipped his wife to ride and drive. Visitors to Bellerby
Manor had the freedom of the stables and the fells. For Dorothy
it was escape, release from her increasing tension. Rachel tried to
talk to her about her coming marriage, but found Dorothy was
distressed and avoided the subject. She told Rachel nothing, but
she was clearly not happy at the prospect.[23] At the end of July
Dorothy left, without saying any more, and went to join Mark
for their promised summer holiday. Mark had hoped to lure
Rachel away too, but she met this challenge to her loyalty with
gentle firmness, sending him the message, 'I would never be
happy away from home, and half the pleasure would be to have
him here with us.'[24] Instead, she asked him to stand godfather
to her baby.

Mark intended this holiday in 1860 to repeat the idyll of the
past two summers. He arranged to take charge of a country
parish, while its vicar was abroad. This was at Knightwick, on
the River Teme near its junction with the Severn which offered

good fishing and an economical holiday, 'total expenses £50'. For himself he provided his usual box of books, his fishing tackle and a dozen bottles of sherry; for Dorothy he hired a pony, so that she could ride on the Malvern Hills, to the South.[25] It is not clear how long they stayed at Knightwick, but the time was shorter than Mark had intended;[26] Dorothy was restless and anxious; she slept badly and was troubled by dreams. One night, according to her own account, she dreamt her mother pulled back the bed-curtains, and called her by her pet name, 'Dora, Dora, Dora!' She woke and could not sleep again. One of the oldest Wensleydale superstitions is the appearance, on St Mark's Eve, of those about to die. She had spent hours of her childhood in the kitchen and the stables, listening with enthralled terror to tales of ghosts and changelings,[27] and she never cured herself of being absurdly superstitious. She did not dare to tell Mark of this frightening dream, for fear of his sharp tongue, but tried to put it out of her mind, without success.[28] The dream came again; this time her mother appeared worn and ill and called her urgently. The return of the dream frightened her. Next morning at breakfast she described it to Mark, saying, 'I am sure our mother is in danger and wants me.' He laughed at her as usual. 'It is only one of your silly north-country superstitions.' 'We must go to the town to fetch our letters,' said Dorothy at her most obstinate, 'nothing else will satisfy me.' They drove to Worcester and found at the Post Office a letter from Hauxwell saying that Mrs Pattison was now dangerously ill. 'On Sept 30,' recorded Mark in his diary, 'they wrote to say she was sinking fast and if we wished to see her we must go at once. Dorothy left by the evening train.'[29] He did not accompany her. This curious episode was seen by some people as the first instance of Sister Dora's supposedly miraculous powers. It is true that she later showed an extraordinary sensitivity to the least change in a patient's condition, and an ability to foresee complications; but many highly experienced nurses do the same every day of their working lives. What seemed miraculous to others was in fact the result of her exceptional skill. The dreams and anxieties on this visit to Mark may have been the first dawning of this skill, or they may have been caused by an unquiet conscience. Dorothy had been brought up to an intensely high standard of duty and self-discipline, which she consistently showed in her work. Yet, on this occasion, she had allowed herself to be persuaded away for the third summer in succession, although her mother was seriously ill and Sarah needed her help.

On 30th September, Dorothy had an anxious and sleepless cross-country journey, with many changes of train, and drove up the lane after midnight, to find her mother awake and asking for her.[30] She did not leave the bedside again, except for brief rests, during the remainder of Mrs Pattison's life. Once bedridden, the patient was doomed. She was totally immobilized by arthritis and Dr Bowes warned them of the danger of bed-sores; 'if these sores could not be stopped, she was going fast.'[31] Mrs Pattison lay inert and for the most part silent; 'you know how reserved she was,' wrote Dorothy, 'she says nothing.' She was shrunken to skin and bone, and before long the skin broke down. 'She is sinking fast,' wrote Jane in general terms, but Dorothy added, with the shock of first experience, 'the sores are frightful, the dressing of them agony'.[32] She watched constantly by her mother, feeding her with sips of wine and water; she felt deeply grieved by her own lack of training, and that 'a real nurse' should be able to relieve suffering more effectively. Yet her presence seems to have been some comfort; 'she has taken a great deal of notice of myself,' reported Dorothy, with touching gratitude, 'sometimes she says "Good night, dear" quite in her old tones.'[33] Both she and Rachel forgot all past grievances when faced with the spectacle of their mother's suffering. 'Poor little Mother,' exclaimed Rachel. 'How the past comes back before me. She never had much warm affection, but I believe we had what she had to give.'[34]

Mrs Pattison had left her affairs in perfect order and had only two wishes, to see her absent children, and to receive Holy Communion. 'Her greatest desire,' wrote Jane, 'was to receive the Communion in peace.' Her husband knew of these wishes, but had already refused them both; he intended to be revenged because she had not altered her will at his direction and disinherited their married daughters. Now he asked, rather irritably, as Dorothy stood by, 'Do you want anything?' 'I have asked you but two things,' said his wife, 'to see Mark and to receive the Holy Communion. You have refused me both.' 'You may have anything you like,' he answered angrily, 'Cardinal Wiseman if you like, but not *that*.'[35] After this he seldom entered her room and hardly saw her, though Dorothy and Sarah noticed how she trembled if she heard his loud, angry voice near her door. To their infinite relief she did not ask for him again. Edward Wyvill attempted to visit her and her daughters, but Mr Pattison slammed the Rectory door in his face. The dying woman was thus left entirely to the spiritual care of her husband. He continued to deny his wife the sacraments, unless she altered her will at his dictation. She refused, steadfastly, to the last, and died unshriven.[36] His family had grown accustomed to hectoring, threats, acts of violence, but this abuse of priestly authority for vindictive personal ends seemed a final blasphemy. To his Tractarian daughters, in their loving reverence for the sacraments of the church, it was a sin against the Holy Ghost. To Dorothy, her father seemed beneath contempt. The Rector, chronically deluded, was now seventy-three years old, feeble, almost blind and becoming senile. Ultimately, he was deeply to be pitied, for by this last act he completed the alienation of his own children for ever.

Mr Pattison also intended to deny his wife the sight of any sons and daughters who had dared to challenge his authority. Here he was less successful. Frank was sent for from London and his kindness was a great comfort to his sisters. Eleanor and Mark either could not, or would not come, though Mark gave practical help by taking charge of Anna, to lessen the burden at home. Rachel drove down from Bellerby for the first time since her marriage. 'I never did and never would have asked *his* leave to see her,' she wrote. She found her mother on 22nd September, 'as if death were written on her face'.[37] Mrs Pattison recognized all her children and seemed comforted to see them. Now, when it was almost too late, she allowed herself to show the spontaneous affection she had suppressed all their lives. 'My poor girls . . . my dear children,' she whispered. They were very moved by this.[38] Yet this tenderness seemed to their mother a sign of weakness. She intended to die by the same inexorable creed in which she had lived. One evening she said to Dorothy, 'This has been a dark day with me, child – come here and give me your hand.' Dorothy thankfully took the wasted hand in her own, but her mother withdrew it saying, 'No – that is trusting too much to an arm of flesh. I will trust in my God alone.'[39] Two days later on 4th October she died. Dorothy wrote five minutes after, to Mark, to break the news. In an age which loved to surround death with a halo of sentimental religiosity, she gave a stark, factual account of their mother's end.

> 2 p.m.
>
> It has been a long struggle, but now it is over. She had never spoken since Tuesday night and indeed most of Tuesday we could not make out what she said. She longed to explain herself, but knew we did not understand her. She suffered agonies from her wounds and it was so hard to stand by and not be able to help her. Last night at 10.30 Frank went to Richmond to get some relief. Mr Bowes sent Morphia to be applied to the wounds on either side, but not the heel ones. She found relief from this and slumbered till 6. Then she changed and [word illegible] till five to 2 when she died. Oh Mark, what it costs us to put off our mortality! Her sufferings were so great and one felt so powerless to help. Our Father never entered her room the last two days, but she never asked for him, so this last neglect cost her no pain. Owing to the state of our poor mother's body the funeral will have to be *very soon*.'[40]

The cause of death was certified by Richard Bowes as bed-sores. Mrs Pattison was only sixty-seven, but emaciated and totally exhausted. Looking back over her life, her children could find very little comfort. 'All her dreary life', said Rachel, could form her epitaph. 'A sorrowful life closed by a painful death,' wrote Mary. Jane, searching for consolation, could only find words that might have come from the dead woman's own mouth, 'The ways of God are dark indeed.'[41] Dorothy had at least one comfort. She helped to lay the body out, and watched by it 'for it gave one such comfort to think of all her miseries over'.[42] The experience of the past weeks had left her with a fierce determination to learn whatever practical skill she could for the relief of suffering.

Jane took their mother's commonplace books and locked them away safely for Mark;[43] they feared their father might destroy them. All agreed to have 'everything very quiet and plain' at the funeral. Dorothy longed for Mark to come. Since he would not enter Hauxwell Rectory, Edward Wyvill wrote, with the greatest kindness and tact, offering him hospitality.[44] He still felt unable to attend the service.

Mrs Pattison was buried on a soft day in early October. Her coffin was borne up the avenue of beech trees leading to the church, and after the service, into the corner of the churchyard where Mr Pattison had decreed that his family tombs, like those of the Hauxwell Hall family, should be railed off from the villagers' graves. The people of Hauxwell village attended, and Dorothy found great comfort, as often before, in their kindness. 'The churchyard was full,' she wrote, 'not of curious eyes, but of people mourning for a friend.' Standing by the grave, she found herself thinking, 'I cannot yet believe I shall see her no more.'[45] Around her, yellow leaves came floating slowly down. It reminded her of verses from Keble's *The Christian Year*, most loved of all Tractarian poetry.

> *Red o'er the forest peers the setting sun,*
> *The line of yellow light dies fast away*
> *That crowns the eastern copse; and chill and dun*
> *Falls on the moor the brief November day.*

> *Now the tired hunter winds a parting note,*
> *And Echo bids good-night from every glade;*
> *Yet wait awhile and see the calm leaves float*
> *Each to his rest beneath their parent shade.*

Mark's absence left his sisters and especially Dorothy bitterly disappointed and hurt. For the first time in all their correspondence she criticized him. 'You say you thought of coming to the funeral. *I expected you* and hoped you would and still think if you had come with me you could have given and received some comfort.' He had acted responsibly in taking charge of Anna, but had clearly been unable to disguise his dislike of neurotic female invalids. 'From Anna's account,' wrote Dorothy, with unheard-of frankness, 'you must have been in one of your freezing moods. . . . Now you ought to have been very good and forbearing to poor Anna, whom you must have found strangely altered since you last saw her.'[46] Not one of Mark's sisters had dared to write to him in these terms before, and he was not the man to submit to it. He simply ceased to answer her letters. 'Dear Brother,' she wrote despairingly in December 1860, 'am I never going to hear from you – at least tell me why you do not write!'[42] In January he did at last write, perhaps for her twenty-ninth birthday, a letter so cold that to read it froze her 'into an icicle'. Trying to answer it, she found her fingers so numb they could hardly hold the pen; the ice was at her heart as well as at the window-panes. She did her best to rekindle the old affection, rejoicing warmly when Mark was at last elected in the same month to the Rectorship of Lincoln College. 'I know you will say that I know nothing about these matters,' she wrote, 'I know one thing, that I wished you to get it very much.'[48] Mark was not to be won over. He was, of course, pleased to be elected Rector, but characteristically his pleasure seemed less vivid and intense than the pain of disappointment ten years earlier. He continued to treat his youngest sister with reserve. 'I know I never came before R[achel],' she wrote, sadly. 'I never expected to, because indeed I was not equal to her, but I used to have a corner in your heart and now I am afraid I have lost it.'[49]

Dorothy was lonely and uncertain. The question of marriage, gladly put on one side during her mother's illness, now had to be faced. An invalid mother had been the unanswerable reason why she could not leave home. James Tate had agreed to prolonging their 'understanding' for as long as her mother lived. Her father had always angrily refused his consent to a formal engagement, but everyone else in both families expected them to marry. There was now no reason to delay any longer. Thousands of her contemporaries married every year without real love, for security, for social status, sometimes merely to escape from home. Why should not she do the same?

In January 1861 the Tates wrote, apparently demanding some definite decision, and Rachel warned Mark in a worried, ungrammatical note, 'I fear things are not going smoothly between J.T. and Dora but I don't feel at liberty for any more. I only mention it to let you know I wish for no concealment between you and I.'[50] Rachel knew more than she would admit. In March Dorothy, very unhappily, said that she could not marry James and broke off all relations with the Tate family. Mark wrote to Rachel demanding an explanation. In reply he received an account of all that Dorothy had so carefully concealed from him since 1854 or '55. He learnt for the first time that Purchas Stirk had loved her, 'and I believe,' added Rachel, 'he has never ceased to do so.' He learnt of Dorothy's fickleness towards the young farmer, her first engagement to James and its breaking in 1858, her meetings with Purchas at Bellerby, yet her renewed engagement to James Tate. 'What was my surprise', wrote single-hearted Rachel, in bewilderment, 'to hear of her visits (to Richmond) and the prospect of her marriage!'[51] Everything fitted only too well; now Mark understood Dorothy's reluctance to talk about the subject of her future, her strange willingness to leave everything and seek his own company. The worst blow to his pride came last. Dorothy was too honest, after her long hesitation, and too passionate to compromise in a marriage of convention. She would not marry James, because 'now she tells me she fears she prefers P.S.',[52] explained Rachel at last. Mark, beside himself with anger, wrote attacking Rachel, as he had attacked Fanny in 1856, for concealing the affair. In reply he got a letter from Dorothy, as cold and hard as flint. She was not afraid to demand freedom. She took entire responsibility for her own affairs, and did not admit a brother's right to interfere. 'Rachel knew nothing,' she wrote, 'though I know from experience how hard you are to convince. Nothing has grieved me so much as that my darling sister has suffered on my account.'[53] Mark's anger was transferred to Dorothy; there are no entries in his diary for this date, but it is clear from his actions that he never fully forgave her for the rest of their lives.

Mark was indeed deeply hurt. He did not love easily, still less believe himself loved. Yet for the past twelve years he had loved Dorothy, against a remembered background of hill and cloud, valley and waterfall. He may even have felt in their devotion an echo of his favourite poet, Wordsworth and another sister Dorothy:

> *She who dwells with me, whom I have loved*
> *With such communion, that no place on earth*
> *Can ever be a solitude to me.*

Now the purity of this communion was tarnished in retrospect. For years, while he had trusted her, she had deliberately hidden her inmost feelings from him. He had taught her, spoilt her, even revealed himself to her, while all the time she had been making a fool of him. There was even some primitive jealousy in his resentment. This surely explained his later accusations that Sister Dora was 'false' and her goodness a self-glorifying fantasy.[54] In fact, his morbid suspicion and her instinct for concealment were two sides of the same coin. Both owed it to their unhappy heredity and upbringing.

Everyone blamed Dorothy. The Tates, who had been to her a second family, could not bear even to hear her name mentioned, 'not that I blame them,' wrote Rachel candidly. The Pattison sisters were frigidly scandalized. Dorothy had done nothing remotely immoral; but by the standards of a provincial clergy family in the 1860s she must have appeared compromised. Rachel, who was extremely sensitive to any slight upon her husband's family, felt Dorothy had 'used P.S. ill'. No one however blamed Dorothy as harshly as she blamed herself. Her nature, warm, impulsive and generous, was ready to accept the whole burden of guilt. At first perhaps she had enjoyed power, the only power she had ever experienced in her life, over two such contrasted men: one so delightful in family and background, the other, rougher in speech and bearing, who had nevertheless the power to stir her deeply. She was reluctant to give up either; in the end she had brought unhappiness to a whole circle of people she loved, to her family, to the Tates, to the two young men themselves, and to Mark, who had meant more to her than either. Those who met her in later life noticed that she bore the scars of fierce battles with herself, some of them to her death-bed.[55] They were puzzled that someone so unselfishly, transparently kind, would sometimes exclaim, 'I have done very wrong. I have been very wilful, let no one be as I was!' Various bizarre explanations, as will emerge, were offered for this self-blame, and for the harshness of Sister Dora's self-discipline. It seems clear she feared that her own power over men, and their power over her, might overcome her judgment. She had still a lifetime of struggle ahead.

In 1861 everything seemed to have come to an end, her mother's life, her nursing duties at home, her love affairs, her brother's love. 'This has been a sad year,' she wrote to Mark, in the birthday letter she never failed to send him even now they were estranged,

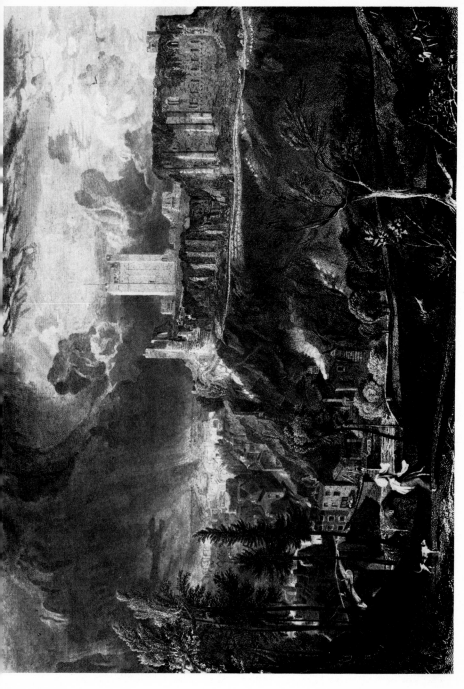

6b. Richmond, Yorkshire, from an engraving after J. M. W. Turner

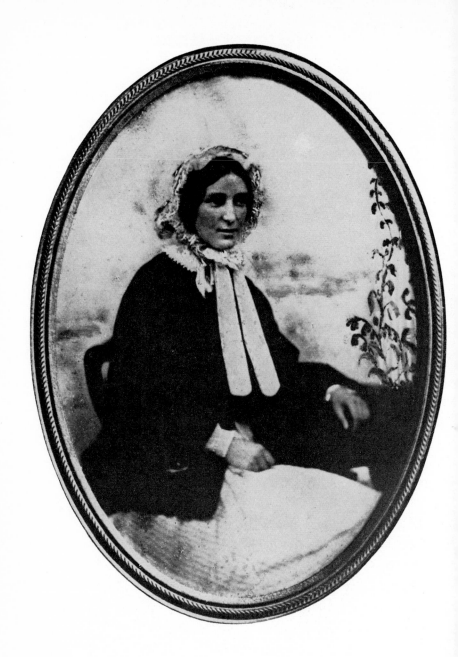

7. 'The Hat has gained great admiration.' The first photograph of Dorothy Pattison, taken on a visit to Mark Pattison at Oxford in 1859 when she was twenty-seven

'but I trust it has left me "a wiser tho' a sadder" person.' She never spoke of Purchas Stirk. She had no intention of looking backward, or lingering over regrets. The fight for freedom was now in the open. 'I have made up my mind to leave Hauxwell and work my own way.'[56]

NOTES

1. Will of the Reverend Mark James Pattison, P.P.R. 1866, f. 49.
2. Pattison, 53, f. 230.
3. Will of Jane Pattison, P.P.R. 1861, f. 546.
4. Pattison, 53, ff. 94–102.
5. Ibid., ff. 235.
6. W. S. C. Copeman, *A Short History of Gout and the Rheumatic Diseases*, 151.
7. Pattison, 53, f. 102.
8. Ibid., 53, ff. 94–102.
9. Ibid., 52, f. 618.
10. Ibid., 52, ff. 618–21.
11. Ibid., 53, f. 379.
12. Ibid., 53, f. 203.
13. Ibid., 53, ff. 179–81.
14. Ibid., 53, ff. 94–102.
15. Ibid., 53, ff. 94–102. In fact this practical experience of cooking and housekeeping proved most valuable to her.
16. Ibid., 53, ff. 133–5.
17. Ibid., 53, ff. 133–6.
18. Ibid., 54, f. 281.
19. Ibid., 53, f. 181.
20. Ibid., 53, ff. 188–91.
21. V. H. H. Green, *Oxford Common Room*, 266.
22. Pattison, 53, f. 235.
23. Ibid., 54, f. 28.
24. Ibid., 52, ff. 210–12.
25. Ibid., 40, f. 38 and 130, f. 23.
26. Ibid., 40, f. 136.
27. *Memoirs*, 37.
28. Lonsdale, 16. 'She told her old servant.' This may be a confusion with Jane Bowe at Builth; Dorothy had no personal maid.
29. Pattison, 130, f. 25.

30. Ibid., 53, f. 474.
31. Ibid., 51, ff. 275–6, bound among 1856 letters but clearly 1860.
32. Ibid., 53, f. 302.
33. Ibid., 53, f. 308–10.
34. Ibid., 53, f. 298.
35. Ibid., 53, ff. 308–10.
36. J. Sparrow, *Mark Pattison and the Idea of a University*, 36.
37. Pattison, 51, ff. 275–6.
38. Ibid., 53, ff. 338–40.
39. Ibid., 53, f. 309.
40. Ibid., 53, ff. 310–12.
41. Ibid., 53, f. 320.
42. Ibid., 53, ff. 338–40.
43. Ibid., 53, ff. 66–9, 73.
44. Ibid., 53, f. 312.
45. Ibid., 53, ff. 338–40.
46. Ibid., 53, f. 379.
47. Ibid., 53, f. 429.
48. Ibid., 54, f. 7.
49. Ibid., 54, ff. 457–8.
50. Ibid., 54, f. 27.
51. Ibid., 54, f. 280.
52. Ibid., 54, f. 281.
53. Ibid., 54, f. 283.
54. V. H. H. Green, *Oxford Common Room*, 304.
55. Lonsdale, 13.
56. Pattison, 54, ff. 457–8.

CHAPTER EIGHT

A Village Schoolmistress
1861–1862

The summer months of 1861 were the loneliest in Dorothy Pattison's life. She was cut off from every source of companionship, from her disapproving sisters, from the Tates' cheerful household, from Mark himself. This last, deepest severance was brought home to her in September,[1] when Mark at the age of forty-eight, used the privilege of an Oxford head of house, and married a girl of twenty-one, Francis Strong. His sisters found it almost impossible to imagine him a bridegroom. 'If your sisters plagued you, what will a wife do?' wrote Rachel, with more pertinence than she knew. Indeed it is difficult to picture the thoughts of this confirmed and parsimonious bachelor, entering in his account book, 'Clothes brush 4/6 Soap 4/- Braces 1/6 Umbrella 8/6 cabs various 2/6'.[2] Such items, repeated over the years, gradually brought home to him the unwelcome change in his habits which marriage must entail. Predictably, the marriage of this strangely-assorted couple was unhappy; ill-matched in body from the first, they became increasingly so in mind, until Mark came to feel that 'a wall of ice has been built between us'. For the present, however, he was undoubtedly in love, and his young wife bound to him both by the powers of intellect and his elusive personal charm. Generously Dorothy rejoiced in Mark's happiness and wrote 'to greet you on your arrival *home*, which indeed it will be now you have a dear companion by your side. . . . I long to hear all about your tour. Did Francis enjoy your favourite haunts?'[3] She would have liked to know her sister-in-law, who was intelligent and beautiful, with a striking personal style of her own; it appears that she was never asked to do so, and that they never met. Nevertheless Francis eased this turning-point in Dorothy's life. She was a believer in employment for women[4] and without her influence it is most unlikely that cautious, conventional Mark would have smoothed the way for his sister to escape.

Dorothy saw her one hope of freedom in work. She had put all depression and doubt behind her. Week by week she scanned the newspapers and answered every possible advertisement. It was pitifully easy to deceive the Rector, now too blind to see any letters that entered or left the house. Later the memory of this was to cause his daughter pain, but for the present it was merely another practical consideration. She lost one post in the Isle of Wight because she could not attend an interview, but promptly applied for others.[5] In the end she was not the first to leave Hauxwell. Most unexpectedly, Elizabeth, quietest and most domesticated of the family, whom Eleanor had once described as 'Betty without an idea', preceded her. In the autumn of 1861 she took a job far from home as nursery governess. Dorothy travelled on the branch line to see her off on the express train from North-allerton Junction, apparently for ever. Mr Pattison, in helpless senile rage, alternated between saying Elizabeth should never enter the house again and threatening to fetch her back; in fact he never succeeded in discovering her whereabouts.[6] Dorothy prepared to follow her.

As always, this unhappy family could not agree on any course of action. Mary and Jane disapproved of Dorothy's plans, Sarah sympathized, Anna could no longer understand, while Fanny appeared too weary and depressed to care. Rachel, who was at this time much more devout than Dorothy, was concerned for spiritual reasons. 'There is a deal of worldliness in it,' she wrote to Mark, 'her wishes and desires tend that way. I do fear for D. I care so much for her and feel she needs teaching and discipline, a fine character untrained.'[7] This is of interest because many of Sister Dora's later admirers flatly refused to believe there was any ordinary human ambition in her character. 'It has always seemed to us evident,' wrote one of them, 'that she was called from a child to the work to which she was eventually led. . . . She heard the Master's voice in early life, inclining her to the work which He had marked out for her, and rejoiced to obey it.'[8] The opinion of Rachel, who was so close to Dorothy, suggests the contrary at this date.

Nothing ever destroyed the affection between these two sisters, but life was preparing to carry them apart. As well as the twins who had died Rachel had five daughters, Mary, Jane, Dora, Rachel and Philippa, born in rapid succession.[9] She loved her husband, but was never strong, and the struggle to win a living for so many from that harsh climate and soil exhausted her. Dorothy was anxious on her behalf. For herself, she knew that under Mark's influence, she had read, thought and seen too much to settle to life on a Wensleydale farm. Though her attraction to Purchas Stirk had ended her engagement to James Tate, the idea of marriage between them was not apparently in Dorothy's mind. This may well have caused Rachel some regret; she felt, with justice, that her brother-in-law had been badly treated.

On 23rd October 1861 Dorothy wrote to Mark in a mixture of triumph and perplexity.

I told you I was trying to get some situation by which I could help myself. I seem to have got the very thing, that of Lady Teacher in a village school at Woolston. Work, stipend, a pretty house, everything suited me and I am hoping to enter on my duties; but a difficulty has now arisen which I know not how to meet and you seemed the only person who could help me. The Trustees are desirous of a testimonial as to character and fitness for the place. You must see nobody could furnish it in this neighbourhood, without informing my Father. Now if he got to know of it he would put a stop to my intentions as he is trying to do to Elizabeth's, only he has not been able to discover her whereabouts. . . . Mr. Hill (the Vicar of Woolston) also wants to know if my Father approves of the course I am undertaking and that I go out into the world 'with his blessing'!!! Now what must I answer to *that* – for it seems to me impossible to make Mr. Hill understand our case? I am sure if I only obtain this situation I shall be a better and happier person; working and labouring and being dependent on my own resources will do me good. Time is precious. They had twenty-five applications for the post and there are many longing for it.[10]

In this crisis Mark's action was decisive. He wrote personally on Dorothy's behalf to the Vicar of Woolston, though it cannot have been an easy letter for him to write. His explanation was satisfactory, for she was appointed village schoolmistress at Little Woolston, near Newport Pagnell in Buckinghamshire. She wrote on 16th November: 'Today I have heard that I am the successful candidate – oh my dear Brother, I do indeed trust that this may be the beginning not only of a new life, but a better, more useful one. . . . How proud I shall be when I first receive money of my *own earning*.'[11] This was the last of many great services by Mark Pattison to his youngest sister. He grew gradually to view her with coldness, even with actual dislike, but she never forgot that she owed everything to him. Without him she could never have won her long fight for personal freedom. To the end of her life she read everything that he published, books, articles, even letters to the press. She could not imagine, and indeed it is impossible to imagine now, what would have become of the ignorant, impulsive girl she was, if he had not come home in 1848, to take her into his exacting but formative affections.

Dorothy left Hauxwell for the last time, in a snowstorm, about a month before her thirtieth birthday. She was never to return. Her sole possession was ninety pounds, which she had received from Frank as executor of her mother's will. but it was enough to release her from total dependence. She had invested seventy pounds, 'a bright idea', as she claimed, and carried twenty in cash for removal expenses;[12] indeed she could not have bought her own railway ticket without her mother's legacy. She was met at Bletchley station by the Reverend Edward Hill, who drove her to the Vicarage, where she stayed with his wife and family until the paint in the minute school cottage was dry. They were 'most kind' she said, and she grew fond of them. The vicar, who was now about thirty-five, had come to this parish straight from Wadham College, and was to remain until his death; he was totally devoted to his village church and people. He had just restored the ruined chancel of the church, and raised money locally for the first school in the village's history. Great and Little Woolston was a joint parish consisting of two hamlets, about three miles from Newport Pagnell. The total population in 1861 was less than two hundred people.[13]

Although it is now within a few miles of the huge railway workshops at Wolverton and the main motorway to Birmingham and the north-west, Woolston is still uncannily quiet. It is a deep and sleepy countryside, with lush meadows, interlaced by the winding, willowy River Ouse and the straight Grand Junction Canal. The contrast with the hard clear uplands of Yorkshire was as great as Dorothy could imagine. A narrow lane, muddy in winter and half-buried in cow-parsley all summer, led through drowsy fields, under innumerable elm trees, from Newport Pagnell. At the entrance to the hamlet it crossed the canal, moving slowly between its sedgy banks. Traffic on the canal was heavier in 1861 than on the road; barge horses plodded along the footpath, the tow-rope dipping and rising behind them on their way to Birmingham. On summer evenings the watermen sat outside the Barge Inn with their mugs of beer. There was a triangular green, one farm-house, a few labourers' cottages and nothing else.

Dorothy was enchanted by her first sight of the school beside the green, with its red-brick Gothic gables, diamond-paned windows, and white wooden bell-cote. One end formed her cottage, small as a doll's house. Behind lay a paved yard, which she scrubbed with vigour, a wash-house where she boiled her own sheets in the copper, and a cellar where she shovelled her own coals. Her only possessions of any value were her forks and spoons and a little silver tea-pot which had belonged to her mother. She was fond of this and polished it to perfection. She could not afford, nor did she want a servant; middle-class visitors were 'astonished to find Miss Pattison blacking her own grate when they came to see her'.[14] Her minute kitchen was kept in spotless order. The 'big boys' of her school helped to dig and plant her vegetable patch. She was poor and quite alone in the world, but happy; for the first time in her life she was free.

Her new job presented many problems. For various reasons the year 1861 was a somewhat bleak time in which to begin work as a teacher. It is of interest as the first year for which we have a comprehensive survey of English elementary education. This was the work of a Royal Commission under the Duke of Newcastle to suggest measures 'for the extension of sound and cheap elementary instruction to all classes of the people'. Dorothy was well acquainted with the details of the Education Commission, for Mark had served since 1859 as one of the assistant commissioners of inquiry, travelling to Germany to make a comparative survey of schools and colleges there. The commissioners found that one in seven English children attended school, and of these only nineteen per cent stayed after the age of eleven. Education was not compulsory, as in France or Germany, since compulsion was 'opposed to the feelings and in some respect to the principles of this country'.[15] In rural districts, like Little Woolston, children were continually taken away from school to work at low wages on the land during harvest seasons. No schools were provided by the State. Buildings and funds were dependent half on private subscriptions and half on grants from religious bodies, either the undenominational British and Foreign Schools Society or its rival the National Society founded in 1811, 'for promoting the Education of the Poor in the Principles of the Established Church'. At Little Woolston a local landowner, William Smith, had given the site for 'a handsome new National School' built in 1861,[16] of which Dorothy was the first headmistress. It was therefore her duty to teach all her pupils the liturgy and catechism of the Church of England and to take them regularly to the parish church twice every Sunday. Woolston lay near Newport Pagnell, centre of the Buckinghamshire lace-makers, with their inherited Calvinist tradition. Dissenting parents were forced to sacrifice their scruples about Church doctrine for the sake of getting their children an education. Cases like these were recognized by the Education Commission as a serious injustice, but nothing was done to take the schools out of denominational control.[17] Elementary school teachers, of whom Dorothy now became one, were a somewhat subdued class, with good reason. They were trained either by apprenticeship as pupil-teachers, or in denominational Colleges, in 'a simplicity of life not remote from the habits of the humble classes'.[18] In National Schools they were expected to be subservient to the managers, the incumbent and the inspector appointed by the Church, a social superior, who 'moving in the same class of society, understands the objects and feelings of the managers. It would be a great mistake to introduce a person of inferior manners and education as an adviser or an authority into the schools'.[19] School mistresses were drawn from the poorer classes; 'and in becoming a teacher a lady was held to have lost caste'. To take examples from fiction, Hardy's Fancy Day was a gamekeeper's daughter, while Cherry Elwood in *The Daisy Chain* had been a domestic servant until an accident unfitted her for anything more arduous than education. 'Of pupil teachers,' wrote a contributor to *The Edinburgh Review* of April 1862, 'the greater number would otherwise now have been domestics.' The average yearly salary of a woman teacher in the 1860s was twenty-six pounds. Dorothy later admitted that she had found it a constant struggle to keep out of debt.[20] As a clergy daughter and sister of the Rector of Lincoln College she was an anomaly in the school system. Happily, she was the first of many; in 1872 Bishop Otter College at Chichester was re-founded to train girls of the professional classes or 'reduced ladies' as certificated teachers.

She had wondered what she would have to teach. Mark had exclaimed impatiently, 'What nonsense that silly girl attempting to teach others when she knows nothing herself!' Dorothy replied, 'I have weighed my own powers, considered my duties and I think I have undertaken nothing that I cannot do. *I like teaching* and think I am competent to teach all that village children require.'[21] In fact she could teach far more. The Education Commission's report makes clear how limited, and how deadly dull, a child's everyday lessons were likely to be. 'It is quite possible', wrote an assistant commissioner, later to be a bishop, 'to teach a child soundly and thoroughly, all that is necessary for him to possess in the shape of intellectual attainment, by the time that he is ten years old. He shall read a paragraph in a newspaper with sufficient ease . . . if gone to live at a distance from home he shall write his mother a letter that shall be legible and intelligible; he shall know enough of ciphering to make out a common shop bill.' The religious education of this ten-year-old was confined to the catechism, and ability to follow 'a plain Saxon sermon. I have no brighter view of the possibilities of an English elementary education than this,' concluded the reverend gentleman rather glumly. 'If I had more sanguine dreams before, what I have seen in the last six months would have effectually and for ever dissipated them.'[22] It was not easy for a young schoolmistress to teach with intelligence, spirit or inventiveness within this dreary mechanical framework. The new system of 'payment by results', which followed the Newcastle Report, put increasing pressure on teachers to do mechanical work, for their jobs now depended on examination results and attendance registers.[23] Clearly Dorothy Pattison could never have made a subservient, mechanically efficient teacher, drumming the three Rs by rote into classes of bored and fidgety small children. There is evidence that she used every inch of free play the system allowed.

The school was built for fifty children of all ages from five until twelve; the school attendance was usually about thirty children, nearly all under ten. Dorothy treated them like a large family party. In this she had the intelligent support of the Vicar, who explained that he wanted her to influence the children by tone and principle, rather than mould them harshly on a rigid and hard system of school keeping.[24] She was allowed to tell them, she said, 'the interminable stories in which children delight'.[25] Sometimes these were tales from the Bible, from history, fairy-stories and folk-lore, which she told in dramatic form, acting all the parts herself, as she had done in her own childhood. Sometimes they were serial stories of her own inventing, which went on from week to week, adding characters and incidents from her fertile imagination. She was already an experienced choir trainer and a competent organist; it was a pleasure to hear her children's confident singing in church. The summer of 1862 seems to have been fine and warm. Whenever she could Dorothy took her children out of doors. She had remained childlike herself in her love of country pleasures, and admitted she shared their delight 'in animals, flowers, a sunshiny day, a roll in a haycock or a game of play of any kind'. The very little ones were secretly her favourites, but she taught herself to manage a mixed group of boys and girls of all ages, engaged in different activities in her one big schoolroom. This, as every teacher knows, is a real test of skill and patience; she found it of practical value later on. After the little children, her sympathies were for the 'big girls', at ten or eleven destined to a future of drudgery as farm servants or labourers' wives. She tidied their clothes, and brushed their tangled hair in a motherly way; when she finally left the school, she continued to ask after them by name.[26] If any child was absent through illness, she went after school, to visit the parents and offer help with nursing the small patient. The parents were touched by this care. Eleanor, who visited her briefly, wrote, 'She is well off, being almost worshipped by the farmers and their wives, and happy in her work.'[27] She was respected as 'a highly-bred lady', but this was apparently no barrier to affection. In 1862 Fanny reported 'From D. at Woolston we have very good accounts, she has certainly fallen among kind friends; she seems to take great pleasure in her work and is succeeding well. She writes most cheerfully and surmounts all her difficulties with great spirit.'[28]

To the school managers and the local gentry, their new head-mistress was an enigma. Nothing was known about her, and she volunteered no information. They agreed she was 'Every inch a lady', but got no further. Some made overtures of friendship. Visiting the splendid Decorated Church at Milton Keynes, she met the daughter of George Finch, Lord of the Manor; they exchanged visits and letters, but the relationship remained impersonal. An elderly and well-to-do couple near Woolston, who were childless, wanted to adopt her as their daughter. She later said they had offered to make her their heiress. She refused, but agreed to accept from the husband a gift of ten pounds every year 'to do as she pleased with'. This she used to give away, since it was difficult to save 'even sixpence out of her income' for charity. The donor was surprised and hurt by this use of his gift; when eventually in 1864 Dorothy left Little Woolston, he sent it no more.[29] Now that she could move about in the world independently she was discovering what had remained largely hidden at Hauxwell, the strength of her power to charm the most casual acquaintances. Her vitality made them feel alive. Where she chose, she could bind others to her strong will as though by some magic spell. At Woolston she began to develop what an observer called her extraordinary 'power of personal influence – that subtle, many-sided, most doubtful of blessings to the possessor'. The only check on it was her constant ideal of 'using all the talents God has given me in his service'.[30] Although she enjoyed teaching and made a success of it she never wavered in her determination to nurse. From visiting sick school children she progressed to visiting any cottage in the parish where there was illness. Wages were too low for doctors' bills, there was no apothecary or chemist's shop nearer than Newport Pagnell, and people were glad to send for the schoolmistress, with her light step, firm, cool hand and shrewd glance which already inspired confidence. Privately, Dorothy was deeply dissatisfied with her own standard of nursing; she knew enough to know that she knew nothing, but hoped to learn by experience. Florence Nightingale's *Notes on Nursing* were published in 1860; Dorothy clearly studied and used them, and it seems likely, though not certain, that she first read them at Little Woolston. She was not free to nurse in the daytime, because she was on duty in the school, but volunteered to stay up all night with anyone who was seriously ill or dying. This offer was thankfully accepted, and she trained herself to take rest in short snatches.

It was lonely in the little schoolhouse, lonelier still sitting up by the light of one candle in strange cottages. Dorothy was not nervous of the country people, all of whom she knew, but barge traffic on the canal sometimes brought rough strangers. One day a ragged man called at her door to beg, and looked round her little kitchen with ferret-sharp eyes. That night she went to sit with a man in the village, who was dangerously ill. He died about midnight; she laid out his body and set out for home. As she walked through the fields between one and two o'clock in the morning, she saw from a distance a light burning in her kitchen. Snatching up her skirts she ran, and burst open the cottage door, just as the beggar escaped through the schoolroom window with a sack. One glance at the kitchen dresser was enough; her forks and spoons, above all the little silver tea-pot she cherished, had gone, never to be found.[31]

In spite of poverty and loneliness, Dorothy still felt herself fortunate to be in her own cottage, as she said 'making her own way in the world'. In October 1862 news from Hauxwell confirmed this feeling. For months, if not years, her sister Fanny had been visibly drifting towards breakdown. She was sleepless from painful sciatica and deeply depressed.[32] Now Sarah wrote in great distress, 'Fanny is seriously ill, and alas, it is not bodily illness but mental'. The first symptom was that Fanny, so deeply devout, refused Holy Communion. She was convinced she had committed a dreadful crime. She must escape from the house and hide where she could no longer bring disgrace on her family. Significantly, she believed that Mark, who had judged her so harshly for a minor fault in the past, would never forgive her. 'It is most distressing to witness her agony of mind,' wrote Sarah. 'The only thing that in the least soothes her is when I agree she is wicked.'[33] Richard Bowes took the case very seriously, but treatment was difficult. Fanny grew worse. She refused to eat or drink, except penitential bread and water, would not dress herself, wash or permit anyone to touch her. She insisted she was impure and her delusions centred on incest; she believed herself to have had 'improper communication with Frank. She has once or twice threatened to destroy herself. . . . I fear that it has been long coming on. Poor F., what a life she has had!'[34] wrote Rachel.

Dorothy was deeply sad. She knew, as all the sisters did, that Fanny had long been secretly and hopelessly in love with their kind friend Mr Wyvill. Mark, characteristically pitied himself, 'Little did I know what horrors were in store for me', and transferred all blame to Sarah, 'the things F. said ought to have roused Sarah to the actual state of her mind'.[35] Sarah's position was desperate. She found herself nurse to a household of six people, three of whom, her father, Anna and Fanny, were effectively insane. Moreover Fanny's threats of suicide were real and dangerous. Fortunately in this crisis the family found the help which had been so lacking at the time of their father's breakdown thirty years before. Richard Bowes diagnosed, in the terminology of the time, Monomania.[36] He removed Fanny from the scene of her miseries, and put her under the care of Dr Forbes Winslow, at the Sussex House Asylum, Hammersmith, London. Forbes Winslow, F.R.C.P., was a former President of the Medical Society of London, and author of a number of standard texts, including one on suicide.[37] Medical treatment in 1833 had left Mr Pattison a mental cripple for life. By 1862 it was able, after some months of care, to restore his daughter to health. The outcome of this last disaster was happy for two members of the Pattison family. Fanny, at the age of forty-five, was able to begin a new life of profound value and fulfilment. What this was will appear later. Sarah's destiny was simpler. On 11th December 1864, at the age of thirty-seven, she married Richard Bowes himself, who was some twelve years older.[38] Mr Pattison, in the last years of his long decline, kept with him, of his ten children, only the two middle-aged spinsters Jane and Mary, and Anna, a helpless invalid.

By the time Fanny had been moved to London, Dorothy herself was struggling with illness. The autumn climate of Woolston was damp and enervating, the fields blanketed with fog from the river and the canal. She caught cold, apparently early in October, but carried on with her work. The vicar, anxious for the success of his school, exhorted her 'not to give way'. Never was advice more unnecessary. Dorothy, brought up in a household of invalids, had a dislike and contempt for invalidism that rivalled Emily Brontë's. She continued teaching by day, and whenever she got a call, went out to nurse at night, walking sometimes two or three miles over soaking field paths. She developed a hard cough, and a sharp pain 'like a stitch' in her side as she breathed, but with iron self-will obstinately refused to acknowledge their existence. One morning the children, coming to school, found their headmistress missing. She lay gasping in her cottage bedroom, and admitted at last, 'I positively could not get out of bed.'[39] The doctor was fetched from Newport Pagnell and diagnosed a severe attack of pleurisy, a repetition of her dangerous girlhood illness in 1846. Neighbours took turns to nurse her, and, as before, her powers of recovery were great. By November 1862, she was well enough to go away on holiday.

Dorothy felt a craving for the strong, salt air of Redcar, which had helped her earlier convalescence; but the fifteen years between had turned Redcar into a conventional seaside resort. She chose instead to go to Coatham, still a fishing village, separated from Redcar by half a mile of open green.[40] Here she found the remembered ten-mile walk along sand so firm that the North Sea, thundering against the treacherous rocks of the Salt Scar offshore, left hardly a ripple upon it. On winter afternoons the sun sank red in the mists behind Middlesbrough, while sailing-ships passed and re-passed in the mouth of the Tees. 'The prospect is rendered pleasing,' said the guide-book, 'by the number of vessels sailing in the offing.'[41]

It seems to have been by chance on one of these solitary winter walks that she met again James Tate, whose parish at Marske was less than five miles away. She was still weak from her illness and perhaps more lonely than she cared to admit. She was delighted to see him. James was kind, considerate, as gentle as ever, and in her present mood she appreciated his good qualities as never before. On his side, he promised never to let anything or anybody come between them. By the end of her holiday their often-broken engagement was once more renewed.[42] James was reluctant to let her go, but she pointed out that she had promised to return to her work at Little Woolston as soon as she was fit. For six weeks they wrote to one another every day. James urged her to give notice and marry him at Christmas. She was just preparing to do this when he wrote to say that he had been to Richmond and told his parents of the marriage. 'They were so much against it, and his mother's aversion was such that he feared it would hasten her death.'[43] His father was already in bad health and in fact died shortly after, leaving James to take care of his widowed mother. The luckless young man was once again the prisoner of his own dutiful character. He wrote to Dorothy, breaking their engagement, this time for ever. 'All is over between us,' Dorothy told Rachel. 'James has not used her well,' wrote Rachel to Mark, adding with some truth, 'had he been more independent everything would have been different.'[44] News travelled fast round the family. Two days before Christmas Eleanor and her husband appeared at the school cottage and carried Dorothy off to spend the holiday with them at Wyham Rectory. 'Her remaining at Woolston to keep it alone under the circumstances was quite out of the question,' reported Eleanor firmly. Playing Christmas games with 'the sweet children', Dorothy summoned up her pride and prepared to return to independence.

James Tate returned to Richmond as curate and lived for the next two years with his widowed mother in the house in French-gate. In 1866 he was presented to the living of Croxton in Lincoln-shire, where he married. In 1869 he moved with his wife to Plaxtol, Kent, where he was vicar for the rest of his life.[45] Dorothy told Rachel when he married that 'she had no regrets, indeed she was glad, his lonely life was no longer on her conscience'. She could not say the same of Purchas Stirk. He moved with his younger brothers Christopher and Edward to a farm at Barden Lane, in the Hauxwell parish; it was local practice to leave a high moor farm, cheap to rent, and move to lower, more fertile land when income allowed. Christopher and Edward farmed down there till the end of the century, and have descendants still farming in the parish;[46] but Purchas died at Barden from some gastric virus, unmarried, only thirty-one. He was buried among his family's graves at Aysgarth on 8th March 1865.[47] Dorothy had long since ceased to be in love with him, but with him was buried a large part of her youth, that time when 'life looked very bright and there seemed so much to attain to'.[48] What remained in maturity was the knowledge that she had caused pain.

In January 1862 Dorothy Pattison was thirty. In looks and bearing she appeared more like a girl of twenty, and to outward view she had led a life sheltered from the world. In fact she had passed through experiences that steeled her for the best and the worst life had to offer. These experiences were largely unknown to her contemporaries and have remained unrecorded and unaccounted for until now. As a child she had wandered untaught through a landscape of matchless poetry and power. Below the surface respectability of Victorian provincial life, she had seen madness, hatred, revenge, suffering and death. She had known the angry bitterness of religious strife and questioned her own faith to its foundations. An ignorant girl, she had been guided in reading and conversation by one of the most distinguished minds of the day, and suffered the shock of rejection when she fell from Mark's favour. She had felt the frustration of talents and energies rusting unused, while the years passed by in deadly sameness. She had been youthfully loved and in love, learning too late the double-edged and dangerous power this gave her. She had fought and won the battle for personal freedom. Gradually under the stresses of life, the circle of family and friendship broke. The scenery of her youth became, in Mark's words, 'the shell in which home love once was, and *is* no longer'. She was now quite alone. Dorothy Pattison's life was ending; Sister Dora was about to take her place.

NOTES

1. Pattison, 55, f. 457. College Fellows were still compelled to remain single.
2. Ibid., 55, 14.
3. Ibid., 54, ff. 457–8.

4. Later, as Lady Dilke, she was to be a patron and supporter of the Women's Trade Union League.
5. Pattison, 54, ff. 457–8.
6. Ibid., 54, ff. 485–8.
7. Ibid., 54, f. 460.
8. Ridsdale, preface.
9. Will of Dorothy Wyndlow Pattison, P.P.R., 1879, f. 39.
10. Pattison, 54, ff. 484–8.
11. Ibid., 54, f. 582.
12. Ibid., 54, f. 502. Lonsdale, 17, says 'Her father told her he should merely give her the allowance she had always had and this added to the schoolmistress's salary was all she had to live on'. She had never received an allowance and her 'private income' appears to have been the interest on seventy pounds.
13. Casey, *Directory of Buckinghamshire: 1863*.
14. Lonsdale, 20.
15. W. S. Maclure, *Educational Documents: 1816–1963*, 70.
16. Casey, *Directory of Buckinghamshire: 1863*.
17. Pattison, 14.
18. H. C. Barnard, *A History of English Education*, 102.
19. J. S. Maclure, *Educational Documents*, 73.
20. Pattison, 56, f. 177.
21. Ibid., 54, ff. 485–8.
22. J. S. Maclure, *Educational Documents*, 75–6.
23. It came into force on 1st August 1863, and may well have confirmed Dorothy Pattison's determination to move from teaching to nursing as her life's work.
24. Pattison, 54, f. 497.
25. Lonsdale, 19.
26. Ibid., 24–5.
27. Pattison, 55, f. 250.
28. Ibid., 55, f. 262.
29. Lonsdale, 20.
30. Pattison, 54, f. 502.
31. Lonsdale, 19.
32. Pattison, 130, f. 23.
33. Ibid., 55, f. 191.
34. Ibid., 55, f. 199.
35. Ibid., 130, f. 35.
36. Ibid., 55, f. 191.
37. Medical Directory, 1860.
38. Hauxwell Parish Registers.

Dorothy Pattison

39. Lonsdale, 21.
40. White, *Directory of North Riding:* 1867.
41. Slater, *Directory of Yorkshire:* 1855.
42. Pattison, 55, f. 220.
43. Ibid., 55, f. 250.
44. Ibid., 55, f. 220.
45. Alumni Oxoniensis.
46. Spennithorne and Hauxwell Parish Registers.
47. Aysgarth Parish Registers.
48. Pattison, 53, f. 179–81.

PART TWO

Sister Dora

CHAPTER NINE

An Anglican Novice
1862–1864

There was no sudden or dramatic conversion in this change. Rather the elements which had crystallized in thirty years of Dorothy Pattison's life, slowly dissolved and set themselves a new pattern. The personality of Sister Dora remained to the last both like and unlike her old self. She went back to Woolston, to the doll-sized schoolhouse and the village children. For the next year and a half no one visited her and she wrote few letters. Slowly an inner transformation was taking place in her life, and these eighteen months formed a hinge between the past and the future. All through her early years bitter religious prejudice had turned home into a battleground; the result for her had been weariness, a purposeless confusion, and a final withering of belief. The difficulties which assailed her, she later said, were 'of the intellectual, not of the imaginative order . . . her mind was filled with doubts relating to the authenticity and inspiration of Holy Scripture.'[1] She had not been Mark's pupil for nothing. She could not let such questions rest without reading and study. Now, in the solitary evenings by the cottage fire, she took up her books again. Slowly belief returned, quietly, unasked, as something distilled from daily experience. Chance echoes, in letters or conversation, give some idea of what passed through her mind. 'Have I given my heart to God? Is every action of my life done, with a single eye to God's service?'[2] She returned often to the image of the single eye. 'It is that,' she said, 'which gives beauty to a character.'[3] In the course of 1863 she decided, quite deliberately, to change her way of life.[4] The result was summed up, almost entirely incorrectly, in the *Dictionary of National*

Biography: 'In the autumn of 1864 she became, in opposition to her father's wish, a member of the Sisterhood of the Good Samaritan at Coatham near Redcar and adopted the name of Sister Dora. In accordance with the rules of the order she became a cook in the kitchen. In December 1865 the Mother Superior at Coatham cruelly refused her permission to attend her father's deathbed.'

The only certain fact in this account is that the winter visit to Coatham in 1862 was crucial in Dorothy's life, for the little sea-side town was the scene of an experiment unique in the north of England. Not far from Coatham, at the foot of the Cleveland hills, among woods and parklands, stood the vast, battlemented mansion of Kirkleatham Hall. Theresa Turner, lady of the manor and heiress in her own right of the whole estate, had married her cousin Arthur Newcomen, and at his early death, buried him in the baroque mausoleum of her own ancestors. She was very rich, autocratic and pious, and, in her widowhood, developed strong Tractarian leanings. In 1854 she built, for her tenants at Coatham, Christ Church, a genuinely beautiful Gothic revival building of chiselled Caen stone, with lofty clerestory, tower and spire. The church, standing among open fields, was a landmark from the sea, and became famous among summer visitors for its 'solemn religious services'.[5] Mrs Newcomen endowed the living and presented it to a young Cambridge man of High Church convictions, John Postlethwaite.[6]

At this church in 1858 Mrs Newcomen founded what she hoped would become an Anglican religious order for women, the Christ Church Sisterhood, with Mr Postlethwaite as Chaplain, and herself as Mother Foundress. This was a step of almost unimaginable boldness. In the whole of the Anglican Church by 1861, there were only eighty-six individual Sisters and these were gathered in established centres of the Oxford Movement at Wantage, Clewer, East Grinstead and Regent's Park. There were few experienced clergy to direct the spiritual lives of nuns, and the 'Ritualist' controversy was becoming increasingly bitter. Low Church tracts related tales of young girls lured into convents and forced to sign away their property. All this Mother Theresa Newcomen swept aside, with magnificent courage and devotion, backed by the assurance that comes from centuries of unquestioned privilege. She gathered her little body of Sisters and novices around her, calmly proposing among other things, 'a devotion to the Sacred Heart, one to which I think no one can object.'[7] If anyone did object, no one, at least in Coatham, ventured to say so. Professed Sisters remained few, never more than eight or ten in the early years, but an order of tertiaries, called Associate Sisters, soon passed the thirty mark.[8] Prayers and parish visiting were not enough to satisfy their enthusiasm. Anglican Sisters of Charity in the south of England were doing rescue work, teaching, nursing. Some had already nursed in the Crimea. Soon the Christ Church Sisters were to find equally urgent work waiting for them near at hand.

From the sands and fishing-boats of Coatham to Middlesbrough was a drive of eight miles. Socially the two places might have been in different worlds. Middlesbrough had started life as an estuary village like Coatham; in 1801 it had four houses and twenty-five inhabitants, in 1831 only a hundred and fifty-four. No other English town grew faster in the nineteenth century and by 1861 the population was nearly nineteen and a half thousand.[9] Middlesbrough, it is said, was rocked in an iron cradle. Its first development had been as a coal port, but its fast growth dated from 1850 when a colossal lode of high-grade ironstone was discovered at Eston in the Cleveland Hills. Within a few years this mine was producing three thousand tons of ore a day, and forty blast furnaces were flaring day and night on Teeside. Day shift and night shift men slept alternately in the same beds. Middlesbrough had all the characteristics of a pioneer boom town. Men outnumbered women by ten to one and it was said to have 'sixty shops for rum and beer' to one church, of which the rector was non-resident.[10] Among the rows of smoke-grimed back-to-back houses the public bar was the main social institution and drunkenness the most common offence. The death rate in the heavy industries was high; the cemetery received their 'steam destroyed sacrifices'. Here in 1858, a field of practical work for the community at Coatham was suddenly revealed. Just before the night shift started at Snowden and Hopkins ironworks on the Tees, a boiler raising power for the steel-rolling mills burst, with a crash which could be heard for miles. Mercifully, as the shifts were just changing over, only seventeen men and boys were near. Of these two were blown clear into the river, to be picked up by passing boats; all were injured by blast and scalding steam. The town had no resources to cope with this disaster; the nearest hospital was at Newcastle, thirty-six miles away. The wounded men were laid with their open scalds on beds of straw in an outhouse, while a local business man rode over to Coatham to ask Mother Theresa for help.

Among the Associate Sisters staying in the convent at the time was Sister Mary Jacques, who, like Florence Nightingale, had spent some months in the Deaconess' Institution at Kaiserwerth near Düsseldorf.[11] She returned at once with the messenger to Middlesbrough, transferred the casualties to a hastily-rented cottage and nursed them there. She was a devoted nurse and a woman of great force of character. As soon as she could be relieved from full-time nursing duties, she explored living conditions in Middlesbrough for herself, and reported what she saw to Mother Theresa. Mother Theresa, always deeply moved by suffering, rented two houses in Albert Street and opened a small voluntary hospital, staffed by untrained Sisters under Sister Mary's direction. From the first it was overcrowded with patients. In 1859 a piece of land was offered for sale at North Ormesby, on the outskirts of Middlesbrough in the direction of the Eston mines. Mother Theresa bought the land, and at her own expense built a hospital with thirty beds, to be supported by voluntary subscription.[12] Here it was possible to give the Sisters an elementary training. Nursing techniques were primitive, but the devotion of the staff was inspiring. The next year the vicar, Mr Postlethwaite, with Mother Theresa's support built a large red-brick institution on the sea-front at Coatham, the Coatham Home, a convalescent home supported by charity. The Sisters and Associates of Christ Church undertook the nursing here as well. Later a seaside home for children was added to the little group of institutions.[13] There were never enough Sisters for the work which lay waiting to hand. They were to be seen every day, hurrying from one building to another, or filing along the field path to Church, in their black cloaks and gloves, with poke-bonnets of straw and black gauze veils.

Dorothy first saw these women, so unlike anything in her experience, during her winter visit of 1862. She heard the

Coatham people praise them warmly as 'reet good samaritans'. Increasingly in her solitude at Little Woolston she thought about their life and work. By the following summer Fanny Pattison had recovered from her breakdown, and travelled to Coatham to convalesce, with Dorothy as nurse companion.[14] Together they went to services at Christ Church, where they heard the Sisters sing. Walking on the pure, white sands, they saw the nursing Sisters at work among beds and wheelchairs on the balcony of the Home.[15] Their life seemed to offer everything for which the two lonely young women hungered, a shared ideal, faith, the care of children for Fanny, for Dorothy real nursing at last. Dare they offer themselves as postulants? They were in no doubt about their family's attitude. '*Not one* of them approved,' said Dorothy bluntly, and with the exception of Sarah, they never ceased to show their hostility. Fanny remained at Coatham while Dorothy went back to the school. 'I am not doing my utmost. I could do more, and I could do it better as a Sister.'[16] Fanny, for the first time in her life, took an independent decision, and applied at the age of forty-three for admission as a novice. 'I am altered very much in some things,' she wrote to Mark with a touching mixture of pride and humility.[17] During the summer holidays Dorothy visited her, and had an interview with the Chaplain, who constituted himself her adviser.[18] She was frank about her crisis of faith, and the questions left unanswered by her textual studies in the Bible. The Oxford Movement, unlike the Evangelicals, did not insist on fundamentalist belief or personal 'conversion'. The Chaplain gave the standard Tractarian advice in cases of troubled faith, based on Keble's words to Thomas Arnold, 'to turn oneself more strongly than ever to the practical duties of a holy life.'[19] Nothing could have appealed more to Dorothy's natural temperament. She went back to Woolston, gave notice, packed her trunk, and said goodbye to her friends. In September 1864, when she was thirty-two she entered the Christ Church Sisterhood, under her childhood's pet name, Sister Dora.[20]

She found herself taking part in one of the great movements of English Church history, the revival of the religious life for women. The Sisters at Coatham were pioneers, the only Church of England community in the north country. An early photograph shows them grouped round a baize-covered table on the gravel path outside an ivy-covered house with Gothic-revival windows. The evergreen shrubberies, the lawns, the black cross-bred spaniel at their feet, all suggest some large Victorian family of a clerical sort. At the centre, looking out upon the little world she rules, with the long, shrewd, rather equine, regard of the Yorkshire county families, sits the Mother Foundress. Mother Theresa, always coldly referred to by the rest of the Pattison family as Mrs Newcomen, was a woman of outstanding courage and generosity. She never showed it more clearly than in accepting Frances and Dora, with their difficult temperaments and troubled family history, as members of a working community. Mother Theresa made herself responsible for the two new Sisters in the most direct sense. The Church of England was still entangled in the idea of class distinction, and in deference to middle-class opinion the Sisters took no vow of poverty. Instead, each retained possession of her own property and paid a monthly contribution, assessed by the Mother and Chaplain, to the household expenses.[21] This equivocal rule meant that poverty continued to harass Frances and Dora, whose incomes, they ruefully said, 'can do little more than pay our washing bills, which are necessarily heavy.'[22] Nor could they afford to take the month's holiday 'to visit relatives and friends', ordered by the constitution. In practice they were living on the community's charity, gladly given and thankfully accepted by Frances, who found in her Superior the affectionate Mother for whom she had always hungered. Dora was too proud to submit easily to being Mother Theresa's dependent. Secretly, she resented the need to accept kindness, which was offered, however graciously, by the lady of the manor, *de haut en bas*.

In giving up her independence Dorothy was making the greatest sacrifice in her power. She had grown up, as she said, 'almost a prisoner'. For thirty years she had lived under the weight of her father's tyrannical will-power and her mother's helpless suffering. She had waited, worked and fought to make her escape to a freedom of action most people took for granted. Through poverty and illness she had clung to it. It was hard now to surrender her hard-won independence to the claims of religious obedience, and in the end the sacrifice was to prove too great for her. Again in deference to public opinion, no vow of chastity was taken; a Sister was free to leave or to marry at any time. For Dora this meant that her emotional life remained ambiguous and insecure. Even more seriously the Constitution made no provision for Chapters to be held. Thus the sisters had no share in decisions concerning the work they were to carry out. This profoundly affected Sister Dora's future career at Walsall. No one person can be blamed for these defects. Mother Theresa, as her papers make clear, read, studied and prayed over her Rule, but she was trying to re-create a way of life unknown in England for three hundred years. Her Chaplain, a kindly and inoffensive young man, lacked the force of character to guide a community, though under his successor matters were to be very different. Meanwhile the Sisters tried to satisfy both conviction and convention, with varying degrees of success. Although the Sisters took no formal vows until 1871, their daily rule of life was austere. The whitewashed rooms and polished corridors of the convent were silent, bare. The day began while it was still dark.

Dora woke every morning at half past five, when a lay-sister knocked on her door saying 'Let us praise the Lord'. It was a shattering discipline to leap to her feet in that icy winter air for the response 'Thanks be to God'. They took the path across the frozen fields to Church for the first of the day's offices. By six-fifteen the Sisters were in their places for Prime and meditation. At seven came Holy Communion, and after breakfast Terce, followed by morning assembly, at which 'the duties of each sister will be assigned by the Mother and they must hold themselves ready to accept their allotted tasks'. Where two Sisters worked together, silence was the rule. At noon they attended Sext, at three p.m. Nones, at five forty-five Vespers, and at six-thirty tea, during which they listened to a spiritual reading or conference. At eight, walking single-file with a lantern, they made their way to Church for the last time, to say Compline and by ten, the last light in the house was extinguished. During the day there was one hour of rest, which Dora used to walk on the sea-shore. This rigid time-table, adapted to the needs of the hospital, remained the framework of her daily life for the whole of her working career. The call of the bell was obeyed 'as the voice of God'. Undoubtedly this early training in planning the day's work added greatly to her later effectiveness as a Sister-in-Charge.

Another lasting influence was the courtesy of the Sisters towards each other, and for nursing Sisters, 'the courtesy and kindness of manner, *compulsory* towards each patient'. This was always maintained by Sister Dora, and taught to her own student nurses, as 'the foundation of duty'. Above all, the recurrent pattern of the church services was a source of unfailing joy to her. The day hours of the Church of England are exquisite and deeply satisfying; their subtle variations engage the mind, while the ordered repitition stabilises the character. To the end of her life Sister Dora turned to them for sustenance.

In the convent a mixture of simplicity and formal decorum was maintained. The Dormitories were partitioned into cubicles, with 'furniture of the plainest kind and nothing unnecessary allowed'. Strict silence was observed from Compline until after Terce. Only one main meal was taken in the twenty-four hours, a midday dinner. The novices undertook hard manual work, yet the meals were served and doors opened by Lay Sisters, so unthinkable was it for ladies to wait upon themselves. Mother Theresa insisted that the Lay Sisters must always wear starched caps and aprons, like the parlourmaids of her youth; she even debated whether the aprons should be formally blessed as part of the habit. The Rule demanded unquestioning obedience. 'I do not ask whether you will or will not do this, but lay it on you as an obligation,' said Mother Theresa one evening in a conference to the Sisters. 'Sisters are to obey the Mother Superior as holding her authority from God. They are to accept without hesitation all her directions, whether agreeable or disagreeable.' Every letter was read by her. Sisters coming to her room had to knock, push a note under the door and wait humbly for an answer in the chilly passage. Frances obeyed these rules lovingly and gladly, but it would have needed long and arduous discipline for Dora to accept them with a good grace.

For the present she was fully occupied by the rule which stated that 'the novices shall be fully trained in all household duties'. She made beds, scrubbed floors, polished grates, and finally became a cook in the kitchen. Ten years later she could still recite the list of her duties to young Eliza Ridsdale. 'My work,' she said, 'consisted in washing, baking, scrubbing, blackleading and all sorts of household work. I remember on one occasion I was in the kitchen peeling potatoes, when a gentleman whom I knew came and was shown over the place. I turned aside lest he should recognize me.'[23] The Pattison family and her friends expended a good deal of indignation over this useful practical training. They described her as 'aching in every limb from the unaccustomed strain' of making her own bed, and wrote, 'It is painful to imagine the high-born lady reduced to a toil the poorest drudge in the land could have accomplished'. Dora herself, though she sometimes embroidered details, was always honest about essentials. She admitted that what ached was less her limbs than her self-will. Each household job, as in any nursing training, had to be done by a set method, to an approved standard. When she made a hospital bed with imperfectly mitred corners, the Sister in charge dumped the sheets and blankets on the floor and told her to begin again. 'At first,' Dora admitted, 'I literally sat down and cried with vexation' but she learnt fast and seldom needed to be told anything twice. Later, passing through a ward, she could make up a fire, lift a saucepan lid, straighten a bed cover, or shake up a pillow, almost without pausing in her swift, gliding walk. '*Nothing* escaped her accurate eye,' remembered a junior nurse with a reminiscent shudder, 'and with her, to see was to do.'

One of the hardest things for Dora to learn was the gravity and decorum of manner considered essential for a Sister. The air of Coatham, as Spede noticed in 1629, 'is subtle and piercing'. 'The sea', wrote Dora, 'is an everlasting amusement.' Clean white sand drifted over the village street and the firm, smooth strand stretched for eight miles. Sister Dora's spirits rose with her health; on her daily walks she watched with longing the heads of swimmers bobbing in the sparkling sea or the riders galloping along the shore. Later she taught herself to swim, but for the moment her temptations centred on a large, very handsome donkey, with a reputation for bucking off anybody who tried to ride him. At last she could resist him no longer. 'Do let me try – he won't kick me,' she said to the astonished donkeyman and, still in her novice's habit, vaulted on bareback. The donkey reared and plunged; she had not ridden for four years, and finally was thrown off on to the shingle. Her knees were so bruised and swollen that for days afterwards it hurt her to kneel in chapel. 'I dared not confess the reason,' she said, 'for the horror of the

Chaplain and Sisters at such a prank would have known no bounds.'[24]

Another misdemeanour could have been more serious. One night, without permission, she slipped out for air, when a drunken man, seeing the pretty Sister alone, lurched towards her, grabbing clumsily and growling, 'I'm coming to get ye.' In a panic she snatched up her skirts and ran full-tilt across the fields towards the church and convent. She lost a shoe in the mud, one of her only outdoor pair. Since she could not afford to buy others, and was ashamed to admit what had happened, she stole round for weeks in slippers, trusting to her long black skirts to hide the evidence of her crime.[25] In fact, the authorities would not have been too severe with her. The atmosphere of the community was, and still is, full of humour and humanity and Sister Dora was a universal favourite. The Sisters, women of all types and all ages, found her intensely captivating; her sense of humour enlivened the day's work, her charm and courtesy disarmed all criticism. She herself was honest enough to see the danger in this. 'Everybody here is so kind to me,' she wrote to Miss Finch at Woolston in January 1865, 'that I am only afraid I shall get spoilt.' She could not help, too, being naïvely pleased with her appearance in the novice's habit. The long, black frock fitted perfectly, the white apron set off her small waist. The frilled muslin cap with a butterfly bow under the chin made her face round and youthful; her cuffs were always immaculate. Since, for reasons which will appear, she never became a fully professed Sister, Dora wore this dress for the rest of her working life. As a woman of forty-five, she confessed with disarming frankness to a young friend, 'You know, I never could have joined one of those Sisterhoods who make themselves hideous frights with bibs and bands across their foreheads!'[26] 'She was at no pains to conceal, at any time of her life that she disliked the sole company of women,' said the same friend ruefully. In many ways Dora's new life changed her less than she expected. Those who knew her best in later years remarked that 'there was more of nature than of grace' in her devotion, her strong will, her passionate possessive love of her patients. 'Charity', a theologian has written, 'is the gift of God's grace and must be understood as different in kind from human love. Human love is directed to the other person for his own sake, spiritual love loves him for Christ's sake.'[27] These two loves existed side by side in Sister Dora, and sometimes it is clear they were at war. It is easy to see, with the advantage of hindsight, that her vocation was to be a nurse, not a nun. Her feminine instincts were too powerful, her nature too wayward and impulsive to permit detachment from the world; sometimes they were to lead her into painful conflicts of feeling, when the old Dorothy Pattison, who still existed, rebelled at the life of the new Sister Dora. Yet nothing was allowed to interfere with her work. All her energies and will power were directed towards the nursing she hoped to do in the future. She viewed her months as a novice at Coatham solely as preparation for this. 'I thought some of the rules very strict,' she said with her usual honesty, 'but they were good for me.' And even at the end of her life, her face would soften at the memory. 'Yes, I *was* happy there.'[28]

Her happiness increased with the next stage of her training, when she was sent to work in the Coatham Convalescent Home. The Home stood on the greensward, facing the open sea, and high tides came nearly up to the windows. It had beds for forty-five men, women and children, each staying for about a month, at the expense of subscribers who sponsored them. By an extraordinary regulation, 'when patients require medical attention, the subscribers who send them have the liberty of choosing the system of medical treatment under which they shall be placed'.[29] Fortunately the place was too healthy for this need to arise very often, and the institution, in every other way, was a model of its kind. Sister Dora worked first in the kitchen, with its huge iron boilers and the cooking range, which it was her duty to burnish every morning until it shone. Next she went on duty in the laundry where an engine turned large washing, wringing and mangling machines in an atmosphere cloudy with steam. From here she was promoted to the convalescent children's ward, where she really came into her own. She bathed the children in the hot sea-water baths which formed part of their cure, she pulled their beds on to the long balconies to see who could count the greatest number of passing ships, she devised endless games for keeping them out of mischief. The Sisters and Associates were all struck by Dora's love and understanding of children of all ages. Pale, fretful convalescents grew brown and firm-cheeked under her care, and the children's ward when she was on duty echoed with cheerful shouts and laughter. Towards the end of her time at Coatham a man who had seen her at work there asked her to marry him. The Pattison sisters, hoping to rescue her from manual work they considered degrading, wrote urging her to accept. Rachel even came over to Coatham for the day and pleaded with her personally.[30] Several of the Sisters, seeing her great love for children, gave the same advice. Her closest friend, an Associate Sister who worked in the kitchen and shortly afterwards herself married the Chaplain, John Postlethwaite,[31] was sure she would find her greatest happiness as mother of a family. Sister Dora rejected the offer without a day's hesitation. She was sincerely delighted to learn in December 1864 that Sarah, at thirty-seven, was marrying their family doctor, Richard Bowes,[32] but she herself would never consider marrying except for an over-whelming love. For the present all her being was concentrated on exploring the implications of her faith. These proved to be revolutionary, beyond anything she had imagined.

Every morning, as she entered the Convalescent Home, its red brick picked out with ecclesiastical blue and white decorations, she looked up at the stone lintel above the door. There, in a rather pinched Gothic script, was engraved 'Inasmuch as ye have done it to the least of these my brethren, ye have done it unto me'.[33] The architect who designed that text and the mason who chiselled it could hardly have realized that they were determining the whole course of another human being's life. For Dora, always given, as she admitted, to 'restless longings', took these words to heart as simply and directly, as though she heard them spoken 'in the voice of the master I serve'. For the rest of her life they recur constantly in her speech and writing, and she firmly pointed out their full meaning. She had been brought up to charity, it was true, but to an intensely individualistic philanthropy, which never ventured to apply Christian standards to society as a whole. Her parents would probably have agreed with Wilberforce in telling the poor that poverty 'has been allotted to them by the hand of God; that it is their part faithfully to discharge its duties and contentedly to bear its inconveniences'. They might even have seconded Hannah More, who informed cottage housewives that hunger 'has been permitted by an all-wise

Providence to show the poor how immediately dependent they are on the rich'.[34] Resignation, humble gratitude, to be deserving, all these in Sister Dora's upbringing had been demanded of the poor. Now, in one simple sentence, beginning 'Inasmuch as . . .' a whole, ingrained attitude to life was swept away. Later in life many people were to object that certain of her patients, fighting men, drunken women, thieving children, were 'not deserving'. She always answered vehemently, 'It does not matter. *Whatever* they are, the Inasmuch holds good!' She came to see the Church she so greatly loved, not simply as the comforter of the individual, but as a standard by which to judge life in society. This was one of the great legacies of the Oxford Movement to England; more than any formal discipline of the novitiate, it transformed Dorothy Pattison into Sister Dora.

NOTES

1. Lonsdale, 23.
2. Pattison, 67, fly-leaf.
3. Ridsdale, 46.
4. Lonsdale, 16, dates this decision from her mother's illness, but in 1860 Dorothy was intending to marry.
5. G. M. Tweddell, *Visitors' handbook to Redcar, Leatham and Saltburn 1863.*
6. Alumni Cantabrigiensis.
7. C.H.R.—MS. notes on Mother Theresa's conferences.
8. Ibid.,—Register of Associates.
   There were many clergy daughters, among them Sarah Dodgson of Darlington, sister of Lewis Carroll. The Sisterhood had been variously described as 'large' and 'small'; this is because the distinction between associate and professed Sisters was not clear to the public.
9. A. Briggs, *Victorian Cities,* 247.
10. Ibid., 260.
11. Anon, *Hospitals and Sisterhoods 1855,* 71–4.
12. W. Burnett, *Old Cleveland,* 119–43.
13. White, *Directory of North Riding,* 1867.
14. Pattison, 56, f. 363.
15. Bulmer, *Historical & Topographical Directory of N. Yorkshire,* 1890.
    The convalescent homes by 1890 were known as Homes of the

Good Samaritan. The Christ Church Sisterhood, however, became in 1867 The Community of the Holy Rood, and the 'Order of the Good Samaritan', of the D.N.B. entry, is mythical.

16. Lonsdale, 20.
17. Pattison, 56, f. 382.
18. *Walsall Observer*, 27th December 1879.
19. A. P. Stanley, *Life of Arnold*, 19.
20. Lonsdale, 21. This date is unsupported by documentary evidence; considering the volume of work done by Sister Dora before January 1865 it may well have been earlier, or even the previous year. No community records exist earlier than 1866.
21. C.H.R., Notes on Constitution.
22. Pattison, 50, f. 381.
23. Ridsdale, 20.
24. Ibid., 20–21.
25. Ibid., 21.
26. Ibid., 6.
27. D. Bonhoeffer, *Life Together*, 22–3.
28. Ridsdale, 20.
29. G. M. Tweddell, *Visitors' Handbook to Redcar, Coatham and Saltburn, 1863.*
30. Pattison, 56, f. 322.
31. This outraged Mark Pattison, who was convinced that Mr Postlethwaite had committed the solecism of marrying not merely *a* cook, but *his own* cook.
32. Hauxwell Parish Registers.
33. G. M. Tweddell, *Visitors' Handbook to Redcar, Coatham and Saltburn, 1863.*
34. J. L. & B. Hammond, *The Town Labourer*, 243.

CHAPTER TEN

A Nursing Sister
1864–1865

❋

The days with the children in the Convalescent Home were abruptly cut short by a crisis in the running of the Sisterhood. During the winter of 1864–5 a scarlet fever epidemic broke out in Middlesbrough. Two of the Associate Sisters, visiting in the crowded streets, caught the infection and died.[1] Sister Frances, with a trust in Providence which bordered on the alarming, was sent to take charge of the Branch Hospital,[2] a dispensary near the docks. Dora, with even less experience, was ordered to the Cottage Hospital at North Ormesby. The railway to Middlesbrough ran along the foot of the Cleveland Hills; looking up through their woods and waterfalls, she could see fresh snowfalls glittering on the heights. In the other direction, the whole shore of the Tees estuary was blackened, and the chimneys of the great ironworks flared against a smoke-darkened sky.

The new Hospital at North Ormesby, a bleak, gaunt building, with rows of staring windows, housed thirty beds for the ironworkers and their families. Unlike the Walsall Hospital where Dora was later to nurse, which was devoted entirely to accident and surgical cases, North Ormesby was a general hospital, the first Cottage Hospital in the North of England. The aim was to provide one bed per thousand inhabitants, to which all the local practitioners could send patients. It certainly had its share of severe cases; in the early 1860s, among four hundred and eighty surgical patients, twenty-eight deaths occurred. Working conditions for the Sisters were primitive. It was agreed that 'there should, in every hospital, be a bathroom', but 'commodes, which can be removed as required, are preferable to a water-closet, which in peasant hands soon gets out of order'. A nurse was expected 'to do a good deal of manual work, which a lady might be unwilling to undertake'.³

Sister Dora was willing to undertake it cheerfully, until she in her turn caught scarlet fever. She made a good recovery and was sent back to Coatham to convalesce. She refused to be coddled, which in her opinion never did any good to anybody 'in body or mind'. 'I caught the scarlet fever,' she wrote to Miss Finch at Woolston, 'but if you could see me now, you would not know it. I am blooming! I bathe every morning in sea-water and get a famous blow on the shore every day. Thank God, I keep well and strong and happy in my work.'⁴ By the New Year of 1866 she was back at work in the wards at North Ormesby.

Here she had her first experience of hospital nursing, and encountered one of the formative influences of her life, in the person of Sister Mary. Miss Mary Jacques, founder of the hospital, was a short, plain middle-aged woman, with a large inquisitive nose and sharp eyes. Her normal working pace was a smart trot. 'If you meet a lady at both ends of the hospital at once,' said the patients, with pride, 'that will be our Sister Mary.' The men adored her. Her favourite expression was 'poor things', by which she meant anybody exposed to her formidable will-power. She would descend on successful Middlesbrough business firms and refuse to go away until they had made a contribution to her hospital. 'Poor things!' she would exclaim after these interviews, rubbing the tip of her large nose reminiscently. 'I wouldn't let them off, you know! I made them pay up! They were very good – poor things!'⁵

This lively and masterful personality was not calculated to appeal to Mother Theresa, and although Associate Sister Mary applied several times for profession in the community, she was never admitted. So, as she said, she 'hurried over to Germany' to take, like Florence Nightingale and Agnes Jones before her, a rudimentary training in the Deaconess' Institution at Kaiserwerth. She came back ready to help in the iron-works disaster of 1859, from which all her later work stemmed. The nursing at Kaiserwerth, though devoted, was primitive, and Sister Mary had little in the way of medical or surgical training to pass on to her nurses. Dora always admitted that she was 'utterly ignorant' when she began work at Walsall. Yet the whole spirit in which she cared for her patients was learnt from Sister Mary. All the work at North Ormesby was done in a spirit of service, but it was unsentimental, practical, lightened by cheerfulness and Sister Mary's sense of humour. From her, Dora learnt 'the happy power of making patients cheerful'. 'Talk to the patients as you move about your work,' said Sister Mary. She maintained that the mental atmosphere of a ward affected recovery. General kindness, she taught, was not enough; the young Sisters must show personal kindness to each individual patient. As she hurried up and down the long wards with hods of coal or bowls of washing water, Sister Dora learnt to make friends with the men. She began to think of them as 'my men', the term she was always to use.

Sister Dora saw the change in the patients' outlook, as they discovered 'the hospital considered them as *men*, not as so many hands to work.' This, not any preaching or enforced religious conformity, was always her means of spiritual influence. She learnt here the practice, which she always maintained, of saying a short prayer for each individual patient at his bedside, every night. Sister Mary was known as an ardent 'Ritualist', where Sister Dora was reserved and restrained, with a marked taste for simplicity in worship. Yet it was impossible to mistrust the older woman's faith, as clear and crystalline as a child's. 'I can do all things in Christ' was found written in her prayer-book after her death. Dora, while still inexperienced, was deeply distressed by disease and mutilation. When ordered to dress wounds she asked, 'How can I do it?' Sister Mary answered her briskly, 'It can only be done in the name of Jesus. We see his divine face in the persons of all the poor and suffering, and it is that which helps us.'[6] Ten years later Sister Dora answered the same question by a young nurse, in almost the same words. 'As you touch each patient, think it is Christ himself you touch, then virtue will come out of the touch to you.'

She learnt fast, she was neat-handed, light of foot, quick-witted and unafraid of responsibility. Nevertheless she was frightened to find herself, on 5th January 1865, left alone at night in charge of a man who had concussion. It was bitterly cold; she sat by the ward fire wrapped in a shawl, trying to keep up her spirits by writing to her friend Miss French. The man lurched out of bed,

and began to stumble round the room. She attempted to speak
to him, and coax him to lie down, but he neither recognized nor
understood her. From her very limited knowledge of remedies,
she put a plaster of blistering fluid on the poor man, and watched
anxiously for signs of change in his condition. 'Oh I *do* hope he
won't die,' she wrote pathetically, 'for I am the only Sister here.'[7]
Whether in spite of, or because of the blister, the patient did not
die, and slowly Dora's confidence grew. She knew how ignorant
she was, how handicapped by her neglected education. She was
determined to get regular, hard training; like Agnes Jones she
perceived 'this is no holiday work; there is no such thing as
amateur nursing'.[8]

Already, unforeseen by anyone, a series of personal links was
forging a chain between Sister Dora and the scene of her future
work – Walsall. Walsall lay near the northern edge of the Black
Country, among the coal, limestone and iron ore mines of South
Staffordshire, a town of collieries, blast-furnaces and ironworks.
Accident cases, of which there were many, were sent by rail or
cart, nine miles to Birmingham, often to be found dying or dead
upon arrival. In 1859 the Borough of Walsall sent a donation to
the Birmingham Hospital which cannot have been very large, for
the Secretary replied, 'the hospital authorities would thank the
people of Walsall to send more money and fewer patients'. Local
pride and local rivalry was intense in the Black Country; the insult
to the town was furiously resented, and a group of Walsall
business-men came forward with the proposal to 'open our own
hospital and shun Birmingham'.[9] Two things promptly happened;
a little girl had both legs fractured by a chain in a coal-mine, and a
boy of twelve had his arm torn off in a hide-splitting machine.
These two children achieved more than pages of statistics.

The Mayor of Walsall called a meeting and opened a hospital
fund; a committee was formed with twelve of the town's manufacturers and clergy, and the editor of the newly founded *Walsall
Observer*, an energetic Scotsman named Samuel Welsh. He had
been running a series of articles called *Wants of Walsall*, in which
he proposed a covered market, a free library, a public park and a
hospital. He published an editorial on the proposed hospital and
offered, with great enthusiasm, to act as secretary. In the first year
the committee managed to raise £970 from donations, which

ranged from collections at a Strict and Particular Baptist chapel to a collecting box at a gin shop. Workmen contributed to a penny-a-week fund, a company of strolling players on the Race Course gave £3 and boys from Walsall's ancient Grammar School contributed their fines for bad behaviour. A neighbouring colliery sent a barge-load of coal by canal. Gifts in kind included linen, blankets, beer, potatoes, window panes from the glass works, new brooms and an old harmonium. By autumn 1863 the committee had acquired and furnished a house at 4 Bridge Street, one of a row of shops, remarkably unsuitable for use as a hospital. Many were scornful of the whole project, calling it botched up, or, in the ironic local idiom, 'a Worsall job', but the committee was determined to open before the year was out.

The doctors of the town agreed to form a voluntary medical committee, on which all would serve as unpaid consultants. The new Poor Law doctor, a young Scotsman, Andrew Wyllie, undertook the surgery. The most urgent problem was to find nurses. 'Where in Walsall,' asked a speaker, 'can you find ladies?'[10] Again Samuel Welsh had a proposal. His last post as journalist had been on the Middlesbrough local paper, for which he had covered the opening of the North Ormesby Cottage Hospital and the Coatham Convalescent Home. He travelled at his own expense to visit Mr Postlethwaite, the chaplain at Coatham, who asked Mother Theresa if she could spare a nursing Sister. Mother Theresa's weakness, if it must be called a weakness, was that she could never bring herself to refuse an appeal for help, even though the result pressed hardly on her already over-worked community. Now Sister Mary Jacques, taking another associate, Sister Elizabeth, and later Sister Louisa as assistant nurses,[11] was sent to Walsall, to establish the little hospital. On 12th October 1863 the Walsall Cottage Hospital opened with four beds.[12]

Most cottage hospitals were intended to provide homely nursing for the ailments of village labourers and their families, though, as a correspondent to *The Times* pointed out with sublime complacency, 'the lessons learnt day by day in these hospitals are, in time of need, of value in the ancestral hall. Thus the peasant's misfortune may be the means of saving the life of the Squire.'[13] Walsall Cottage Hospital was quite different. From the first it was an accident centre; no medical wards were added until 1894. Its object was 'to furnish in cases of accident, prompt and skilful surgical aid and trained and experienced nursing and thus supply a want long felt in Walsall.' The Sisters from Coatham were introduced to a somewhat sceptical Black Country public as 'ladies of education, whose services to the hospital are purely voluntary and benevolent and who have been induced to undertake the nursing and internal management of the Institution. The public have therefore a guarantee that everything which Art or the judgment of Experienced Nurses can devise for the relief of patients, will be adopted.'[14] In effect the hospital was to be a sort of casualty clearing-station in the ceaseless assault of fire and steel on human flesh.

During the first year the number of beds was doubled, in 1864 increased to twelve and then to fourteen. In the New Year of 1865 Sister Mary, who had been travelling between Walsall and Middlesbrough since the Cottage Hospital opened, fell ill and telegraphed to Coatham for a relief nurse. It was a rule of the Order that 'Novices should not be employed in any external work except in great emergency'.[15] Only three days before, Sister Dora had been nervous at the prospect of one night's duty alone in Middlesbrough. Yet, whatever her inner fears, she appeared calm, confident, equal to anything. There was no time to consider her state of mind, or her readiness for the work. Looking round the hard-pressed community for a spare pair of hands Mother Theresa selected Dora to be sent to Walsall. In this haphazard, impromptu manner, one of the essential decisions of her life was taken for her. At a few hours' notice she packed, put on the nursing Sisters' outdoor habit of black bonnet and veil, black cloak, funereal ribbons and gloves and set out. It was three days after her thirty-third birthday.[16] She was so fine-drawn, so full of vitality, at a time when women settled early into middle age, that she was commonly believed in Walsall to be twenty-three, not thirty-three. This later led to some confusion in her private life, for she continued to look much younger than her age.

On 8th January, 1865, as the early winter evening closed in and the train swayed and rattled through the darkening landscape, Sister Dora, peering from the window of a third-class carriage, had her first glimpse of the Black Country.[17] For her, as for all strangers, the experience was overwhelming, an assault on the senses by blackness, ferocity, noise and dirt. This industrial landscape was a world apart. Novelists had already dwelt on its horrors in famous passages of description. 'Everything around is blackened,' wrote Dickens. 'There are dark pools of water, muddy lanes and miserable habitations far below. . . . It was the journey's end and might have been the end of everything it was so ruinous and dreary.' Disraeli had described the nights when 'vaults which had been dark all day now showed red hot with figures moving to and fro within their blazing jaws'. A visitor in 1863 felt a sense of 'preternatural power and unearthly desolation as smoke rose from the flayed fields'.[18] Mountains of slag and cinder smoked with sulphurous fumes; sullen clouds through which the sun could hardly burn its way shed black rain upon naked earth and a network of dark canals. Here and there a shallow lake reflected the scene in its black mirror. At sunrise and sunset through the smoky haze, distant shapes of cranes, canal boats or chimneys, wavered like a mirage on the skyline. The Black Country was as light by night as by day, for ninety per cent of the blast furnaces still flared their waste gases away to the sky in a series of crimson clouds, plumes of pink steam and sudden nasturtium flowerings. Day and night, as the shifts came and went, the cough of pumping engines, the thud of steam hammers and the clash of metal battered the ears.[19] Below the ground, in an area less than fifteen miles across, lay coal, iron ore, limestone and fire clay, supporting a population of craftsmen, unmatched in Europe for courage and skill. Moreover, to those who understood it, the Black Country landscape revealed a vein of iron poetry.

Sister Dora had no time to discover this in the next two months, for from her first morning in Walsall, she was overwhelmed with work and the problems of the new hospital. Hard experience had taught Walsall working men and women to expect nothing for nothing, and a free hospital filled them with the deepest mistrust. Some claimed that the doctors would perform experiments on the bodies of helpless patients, others, equally glumly, that the Sisters of Mercy would try to 'convert' them. The committee did its best to counter hostile prejudice. There were to be no formalities of admission for any accident case, no major operation without a consultant's opinion, no sectarian church services and complete religious liberty for all patients. To make sure that everything was above board, the hospital was open every day after two o'clock, but in addition 'a patient may have any visit he specially requires at any time'.[20]

In spite of these precautions, the two Sisters were met by some of the people they had come to serve with suspicion and hostility. In the crowded hospital one small room was set aside for their private prayers, and here on festivals and Sunday mornings, a clergyman celebrated Holy Communion for them.[21] This was still the England in which the Royal Chaplain could write, 'The Dean (of Windsor) likes neither early Communions, nor frequent Communions, nor does he attend either', and the Sisters aroused the deepest suspicion. Some of their early encounters provided a comedy of manners. Sister Mary set out on one of her fund-raising calls upon local clergy. Mr Welsh, who called half an hour later, found her bristling with indignation. 'What is the matter, Sister?' 'Your vicar is the matter! He says I am a Romanist. One look at my garb was enough to convince him. He says we are heading straight for Rome!' The Chaplain, John Postlethwaite, travelled from Middlesbrough to attend a meeting of the hospital committee. 'I have one question to put to Mr Postlethwaite,' said Mr Gordon, the Congregational minister. 'Are you a *Ritualist*?' Poor, inoffensive Mr Postlethwaite replied that he knew no one in Walsall, and felt it very strange he should be asked such a question on his first visit. 'I believe there is good in all religions,' he said, 'and when I see good I try to adopt it.' Mr Gordon expressed himself satisfied.[21] The obsessional suspicion towards Roman Catholics was in reality transferred from the prejudice against Irish immigrants, who were regarded by the native Black Country people with hatred, contempt and fear.

Sister Mary was not the person to make any secret of her beliefs; the Sisters were soon called 'co-workers in the great work of getting the British nation back into the arms of the Pope'. Rumour spread through the town of nameless rites. The Sisters, when they went out into the slums of the town to visit patients, wore black cloaks and bonnets, with black gauze veils. 'Were they to be seen in some of the places to which their duties called them dressed in fashionable attire,' explained a committee report laboriously, 'they would be liable to insult. Hence the need for the simple dress which to some has been a stumbling block, but to the Sisters a protection.'[23] This was wishful thinking. In fact, louts threw stones at them in the streets.

In Sister Dora's first two months at Walsall this hostility reached a peak. She herself was the unconscious cause. While Sister Louisa nursed the bed patients, she was sent to take charge of the old kitchen at the back of the shop, which served as a combined dispensary and casualty department. Here, jostled as she worked by a crowd of waiting patients, she caught smallpox within a month. She took it lightly, and this immunizing attack was later to prove a blessing, but for the present she was ill enough. The surgeon of the hospital, whom she was later to know better, attended her, but Sister Louisa and Sister Elizabeth, harassed and over-worked, had little time to nurse her. The charwomen who came in to scrub were forbidden for their own protection to go near her. She lay in strict isolation in a darkened room, where for a few days she was delirious, and tore up her sheets, in the belief that she was making bandages. As her fever subsided, she began to notice ugly sounds from outside, shouts, cat-calls and the thud of stones and horse-dung flung up at her window. Some scandal-monger had put about a rumour that the drawn window-blinds concealed 'a Popish oratory with an idol of the Virgin Mary with a crown on her head'. The Protestant wrath of the Walsall people was aroused, and they gathered in the street to demonstrate. Even some educated people made suspicious inquiries of the hospital secretary, Samuel Welsh, who finally lost his temper and said, 'Yes, the room is devoted to the honour of the Virgin, but to the Virgin Dora, not the Virgin Mary!'[24] By the time that Sister Dora was strong enough to walk to the window and look out, the angry crowd had vanished. She only found out later what had happened. Her hair, which had hardly had time to grow since the scarlet fever, was once again cropped in tight dark curls against her head. She anxiously scanned her face in the glass for traces of pock-marks, and was passionately grateful to see her unblemished skin. Soon the whole memory of illness faded into the background. 'I had two fevers soon after the start of my nursing life, but I regarded them as necessary seasoning and they did me no harm,'[25] she said carelessly. Her new work was so absorbing, so full of responsibility and interest, that her old life fell away from her, like a cloak.

Both she and Sister Frances used the same expression: 'I feel I am become a different person.'

This new personality was exposed, from April 1865, to yet another new experience. After two months at Walsall she was recalled to fresh duties at Coatham. The Order, to help finance its numerous works of charity, undertook to supply trained nursing sisters for private cases, whose fees were paid into a common fund. Sister Dora had not the slightest desire to undertake this work, but in a comic episode, she found it wished upon her. Almost the whole of her life as a nurse was passed in professional obscurity. Now, however, she had one encounter with the most famous physician of the day, Sir James Simpson of Edinburgh. The occasion was characteristic of them both.

Sir James had been summoned to Yorkshire by the relatives of an immensely rich old lady, who was exercising a senile tyranny over them day and night by threats to give away her valuable jewellery and alter her will. His prescription was 'delicate management and firm control', and he applied to the convent for a Sister capable of supplying it. The Chaplain, flattered, produced his most experienced Sister, but Sir James merely shook his large head, with the dishevelled hair and keen eye, and demanded to choose for himself. They set off on a tour of the Convalescent Home, Sir James, short and stout, as usual almost running on his small feet, while the Chaplain, increasingly nervous, panted after him. They saw Sisters cleaning and polishing, making beds, feeding patients and starching fine linen, but none of them suited the great physician. Finally they came to the kitchen, where Sister Dora, with her sleeves rolled high above the elbows, was making a pudding. Sir James did not hesitate for a moment. He pointed and said, 'Send me that one.'[26]

Sister Dora was sent off at once to take night duty, and gave her distinguished consultant every satisfaction; he pronounced that she 'answered perfectly', but from her point of view the case was a hornets' nest. The old lady first tried to frighten her with a knife, then took a fancy to her and dragged out from a strong-box under the bed rings, bracelets and brooches, which she pressed upon her pretty nurse as gifts. Refusal agitated and distressed her. Every morning Sister Dora returned the jewels to the relatives, who received them with patient resentment and mistrust. A final, ludicrous embarrassment was provided by the footman, who served her breakfast every morning in the housekeeper's room. He very reasonably considered the fresh-cheeked young woman in white cap and apron a fellow servant, and declared himself in love with her. He insisted on bringing her chops, devilled kidneys and kedgeree out from the silver dishes in the dining-room, although Sister Dora, pink with dismay, begged for 'nothing but a cup of coffee'. Next he took to walking with her to and from the Home, and she was reduced to coming by roundabout ways to hide from him. 'An uncommonly unpleasant time I had of it,' she said, laughing, 'what with the mad old lady who was fond of me, and the relations who were jealous of me and the footman who took me for a servant and would make love to me!'[27] Yet, though she made a joke of it later, she hated it at the time, and submitted with secretly increasing resentment to being sent here and there on private cases, all through the summer of 1865.

The position of a private nurse, 'earning her guinea a week in good families', was in fact that of upper servant in the households which employed her. The Pattison family was humiliated by this menial position, and there is no doubt that this aggravated their general sense of grievance against the Sisterhood. Dora herself was enough of a Pattison to dislike it intensely. Her vocation, which grew day by day, was to serve the suffering poor. She found none of the satisfaction of nursing in waiting on rich invalids, and dwelt regretfully on the rewarding drudgery of the wards at North Ormesby or Walsall. She went, dutifully, wherever she was ordered, but inwardly she rebelled. At last, in November, to her intense joy, she was sent back to Walsall. The doctors and the hospital committee were equally overjoyed to see her; they had found no one else with her talent for organizing hospital work.

Now followed a confused series of incidents, which has never been fully unravelled. Her father, whom she had not seen for four years, was eighty and suffering from cancer. 'My father has been slowly sinking all the summer and autumn,' wrote Mark. 'Today a letter from Frank to say it is indeed the approach of the end. He is confined to his bed and is so reduced that he cannot hold out much longer.'[28] The news spread round the scattered family, even to cousin Philippa, living alone in lodgings in Florence. She wrote, with true charity, 'My memory carries me back further

than others can go, to *my uncle's youth*; he certainly had, in his
little world, a brilliant and hopeful youth, and it was strangely
blighted. I feel it irreverent to do more than pray for him
unfailingly.'[29]

Most of his children went to see him during his illness, but
Mark and Dora did not. They might forgive personal grievances,
but they could not forget their mother's tragic end. Moreover
Sister Dora was fighting a battle on her own account. In mid-
December she was ordered once more to take a private case in
Devon, but this time the surgeon in charge was not prepared to
let his best nurse go without putting up a fight. The secretary had
written to Coatham with 'strong remonstrances', demanding to
keep her.[30] At this point on 28th December 1865 Dora heard
from Frank that her father was dying and wrote at once asking
for another Sister to be sent to the private patient, so that she
herself could go home. On 30th December the order to go to
Devon was confirmed by telegram, followed at seven in the
evening by a telegram from Frank, saying 'All is over'.[31]

It is of course possible that Mother Theresa and Mr Postlethwaite, with their knowledge of the Pattison family affairs,
decided to protect Sister Dora from a cruel experience. It would
have been cruel indeed. 'The horror of my father's fearful end
comes over me again,' wrote Eleanor. 'It fills my whole soul with
horror and terror.' It is more likely, though less dramatic, that
letter and telegram merely crossed in the post. The hospital secretary, who saw Dora every day, said roundly, 'This story is very
sensational, but it is fiction.' Whatever the truth she was determined not to give up hospital work again. She received leave of
absence to attend her father's funeral, but replied sharply, 'When
he was alive you would not let me go. Now he is dead I no longer
care to.'[32] The Pattison family, already embarrassed by the fact
that Eleanor, defying convention, refused to wear mourning for
their father,[33] wrote one by one to Dora urging her to come, but
she refused to leave the Cottage Hospital.

The whole episode of Mr Pattison's death, confused as it was,
received almost hysterical treatment from later writers. It was
exaggerated into the central traumatic experience of Sister Dora's
life, which accounted for all the signs of emotional stress later
seen in her. One Evangelical writer described it as 'the punishment

which she brought on herself, terrible as it was' for her sin in joining a religious order, and her refusal to attend the funeral as 'a natural shrinking from meeting her family under such painful circumstances'. With great dignity and restraint, Mother Theresa made no reply to attacks upon herself. Sister Frances Pattison, whose family loyalty was intense, remained devoted to the community. Sarah Bowes, level-headed, warm-hearted and essentially good, became an Associate Sister in 1868,[34] with her husband's full approval. Her two sisters did not feel that Dora had been cruelly treated, nor did she herself ever suggest it. There were differences between herself and the authorities at Coatham, it is true, but they were rational, comprehensible disagreements about her work, which were finally settled in a rational way. Nevertheless a legend had been created, which the nineteenth century exploited for Sectarian purposes. Little stories of Sister Dora's life became, as many second-hand copies bear witness, a favourite prize in Low Church Sunday schools. She became well known to many people who had no conception of her actual work or its value.

The tragic household at Hauxwell was at last broken up. Dora played no part and took no apparent interest in the family negotiations which ensued. True to his threat, Mr Pattison had disinherited his married daughters, also, apart from a small devise of land, his sons. 'A miserable fortnight,' followed for those at Hauxwell. Eleanor quarrelled with her sisters. Mark, even in the privacy of his own journal, had recourse to Latin to record 'iniquissimo Patris testimonio, hominis morosi et perfidiosi'.[35] The sisters searched for a new house at Richmond and answered letters of condolence. 'Your father is gone to heaven and may it be my happy lot to meet him there,' wrote their pious old friend, David Horndon. This prospect must surely have filled Mr Pattison's family with mixed emotions. For the moment, they all existed in an empty trough of time. The Rector's forty-year-old tenure was ended and Mark composed his Latin epitaph. 'Your inscription I do think most neat and appropriate,' wrote Mary. 'Yes – 40 years is correct! I was in the churchyard on Monday afternoon. How quiet and calm it looked. It made me feel as if these last months had been a dream.'[36]

Sister Dora, at Walsall, felt that life itself had been a dream until the waking, purposeful present. She was determined to stay at the hospital, and tacitly ignored recalls to Coatham. The hospital Secretary wrote on 17th December 1865, 'to explain the cause of Sister Dora's remaining beyond the time she was allowed was to oblige the Committee and the Surgeon'.[37] In the end, Mr Postlethwaite, who was a far from forceful character, wrote to the Hospital Committee that, as they were unwilling to accept another Sister in her place, they might keep Sister Dora. This, and not any question of her father's death, was the point at issue between her and the Community. Except for short holidays she never left Walsall again during the rest of her working life. She had found her home and her vocation.

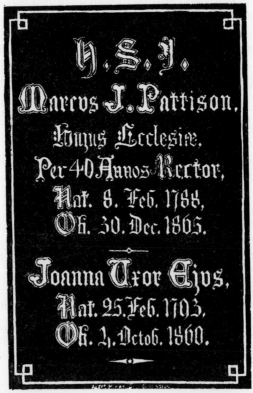

The tombstone of Dorothy Pattison's parents, with
Latin inscription composed by Mark Pattison

NOTES

1. W. H. Burnett, *Old Cleveland*, 142.
2. Pattison, 56, f. 381.
3. E. J. Waring, *Cottage Hospitals*, 23–32.
4. Lonsdale, 24–5, quotes this letter.
5. W. H. Burnett, *Old Cleveland*, 119–48.
6. Ibid., 119–48.
7. Lonsdale, 24–5, quotes this letter.
8. *Memorials of Agnes Jones*, xiii.
9. F. W. Willmore, *History of Walsall*, 429–33.
10. W.P.L. Album.
11. W.C.H.A.R. and C.H.R.
12. W.C.H.A.R., 1864.
13. *The Times*, 3rd January 1866.
14. W.C.H.A.R., 1864.
15. C.H.R. Draft rule.
16. C.H.R.
17. F. W. Willmore, *History of Walsall*, 430.
18. *Edinburgh Review*, April 1863.
19. Ibid.
20. W.C.H.A.R., 1864.
21. Reprints.
22. W.P.L. Album.
23. W.C.H.A.R., 1864.
24. Lonsdale, 30.
25. Ridsdale, 20.
26. Lonsdale, 33.
27. Ibid., 34.
28. Pattison, 130, f. 61.
29. Ibid., 56, f. 48. It is not clear whether or not Sister Frances went home for a visit, but her Rule certainly allowed this.
30. *Walsall Red Book*, 1879.
31. Pattison, 310, f. 62.
32. Lonsdale, 36.
33. Pattison, 56, f. 118.
34. C.H.R. Register of Associates.
35. Pattison, 130, f. 61–2.
36. Ibid., 56. f. 240.
37. W.C.H. MS.

CHAPTER ELEVEN

The Hospital at Walsall
1863–1865

To her family it seemed as though Dorothy had vanished without trace. 'Has D. appeared at all on the scene since her father's death?' asked Frank. 'I have heard nothing of or from her.'[1] Mark wrote for news to Rachel, who could reply only 'I will try if I can elicit any information from Fanny'; but Sister Frances knew nothing. Mary could not even supply Sister Dora's address. In the end Mark's letter, setting out the terms of their father's will, was forwarded via Coatham. At the end of March, three months after the Rector's death, it at last produced an answer. There is certainly no sign of excessive grief or even of family affection in this dry and businesslike letter.

> As regards the land you mention I am willing to agree with whatever they all wish, but should think it best to wait until a better time for offering it for sale. Could you tell me when we shall have a chance of receiving any money? I really am needing some *now*; I should never have owned this if I had wanted to beg from you, but I simply want to know about what is my own. Will you tell me, for I have never heard a word from my sisters, exactly what I may expect and when I may expect it? I have struggled on for five years now, through poverty and sickness, without ever being indebted to anyone, and I can truthfully say it was a surprise to me to learn that I came in for anything,
>
> Yrs affly, D P[2]

This was a declaration of independence, a final slamming of the door upon the past. Mark and Frank as executors sent her ten pounds on account of the estate, and she used it to take a long-overdue holiday that summer. She went on a tour through the Lake District, with the Reverend John and Mrs Postlethwaite. They had often invited her before, but to their distress she had always refused from pride and poverty; now she could pay her own share, she was glad of their company.[3] This was only a brief interlude. Walsall and her work absorbed her utterly. Before its reality, all her past life seemed to waver and fade, like a forgotten dream.

In this century prosperity and civic pride have swept away most of Sister Dora's Walsall. One has to search for its traces in the broken windows of back streets, in ruined foundries awaiting demolition, or among the blackened tombstones and eroded gargoyles of its churchyards. A hundred years ago Walsall was a place of fire and sweat, smoke and thunder. The old borough rode proudly astride a precipitous hill, crowned by the Gothic spire and pinnacles of St Matthew's Parish Church, a landmark for miles around. Below fell a steep, twisting High Street of ancient houses and iron-studded cobblestones. This hairpin-bent hill was part of Black Country folk-lore; it was said to produce a race of bow-legged men and women in Walsall. Standing at the top of the church steps one looked down, through drifting smoke, over a wilderness of slate roofs and crowded streets. Beyond lay blast furnaces, smoke-stacks, rusty spoil-heaps and pit banks with, in the far distance, the wooded heights of Cannock Chase. On clear days the skyline was broken by the great hump of the Wrekin.

Walsall was proud of its long history. It had been famous since the Middle Ages for the manufacture of saddlery and saddler's ironmongery. 'Being tinged with the smoke of a manufacturing vicinity, this town has often been looked upon with ignominy and contempt, but surely without reason,'[4] wrote a local historian defiantly in 1813. During the nineteenth century its growth burst all bounds. The population multiplied by four between 1800 and 1860. Forty thousand work-people lived in overcrowded squalor without drains or water. Walsall had the reputation of a rough town.

By the 1860s the town had clay mines, thirteen blast furnaces and thirty-nine collieries, as well as two hundred and fifty saddlery workshops. Cavalrymen in Europe, cowboys in North America, Australian overlanders and gauchos in the South American pampas, all rode in Walsall saddles.[5] Saddlery was a trade employing a large number of small masters, sub-contractors, handicraftsmen and outworkers, in a warren of little black workshops, containing five or six men each. Work in leather and wood was similarly divided; 'black saddlers' who made harness, were distinct from 'brown saddlers' who made riding saddles. These proud and independent craftsmen could not be controlled, either by employers or trades unionists. There were three sets of unions in the South Staffordshire iron trade before 1867, and disputes between union and non-union men broke out if they found themselves patients in the same hospital ward. Small iron-masters had themselves been workmen, while many skilled craftsmen, miners, puddlers, furnacemen or saddlers, had never surrendered their freedom to work for a regular wage. Master and man stood on an equal footing as in few other parts of England at that date.[6] Local pride in the town's crafts was overwhelming. A speaker told an election meeting, he should like to see 'all the horses in the world harnessed by Walsall saddlers, all the boxes fastened by Walsall locks and all the world's dirt swept by Walsall brushes'. He was cheered to the echo.

Walsall men were fighters, and their political history had been stormy. During an iron-workers' strike against the truck system, blacklegs were thrown into the canal and half-drowned. At the first election after 1832, the Riot Act was read over a pitched battle with sticks and stones, while the people dragged furniture out of the houses and burnt it in the street. After an anti-Corn Law meeting a crowd attacked the Town Hall, while during the great colliery riots of 1842, the dragoons were called out to repress angry demonstrators. As late as the election of 1859, the Riot Act was again read, and the police charged the crowd with drawn cutlasses.[7] Mounted police kept order in the famous open-air market. Labour relations were hard in the blast furnaces and foundries, harder still in the coal and ironstone pits around the town. An old collier explained the custom of 'giving the boards'. 'Ya man is killed and carried home on a shutter, the master give the widow the boards to make t'coffin, and that's all he ever gives.'[8] Destitute Irish families arrived every month to find work,

and lived encamped in shanty towns, like the strangely named
New Invention. In the nineteenth century Walsall suffered
repeated outbreaks of cholera and a lethal smallpox epidemic.
A second smallpox outbreak was contained only through Sister
Dora's personal intervention. As it was, the churchyard was so
packed with corpses that grave-diggers used a boring-rod to work
over the same ground three times in fourteen years.[9]

The little house in Bridge Street was as crowded as the grave-
yard. There was no room to put another bed, and Sister Mary
who had returned to take charge had to send home accident cases
which should have been admitted.[10] At home, reported the
doctors, patients lay in dark rooms, without air, warm fire, bedclothes, clean water or suitable food. In case of death, the body
lay in the one room, where the whole family, including children,
lived and slept.[11] A doctor, visiting the home of a nail-making
family, described: 'The broken panes where pieces of paper fill
the place of glass, pilfered nail bags keeping out the cold, the
mud floor on which are three or four naked children sprawling
unwashed. . . . Enter their sleeping room as I did this morning
and you must hold your breath and rush to the window and
throw it open. There lie husband and wife and two sick children;
a young man of twenty-five in the same bed with a daughter of
nineteen, brother and sister. In a corner a truss of straw covered
by a bag or two is the bed of two more little ones, no blankets,
no sheets, no washing apparatus.'[12]

Sister Mary and Sister Dora appealed for old linen and blankets.
They cooked broth, beef tea, eggs, fish, arrowroot and port wine
for their in-patients, and sent whatever they could spare to starv-
ing households, whose breadwinner was injured and could no
longer earn their living. They went visiting at all hours and in all
places, but nothing could take the place of the extra beds they
needed, or supply the missing bathroom and hot water system in
the Bridge Street house. They would have to move. By the utmost
economy they and the committee saved seventy pounds out of an
income of £970, towards a building fund.[13]

At first sight the hostility of the local people was frightening,
and Mr Postlethwaite several times threatened to withdraw the
Sisters.[14] Walsall people were defiantly proud of their town, and
bitterly resented the criticism of strangers. Work was hot, dirty

and dangerous. Men took their lives in their hands every day they went to work, but they were as tough as their dogs, the famous fighting Staffordshire bull terriers, and proud of it. Many accidents arose from a general dogged determination to ignore new-fangled safety regulations; the workers would take orders only from their own overhands and butties. They neither asked nor accepted concern for their welfare. Among themselves they would fight with broken glass or belt buckles, or hold kicking-matches with their iron-shod clogs. A ballad describes the quarrel at a cock fight between Wednesbury and Walsall supporters:

> *The company rose in disorder*
> *A bloody fight ensued*
> *Kick, bugger and bite was the word*
> *Till the Walsall men subdued.*

> *Ruff Moey bit off a man's nose*
> *It's a wonder no one was slain,*
> *They trampled both cocks to the death*
> *And so made a draw of the main.*[15]

They would face each other and hack away, until one fell unconscious. Strangers shrank away from their black faces and fierce white eyes, sweat rags and moleskin trousers.

Walsall men and women prided themselves on being suspicious, or in their own splendid idiom 'jubous' of strangers intent on reform. The middle classes were intensely respectable, usually low-Church or non-conformist. The workers had little time for religion from childhood onwards. Child ironworkers told a Commissioner of Enquiry that they said 'Our Father' every night. He took this to mean that they repeated the Lord's Prayer; further questioning revealed that they knew only these two words. Churchgoing made no appeal to working men, though in 1863 they had enjoyed performances by the 'Hallelujah Band', a troupe of ex-prize-fighters, gamblers and drunkards who performed at revivalist meetings as dramatic trophies of salvation.[16] The saints' days they traditionally observed were 'St. Monday and St. Tuesday', when they stayed at home to sleep off Sunday's drinking, working fifteen or sixteen hours on the remaining days to make up their wages. Their reputation for toughness and irre-

ligion was a matter of some pride to them. A local rhyme described
a typical Black Country parish:

A tumbledown church,
A tottering steeple,
A drunken parson
And a wicked people.

Walsall supported three hundred and twenty-five public houses
and spent £196,000 each year on drink. Given the harsh living
conditions and the harshness of their work, it was useless for a
doctor to deplore 'the rush of the labouring classes to the gin
shop'. Furnacemen and miners were the heaviest drinkers, and
the butties, who controlled labour below ground, drank on a
homeric scale. Sermons, tracts and quantities of good advice
had no effect whatever. 'In such a society,' wrote a Walsall
clergyman regretfully, 'it is easier to build churches than to fill
them.'[17]

The stock responses for visitors to Walsall was horror and
dismay, but Sister Dora took to it at once. Its crowded, raucous
vitality suited her much better than the solitude of Hauxwell or
the sleepy calm of Woolston. She enjoyed market days, when the
high street was lined with stalls from the church steps right down
to the bridge. She took an interest in the crafts of innumerable
little back-street workshops, and admired the skill and judgment
by which apparently casual hammer blows on a glowing ingot
produced goods finished with the utmost precision. Above all
she liked the people, their courage, their pride, their loyalty to
workmates and their sheer toughness. Their affection, once won,
would last for ever.

She set herself to win them over and first found common
ground in field sports. These industrial workers were still country-
men at heart. Behind and between their towns lay a patchwork
of old farms, sooty wasteland, dark pools and reedy canals. Here
men went fishing and children played, with bad language and
bloody noses. Little boys sitting in holes in the ground, played at
mining with their fathers' old pick-axes. Workshops formed
'gypsy clubs' to go picnicking in the green borders of the Black
Country, among scenes of Rabelaisian enjoyment. There were
still yellow candles and firelight to be seen in cottage rooms, and

winding green walks on the uplands of Cannock Chase. Miners kept pigs in home-made sties or grew runner beans on waste plots.[18] Here cocks fought to the death and bulls had been baited until the sport became illegal in 1825; a favourite local ballad related the misunderstanding when a visit from the Bishop of the diocese was mistaken for a baiting of Bishop the celebrated bull.[19]

Sister Dora, unshaken by the language, entered into the spirit of these robust enjoyments. She told the men, as she moved about the ward at her work, of the sport she had seen in Yorkshire, how, as a child, she had joined in 'anything in the nature of a hunt, whether of fox, hare or rat', with all the enthusiasm of a boy. She described driving the pony cart over the moors and riding across country after the hounds. They listened enthralled to stories of gallops across the wild Yorkshire moorland, jumps over stone walls and wading through streams.[20] Afterwards they were loud in admiration of her daring. 'Her'm a plucked 'un,' was the general verdict.

Gradually this refreshing natural friendliness, and the kindness of the two Sisters, disarmed suspicion. So far as Sister Dora was concerned, an incident in April 1867 ended mistrust for ever. A speaker, whose name rather incongruously was Murphy, toured the Black Country giving what were billed as 'anti-Romanist lectures'. They were received as an excuse to attack the Irish immigrants. At Wednesbury his hearers stormed out of the lecture hall, and beat up any stray Irish they could find in a series of free fights among the slag heaps, the so-called 'Murphy riots'. When Murphy was due to speak at Walsall, two hundred special constables were sworn in and a troop of hussars stood by. There was no large-scale fighting, but gangs of roughs roamed the streets.[21] Sister Dora had been out late visiting a patient and was walking home when she heard a hulking young miner shout, 'There goes one of the Sisters of Misery!'[22] A few days later he was carried into hospital, seriously injured in the pit. She recognized him at once. 'That's my boy,' she said to herself, and nursed him with the utmost devotion. As he grew better, she watched with secret amusement, his hang-dog air. 'I knew well enough what was the matter,' she said, 'but I wasn't going to ask him, because I wanted him to own up to it himself.' At last, wretchedly, it came out. 'Sister, *I* shouted at you.' She laughed. 'I recognized you the moment they carried you in at that door!' He stared at her, shaking his head with puzzlement. 'You knew me – and yet you have taken care of me like this?' Years later she still smiled at the memory of his expression. 'He didn't know what to make of it at all!' Nothing more was said on either side, but from that day onwards no one ever attacked the Sisters. A local writer believed this was due to Sister Dora. 'She melted the icy barrier of prejudice and completely uprooted the suspicions which the novelty (of nursing Sisters) at first aroused,' he wrote.[23] As more practical proof that they were trusted, the number of out-patients doubled in the first two years, and the makeshift pantry-like dispensary would no longer contain them. During 1867 the committee bought a large house, with coach-house, outbuildings and garden at the Mount on the outskirts of Walsall, for conversion as a new hospital. The cost was £2000 to which Sister Dora contributed £10 and Sister Louisa who had again been sent to help, £5, in addition to their unpaid labour.

The hospital consultants welcomed the Sisters from the start. Their chief was a veteran Walsall general practitioner, affectionately known to everyone as Old John Burton. He had qualified in Scotland, and when a young man had served as medical officer at Haddington during the calamitous cholera outbreak of 1832.[24] He was kindness itself to Sisters and patients; reading between the lines, he was also distinctly old-fashioned, if not actually rusty, in his medicine. With him he brought his son, 'young John Burton', newly qualified at Edinburgh in 1865, who was to put in three years of hard, unpaid work as house-surgeon to the struggling Cottage Hospital. Old John Burton was old enough to admit comfortably that he was first attracted to Sister Dora, 'like all men of all classes, by her personal charms'. He found her intensely captivating, gay, courteous and unaffected; her wit and high spirits made his daily visits to the hospital a pleasure. Young John Burton, in and out of the wards at all hours, remarked how skilful she was in the management of patients, and how deeply she cared for their welfare. Finally, in a surgical emergency, when a stand collapsed at the race meeting and several people were injured[25] she revealed her full potential. 'Such coolness, courage and commonsense, I never before found combined in any woman,' said the old doctor. 'I resolved it should not be my fault if she were not thoroughly instructed in her calling.'[26] Sister Dora was to learn accident surgery and nursing from the two hard task-masters of the Black Country, coal and iron.

Black Country towns tended to specialize in particular branches of the iron trade, but were closely linked by a network of canals, and what appeared to the stranger a bewildering tangle of railways leading from nowhere to nowhere across smouldering waste land. So many heavy industries within a few miles of each other, and the constant passing of goods trains, were to face the nursing sisters at Walsall with a wide variety of accidents. There was probably nowhere in the world at this date which could offer a more concentrated experience of accident surgery and nursing. The Childrens Employment Commission reported that in South Staffordshire accidents were so common that the people talked as if the whole population was engaged in a campaign.[27] Each town had its own craft, and each craft its own threat to life and limb. Walsall itself had its tanneries and blast furnaces and was surrounded by coal and iron pits. Nearby, Bloxwich produced awl-blades, Willenhall cast-iron locks and keys for the entire world, Darlaston nuts and bolts, Wednesbury axles and gas pipes, Pelsall railway wheels, girders.

The mining industry was surprisingly primitive. Coal and ironstone were hacked out together in small, ramshackle collieries, of which there were nearly four hundred and fifty. Much of the area was surface mined along the seams, and South Staffordshire was pitted with groups of shafts, six to eight feet in diameter, set six to eight yards apart. The miners were raised or lowered in skips, worked by an old-fashioned beam engine, or sometimes by horse-driven winding gear. They worked in a series of rectangular chambers, which often fell in, causing crushing accidents. Once underground they were entirely under the control of their 'butty', a sub-contractor, who until 1866 was held responsible for all accidents. These shallow workings, according to H.M. Inspectors of Mines Reports for 1860 and 1861, were no less dangerous than the deep pits in the North.[28]

A different set of dangers lay in wait for workers in the blast furnaces producing pig iron. The process, at its simplest, consisted of heating and melting the iron ore in a furnace of local coal; it then flowed out in two molten streams, iron and slag. The blast furnaces were small and isolated, of the old-fashioned 'open top' construction from which waste gases flared, lighting up the sky at night. The labourers worked day and night shifts. A gang of men, women and boys called fillers, under the charge of a 'bridge-stocker' filled the furnace from the top. Below, men under a 'stock-taker' prepared sand moulds, tapped the furnace and weighed the pigs of iron. Young boys of twelve and thirteen were used as 'holders-up' to raise the furnace door for tapping. Slightly older boys wheeled about heavy masses of red hot iron on a sort of porter's barrow. 'They may be seen,' wrote an observer, 'skipping about rivulets of molten metal with more indifference than a tidy housemaid shows to the water with which she is washing the door step.'[29] An American visitor in 1868 described the melting pots as 'terrible crucibles. Their lidded mouths dull the roaring sound of the combustion. When the lid is removed from each furnace and the pot of molten metal lifted out with long-handled tongs, a spectator must have steady nerves to look at it. As the stalwart men, naked to their waists, remove the cover from the pot and pour the fluid, the brightness is almost blinding.'[30] Everyone was struck by the danger to the eyes of the men, who never wore goggles, and Sister Dora developed a special interest in ophthalmic work. Burns and scalds in ironworks provided the most agonizing and by far the most difficult of the cases the accident hospital had to treat.

A continual series of accidents came from the ironmongery and small metal workshops. Black Country cast or wrought iron was famous as the best in the world. Puddling, casing and forging were carried on in the vast number of small workshops, often outhouses in the backyards of the iron-master's house. The puddler, sweating at his furnace with his underhand, was the key man of this industry, the king of metal-workers, not to be deposed for a generation. To serve him he had perhaps eight or nine adult piece-workers, with odd boys and girls. The back yard forge struck an inspector as 'like a coal hole or a little black den', where the children of the family were exposed to showers of sparks, hot cinders, random hammer-blows and white-hot iron. Slightly larger workshops, employing about thirty hands, were often in disused sheds or dwelling-houses up narrow back lanes. 'The rooms are all crowded with dangerous machinery, so close that you can hardly pass,' wrote an Enquiry Commissioner in 1863. 'None of the machinery is boxed off or guarded in any way. . . . There is a constant hammering roar of wheels, so that you could not possibly hear a warning voice. You have but to stumble on your passage from one place to another and you are certain to be punished with the loss of a limb.' The most common accidents in these crowded workshops were from guillotine shears, stamps and presses. Fingers and thumbs were sliced off, or so badly crushed that they had to be amputated; sometimes a whole arm was trapped. Equally dangerous were the shafts and bands used for driving machinery from a central steam engine. These 'drag the unfortunate sufferer under its power. Shawls of females, or their long hair and aprons or loose sleeves of men are frequent causes of dreadful mutilation.' A boy apprentice 'was stripped to the skin, all but his boots', though he escaped with his life.[31]

Dr Burton's annual report for 1866 gives a clear factual picture of the work done during Sister Dora's first year at Walsall. It included eleven hundred and fifty-six minor operations on out-patients, exclusive of suturing and reduction of fractures. The operations included removal of foreign bodies, shot, needles, glass, metal and stone from ear, nose, throat and eye; small abscesses had been incised and small tumours removed in the out-patient department. Dora had helped to nurse a hundred and forty-seven in-patients after major surgery, resection of bones, excisions of extensive cancer, and many, far too many, amputations.[32] She had witnessed six deaths including a railwayman with leg amputated at the thigh, a man with ribs and lungs crushed by a runaway colliery truck and a pitiful child who fell into a boiler and was scalded all over. This last was an agonizing experience; in its mercifully few last hours on earth, the child was hardly recognizable as a human being. The hospital was still primitive and its methods exceedingly old-fashioned. The annual bill for drugs, £35 2s 5½d., was almost ten pounds lower than the expenditure on ale and spirits. Sister Mary, Sister Louisa and Sister Dora worked all day, with no official off-duty hours, but at night they had to hand over their wards to domestic servants, engaged from the town at a cost of £44. Sister Dora was already dissatisfied with this arrangement; if she had a patient dangerously ill, she woke constantly at night and went down with bare feet to 'keep an eye on him', as she said. There was no garden and no fresh air. The converted shop stood in the most crowded and noisy part of the town. Smells of drugs and cooking hung in the air of the close little house, the summer days were stifling. Yet no cases of severe wound infection, erysipelas or pyaemia were reported. The usual death rate among the victims of serious accidents in London teaching hospitals was estimated at six per cent. At Walsall, since the Cottage Hospital opened, it had been less than five per cent, a fact noted in the national press.[33] Voluntary nursing by the Sisterhood, said the Hospital Report, 'notwithstanding the prejudice it has had to encounter and the severe criticism to which it has been subjected, has proved successful beyond the expectations of its most sanguine supporters.' This, said the surgeons' report, was thanks to the zeal, care and intelligence of the Sisters. 'Indeed your surgeons beg to represent to the committee that these ladies merit their warmest, most sincere praise and grateful acknowledgment of their prompt, intelligent and efficient assistance on all occasions.'[34]

On one occasion at least Sister Dora's assistance was rather too intelligent for old Dr Burton. The case, her first to become famous, passed into Walsall folk-lore under the title of 'Sister's Arm'. Very many of the accident cases brought into the hospital were compound fractures of an arm or leg. Coal dust, metal filings, machine oil and mud had often penetrated deeply into the raw, ragged wounds. Old John Burton had a wholesome dread of infection, and a short way with it; in most cases of crushing or compound fracture, without more ado he amputated the limb. By doing this, he probably saved many lives, but Sister Dora, who spent all day with the patients, knew what a black future they faced. They had no workmen's compensation to hope for, no unemployment pay and no prospect of finding work. Either their wives and children would be forced on to the crowded labour market, or the whole family would have to go to the workhouse. She checked dressings, moved stump pillows and smoothed draw-sheets hearing always, 'You might as well have killed me as take off my leg,' or arm or hand, as the case might be. 'I shall never get work again and I don't know what's to become of my wife and children!' These words haunted her.

One night during 1866, a young iron-worker was brought in from the night-shift. His arm had been caught and twisted in a revolving machine; Dr Burton took one look at it and said, 'Nothing can save that arm. I must amputate at once.' Sister Dora had been called from her bed to admit the new patient, who seized her hand as she stood by the stretcher. 'Oh Sister! Save my arm for me, it's my right arm.' She looked at him with the concentration she was beginning to develop, as though, said someone, 'she could look *through* a wound, to the state of the circulation beneath'. The injured man looked questioningly from one face to the other, and this look decided Sister Dora. She seemed to pluck up courage. 'Doctor, I believe I could save this man's arm if you would let me try.' Dr Burton was dumbfounded, as well he might be, to have his professional judgment questioned by a nurse. 'Are you mad?' he said. 'I tell you it's an impossibility. Gangrene will set in in a few hours, nothing but immediate amputation can save his life.' Sister Dora turned to the patient. 'Are you willing?' He nodded, unable to speak. 'Then I will try.' No one had ever seen Dr Burton so angry before. He turned on his heel and walked away saying, 'Well, remember, it's *your arm*. If you choose to have this young man's death on your conscience I shall not interfere, but I wash my hands of it. Don't ask me for help.' Nursing etiquette and ethics alike condemned what Sister Dora had done, but now for the first time she showed that lion-like courage and fighting spirit which was to save so many lives. She irrigated the wounds with cold water, constantly changed the dressings of old, clean household linen, and gently splinted the arm on supporting pillows. During all the time she did not allow herself a whole night in bed. For three weeks she watched and dressed 'her arm', as she called it, night and day.

Her gratitude was as great as the patient's when she saw beyond doubt that the arm was beginning to heal. Rest, free drainage, the absence of strong antiseptic chemicals, had avoided damage to the surrounding tissues and the young, strong patient had natural powers of recovery. Sister Dora waited until Old John Burton was in a particularly good mood, then begged him to come and 'Look at my arm'. Not with a very good grace, he agreed. He stood by, while she unwound the bandages, revealing healthy scar tissue and well-aligned bones. In the 1860s 'conservative surgery' was a novel medical concept. 'Bless my soul, you have saved it!' he exclaimed. 'And it will be a useful arm to him for many a long year!' He was a kind and generous man; he forgave Sister Dora for defying his orders and he admired her moral courage. The patient declared she had given him back all that made life worth living. He had made Walsall history; he was Sister Dora's first triumph.

NOTES

1. Pattison, 56, f. 118.
2. Ibid., f. 177.
3. Ibid., f. 322. She would harldy have chosen to go with them if the Chaplain had treated her 'cruelly' a few months before.
4. T. Pearce, *History and Directory of Walsall*, Introduction.
5. G. C. Allen, *Economic Development of Birmingham and the Black Country*, xviii, 129–30.
6. Ibid, 167.
7. F. W. Willmore, *History of Walsall*, 417.
8. *The Edinburgh Review*, April 1863.
9. P. Drabble, *Black Country*, 119.
10. W.C.H. MS.
11. E. Waring, *Cottage Hospitals*, 8–13.
12. E. Royston Pike, *Human Documents of the Victorian Golden Age*, 258.
13. W.C.H.A.R., 1865–6.
14. W.C.H. MS.
15. P. Drabble, *The Black Country*, 148.
16. Horton Davies, *Worship and Theology in England*, iv, 167.
17. *The Edinburgh Review*, April 1863. These revelations were deeply resented by the respectable middle-classes of Walsall, but they are amply confirmed by the local police court news.
18. E. Burritt, *Walks in the Black Country and its Green Borders*, 116.
19. F. W. Hackwood, *Religious Wednesbury*, 128.
20. Lonsdale, 8.
21. F. W. Hackwood, *Religious Wednesbury*, 89.
22. Lonsdale, 31, claimed that he threw a stone and cut her forehead, but this was denied by the hospital secretary.
23. *Midland Counties Express*, 28th December 1878.

24. J. Burton, *Some Observations on the History and Treatment of Cholera Asphyxia as it appeared at Haddington in* 1832.
25. W.C.H.A.R., 1866.
26. Lonsdale, 38.
27. G. C. Allen, *Economic Development of Birmingham and the Black Country*, Appendix A, Table 2.
The population of the region, roughly two hundred miles square, had multiplied by four and a half since 1800. In 1865 it included 24,000 coal miners, 1500 clay miners and 2500 ironstone miners; there were also some 5500 furnacemen in 147 blast furnaces producing pig-iron, and 21,000 finished-iron workers in 1588 puddling furnaces.
28. G. C. Allen, *Industrial Developments of Birmingham and the Black Country*, 192.
The average yearly number of accidents was eight hundred and deaths were classified as follows: accidents in the shafts or winding gear 150, explosions from fire-damp or choke damp 70, falls of roof 400, miscellaneous, above ground 50, below ground 130.
29. *The Edinburgh Review*, April 1863.
30. E. Burritt, *Walks in the Black Country*, 175.
31. Quoted E. R. Pike, *Human Documents of the Industrial Revolution*, 190.
32. W.C.H.A.R., 1866.
33. E. J. Waring, *Cottage Hospitals*, 14–15.
34. W.C.H.A.R., 1866.

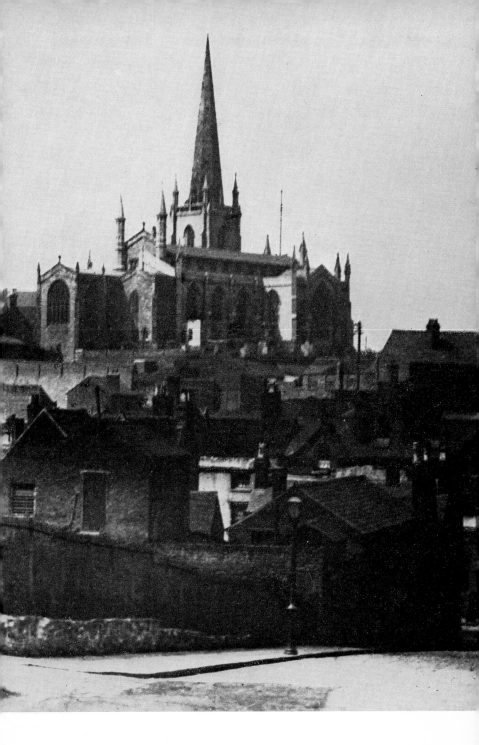

11. Walsall: the ancient borough and the parish church

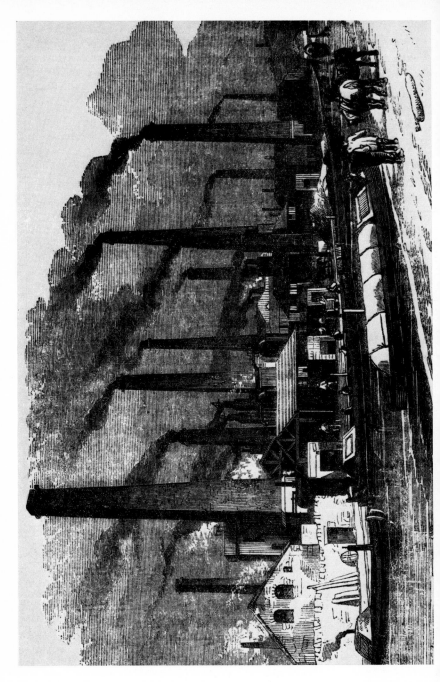

12. Walsall: iron-
works on the
Walsall canal

CHAPTER TWELVE

The Shifting Relation
1866–1868

Sister Dora was always to experience the quintessential Victorian conflict, called by her great contemporary George Eliot, 'the problem of the shifting relation between passion and duty'. She had not been long at Walsall when she met and fell in love with a man of exceptional character; his name and the date of their meeting were suppressed by Victorian propriety.[1] However, a good deal is known about him. They met in the course of her work at the hospital and were brought into day by day contact and 'equal companionship'.[2] In the England of the 1860s this implies that they were of the same social class. The man was near her own age, a man of the world, travelled, well-read and interesting. She was first attracted to him by his conversation, about a 'host of non-professional subjects'. In his society 'she found an ever-increasing pleasure', while he was charmed by her original mind and delicate beauty flowering so unexpectedly among the South Staffordshire slag-heaps. They fell in love, and became engaged, but Sister Dora broke the engagement from a sense of duty and he went away, never to return. Rachel Stirk, writing in 1866, believed him to be 'one of these doctors who seem so fond of her' and hoped that she would marry him.[3] No letters survive to establish his identity, but it seemed worth looking for a doctor who left the hospital unexpectedly at about this date. Sixteen physicians and surgeons in the town visited the Cottage Hospital as honorary consultants.[4] Three of them left during Sister Dora's early years at Walsall; of these one was in his sixties, while the other had qualified as long ago as 1807. There was however a much younger surgeon who left Walsall

G

in 1866, in the middle of a distinguished professional career. His name was Redfern Davies. It must be made clear that no documents more personal than the hospital minutes exist to link Redfern Davies with Sister Dora. The probability that he was her unnamed fiancé is suggested only by a comparison of dates and circumstantial details. In character he certainly fits the known facts.

He had arrived two years earlier in an unconventional way, to help the hospital in a crisis. The young Poor Law doctor, who had done the surgical work, resigned because of disagreements with formidable Sister Mary. The Committee, at a loss, were delighted to receive a letter from 'one of the most able of the younger surgeons in Birmingham', saying 'I should be happy to undertake the duties of acting surgeon free of any fee or reward'. They made haste to accept 'this most kind and generous offer by Mr Redfern Davies'.[5]

John Redfern Davies was the son of John Birt Davies, M.D., J.P., the first Professor of Clinical and Forensic Medicine at Queen's College, Senior Physician to the Queen's Hospital and first Coroner of Birmingham. The family was of Welsh descent. They had farmed at Tirbach, Cardiganshire, until the grandfather, an Oxford man, became a country rector at Nateley Scures, Hampshire. John Birt Davies's brother, another Oxford man, was at this time vicar of Malvern Link. The family home was at 280 Hagley Road, Edgbaston. The eldest son was always known by his mother's family name of Redfern. One of his Redfern uncles was a barrister, another Birmingham's first Town Clerk, while a great-uncle had been the first M.P. for the city after the Reform Bill of 1832. On both sides of his family, Redfern Davies came from able, even distinguished, professional people. No picture of him has been traced, but surviving portraits show his father as tall and dignified, and the women of his mother's family as remarkably good-looking. The three sons of Professor Davies were all educated at King Edward VI School, from which the younger went to Cambridge, while Redfern followed in his father's profession.

As a student Redfern Davies served his five years' apprenticeship to William Sands Cox, F.R.S., founder of the medical school at Birmingham, and author of a series of standard surgical textbooks. From Queen's College and Hospital he qualified L.S.A., and M.R.C.S., in 1855, then took a London M.B., while 'resident clinical assistant' at the Brompton Hospital. For a time he practised with his father at 25 Newhall Street, Birmingham, then decided to specialize in surgery and went for a year to walk the Paris hospitals. It is interesting that, though Sister Dora could never spare time or money to travel, in 1878 when she had only a few months left to live, she made the sole foreign journey of her life to visit Paris.

In 1858 John Redfern Davies published the first of a series of papers in the medical press on various surgical subjects.[6] In 1859 he was appointed Surgeon to the Birmingham Workhouse Infirmary and thereafter published two or three original articles every year. He wrote well, in the forceful, straightforward style of a well-read man. His approach was progressive and hopeful; at this early date he had already insisted on 'the utmost possible cleanliness in nursing'. 'Consult the patient's own ideas,' he told a surprised local meeting of the B.M.A.[7] Like Sister Dora he was the friend of pauper patients; faced with the ignorant, the drunken, the syphilitic, he wrote with intelligent human sympathy of 'the misery attendant upon their condition'.[8] He moved on to the recently founded Birmingham Free Hospital for Sick Children where he was equally popular and successful. In the words of the Chairman, 'he highly distinguished himself'.

Meanwhile he had enjoyed an adventure still possible for an energetic and unattached young doctor. In December 1862 he travelled independently, at his own expense, to the United States to serve as a volunteer surgeon with the Confederate Army in the American Civil War. This of all others was a subject near to Sister Dora's heart. As a girl she had longed to nurse in the Crimea; in 1870 she wanted to volunteer for duty in the Franco-Prussian War, and in 1877 on the battlefields of the Russo-Turkish war in Bulgaria, though each time the Committee refused to spare her.[9] A military surgeon was a natural hero to her. Redfern Davies could tell her of his four months, based on the Military Hospital at Frederick City, Maryland, when he had attended casualties at the great battles of South Mountain and Antietam. She confessed to 'a vivid interest' in politics, travel, adventure outside 'the little world' of hospital. Moreover Davies had learnt a great deal professionally from this concentrated experience. He had ideas about the extraction of bullets, by the use of a probe designed by the great French surgeon Nelaton, and the use of silver wire ligatures which did not form a focus for fresh infection like the old silk sutures. Like Sister Dora he would watch a patient day and night to prevent needless amputation or deformity in a wounded limb, and restore the soldier to active life after 'the prolonged and weakening process of suppuration and confinement in bed'.[10] Perhaps this had suggested to Sister Dora the idea of saving the young workman's arm by conservative treatment, which old Dr Burton found so unexpected and startling in 1866.

The appointment of Redfern Davies revolutionized the Walsall Cottage Hospital, where affairs had been largely in the hands of the lay Committee. He was a good surgeon and a forceful character. He admitted urgent cases for operation, by-passing the rule that the Committee must be consulted. One of his diagnoses was queried by another doctor. He sent the patient, with a bruised, but not fractured arm, by carriage to Birmingham General Hospital, bearing a pre-paid telegram form. There his diagnosis was confirmed by telegram the same day, and he courteously but firmly demanded to have the matter entered in the minutes. He paid particular attention to eye injuries, which later became one of Sister Dora's special skills. He inspected the drainage and informed the Committee 'There is no doubt that the state of your hospital retards the progress of the patients'. He advised them to move to a healthier situation, as soon as possible and offered to inspect possible houses for them. It was he who attended Sister Dora during her attack of smallpox early in 1865, and sent her away from the overcrowded hospital to recover, and he who urged the Committee to keep her 'beyond the time she was allowed' at the end of the same year.

As their friendship deepened their conversations became more serious; in the young surgeon's intelligent sympathy Dora found the understanding which she had longed for all her life and never found. Hesitantly she told him that she had always been seeking for some experience higher than everyday human life could offer, expecting the withering irony with which her brother Mark had greeted such confessions. To her astonished gratitude, he accepted her desires, and sympathized with them. He was, she said, 'the only person she had ever met, who could attempt to understand her strange imaginings and longings.'[11] To her astonishment, he understood both her hunger for love and her fanatical need for independence. He combined a Celtic charm and wit with unfailing kindness; yet there was nothing soft about his character. For once Sister Dora had found a man she was powerless to influence. From their very first meeting he made it clear that he had no belief in the religion which was the inspiration of her work. He may also have had personal reasons for disliking the power of the Established Church which was then very great. The early history of Queen's College was bedevilled by the hostility of Church towards Dissent, and in his student years many lively young medical students were in revolt against two clergymen imposed on them as tutors by the college charter.[12] He looked at the world in the light of the new scientific humanism of Darwin and Huxley, not generally accepted by the rank and file of the medical profession until the 1880s. To Sister Dora this presented a new and fascinating philosophy, or, as her alarmed associates felt, temptation. Eagerly she waited for each fresh meeting to question, discuss, explore his mind and reveal her own.

From these long talks it was only a step to falling in love. These two natures, both passionate and profound, both unconventional, both idealists, seemed made for each other. Even those who disapproved recognized that Davies loved Sister Dora with unselfish devotion; he longed to take her away from a life of hardship and give her the security of mind and body she had never known.

On her side the feeling was more primitive. She was a woman of thirty-four, but loneliness had damned up her emotions. Rachel, who knew her best, was frightened by the force of her sexuality. The nearness of her lover, she admitted, overwhelmed her like a young girl; she trembled, she could hardly swallow, her bones seemed to melt at his touch. The thought of him obsessed her night and day. Nothing in her experience had prepared her for this passionate desire to surrender. Having at last found a man capable of mastering her, she was ready, she said, 'to give herself up body and soul'. When set beside him nothing else mattered. Onlookers watched with bewilderment. 'She seemed suddenly to change,' remembered someone years later, 'and to throw to the winds all consideration, save the satisfaction of this passionate attachment.'[13] She had taken no vow of celibacy. Without consulting anyone, without hesitation or thought for the consequence, she promised to marry him.

This seems to have been the situation in 1866, when Sister Dora, for her annual holiday from the hospital, went to spend a few days with her unmarried sisters in their new house at New-bigin, Richmond, and with Rachel at Bellerby,[14] her first visit to her old home since 1861. Dora told Rachel something, but not the whole story of her love affair. 'This step of hers was without the approval of the Sisters in the Home,' wrote Rachel to Mark later, 'but she did not let me understand the whole matter, and indeed, dear Mark, I confess to you what I cannot to anyone else, her visit leaves a pain in me I cannot willingly touch upon; it was this feeling made me not discuss her with you. . . . I can only say I wish she *could* marry one of these doctors who seem so fond of her . . . then she might live a safer life for her character. But it is useless to write more, dear M. Dora was very reserved this time, so much so that I fancied something seemed to weigh on her; I could only give her my love, should she ever need or could use it.'[15]

Something did indeed weigh on Sister Dora. Once removed from the compelling physical presence of her lover, she was forced to realize what it would mean to give up her vocation and her work for ever. Nursing, with total dedication of self, could never be reconciled with giving herself up body and soul in a passionate marriage. She asked advice from 'an old friend', probably Edward Wyvill. He told her what she already knew, that she would have to give up nursing, and advised her to 'pause and consider what she was about to do'. He also added, from knowledge of her temperament, that if she lived with a man she was so much in love with 'her own faith would not suffice to stand against the power of this man's intellect'. He gave her the advice which was his plain professional duty as a clergy-man, 'to draw back while there was yet time'.[16]

Sister Dora went back to Walsall in extreme anguish of mind. For days, perhaps even weeks, she tried to put off choosing between the two things which meant most to her in the world. She was too impulsive to take advice easily, but she had doubts of her own to ponder. Only four years later, a young woman doctor was to write about her own engagement. 'I do hope you will not think that I have meanly deserted my post. I am sure that the woman question will never be solved in any complete way so long as marriage is thought to be incompatible with freedom and with an independent career.'[17] The future Elizabeth Garrett Anderson, in 1870, already foreshadowed the twentieth century; but Dorothy Pattison belonged to the Romantic Age. For her, marriage meant a total commitment of body and mind. The memory of her parents' wretched marriage and the misery of their children, the chance that her own children might bear a hereditary taint, above all the sacrifice of nursing, which she believed was her God-given work, all passed through her mind in succession. This was, in an intensely personal form, the dilemma of mid-Victorian England, scientific humanism against faith, passion against duty. In the end, she broke off her engagement. She felt the bitterest self-reproach. She knew, she said, 'that she had treated her lover with the utmost unfairness and had given him cause to think meanly of her principles and her conduct.'[18] Once again, in loving a man, she had brought him nothing but grief. She was in despair.

John Redfern Davies resigned as surgeon; he had been violently thrown from a horse and strained his back. He regretted he could not 'perform my hospital duties with that efficiency which your noble charity deserves'. He gave a small donation; 'Sister Dora handed in £2:0:0 from Mr. Davies' and the Committee thanked him. 'His kind and skilful treatment of the patients and his gentlemanly conduct,' they said, 'had secured him the sincere esteem of all connected with the hospital.'[19] Sister Dora never saw him again.

The full facts of their tragic love will probably never be known. What is of public interest is the effect on Sister Dora's work. It has always been a mystery how a woman of sketchy education, brought up in a remote village and working in a rough town, could have acquired standards of nursing so much higher than most of her contemporaries. Everything suggests that Redfern Davies, a surgeon of exceptional skill and intelligence, was a great formative influence in her life. It will emerge over the next ten years how much of his teaching on medicine and surgery she put into practice.

This love affair was quite unlike Dorothy Pattison's youthful attachments. It was a mature passion, and there is no doubt that the pain of its ending scarred her for life. She alone knew how much her decision had cost her. She once told another woman that she would never cease to regret not having children of her own; years of caring for other people's children, though she loved them, never took the place of the primitive maternal relationship. She remained a romantic at heart, a favourite and sympathetic confidante in young people's love affairs. She could write to them charmingly about their mild flirtations. 'I do not know,' she wrote to a girl, 'whether I like your clever friend very much. Somehow he and I do not get on very well, so far. Is he just a little conceited, do you think? Or perhaps he is one of those reserved people who grow upon you slowly? Anyway – mind you always write as if you were talking to me.'[20] As a middle-aged woman she startled a group of young girls by saying dreamily, 'If I had to begin life over again I would marry; a woman ought to live with a man and to be in subjection.' Long after she believed herself immune, she was to experience once more the delight and pain of falling in love.

Nature revenged itself for the intensity of frustration she had endured. One day in mid-November 1866, Sister Dora, while working in the wards, fainted across a bed.[21] This was the beginning of an illness lasting six weeks, which threw the whole hospital and the Pattison family into a state of confusion and distress. Only the patient remained calm, as though the symptoms were indifferent to her. 'Either she does not know or else does not explain clearly what is the matter with her,' wrote Rachel to Mark on 18th November. 'She speaks of the pain or spasms, lasting sometimes for hours at a time and very violent. For myself I believe it is over-fatigue, when she was here it was too evident that she was completely over-strained. I would have gone to her, but she does not wish it, though had she not written today I think I must have gone, I was so uneasy. I can give you no information as to the cause.'[22] Mark was so out of touch with Dorothy that he believed she might have fallen ill on hearing

that her old suitor, James Tate, was married. The Committee
believed she had injured herself in lifting a heavy patient.

A fortnight later she was no better and her sister Mary insisted
on coming from Richmond to nurse her. She found Dora helpless,
with one knee joint fixed and immovable. 'She suffers acute pain
and cannot bear to sit up.' At first Dr Burton assured Mary that
there was no danger 'unless inflammation sets in, but he feared
her weak state might produce it at any time'.[23] On the night of
1st–2nd December she appeared much worse; the hospital telegraphed to Birmingham for a second opinion, and straw was laid
in the street under her window to deaden the sound of horses'
hooves.[24] The verdict was an attack of pyaemia; Sister Dora was
told that it might be necessary to amputate her leg in order to
save her life. She replied calmly that she would refuse her consent
to the operation. In any case, she said, 'I would rather die than
live.' The old doctor was in despair; he was seen to leave the
hospital with tears in his eyes saying, 'If Sister Dora dies, I'll
never enter these doors again.'[25] She did not die, however, and
on 15th December Dr Burton told Mary, 'She has so good a
constitution, she will pull through, though it will be weeks before
she is out of bed, and I doubt she will ever be the same again.'
Mother Theresa sent an experienced nursing Sister from Coatham,
a strong and trustworthy young woman to take care of her,
though Sister Dora was told nothing of this until the last minute
'in case she should dislike it'. Sister Frances had offered to come,
but Dora put her off, with the excuse that there was fever in the
town. She seemed indifferent to Mary's presence also, and her
sister went home. 'I felt sadly dispirited', she wrote, 'with the
fruitless journey I had made.'[26] 'It was useless to think we could
give her pleasure or be of comfort to her,' agreed Frances, rather
wistfully. All Dora wanted was to be left alone. Yet she did
receive one last family visit. Mark was deeply anxious about her.[27]
On 19th December he travelled to Walsall to see her for himself.
He found her, as Mary had, in a town which, to his fastidious
taste, appeared sordid, in a mean little house, where the coming
and going of nurses and the crowded, noisy out-patients continually woke her from sleep. She insisted 'she had quiet nights and
felt easier' and 'they all took very good care of her'. No one will
ever know what other words passed between them, but it must

have been a bitter meeting for them both, to judge from what followed. Mark never visited his sister again, and seems to have written only on unavoidable business.[28] In the remaining quarter of Sister Dora's life they met once only, for five minutes in public. Their last private meeting received only the bare, utterly characteristic record in Mark's diary: 'Walsall (19/– fare).'[29]

Sister Dora's feelings towards her family were numbed, but by contrast she was touched by constant inquiries from old patients. None pleased her more than those of the young man whose arm she had saved. He lived eleven miles away and Sunday was his only holiday, but each week he walked over, pulled the hospital bell, and asked, 'How's Sister?' He listened to the reply, said, 'Tell her that's *her* arm that rang the bell!' and walked back again. Grateful ex-patients brought gifts of touching simplicity, a pound of tea and a laying hen.

Illness brought Sister Dora another visitor who was to become one of her closest friends. This was Richard Twigg, a fellow Yorkshireman who had come to Wednesbury as assistant curate and was to stay there for the rest of his life. He brought with him his schoolgirl daughter. They sat on either side of the sick-bed, and he read aloud to Sister Dora. He was, he said, 'astounded at her fortitude . . . her face was smiling and beautiful as I had never seen a human face before', though he noticed she sometimes turned her head away. Later his young daughter told him how surprised she had been to see sudden tears streaming down Sister Dora's cheeks as he read.

The end of this illness was as sudden as the onset had been. By 29th December 1866 Dr Burton wrote to the Pattison sisters at Richmond that at best 'she would have a long and tedious convalescence. He only hoped that in the end it could be a perfect recovery, but this of course he begged should not be breathed to her'.[30] To the hospital secretary he spoke more frankly about his patient's chances. 'She has blood poisoning and I doubt whether she can pull through.' Yet from force of habit he told her about all the new admissions, among them a man so badly crushed in a pit fall that he was expected to lose a leg. The same day, as the early winter darkness closed in, Samuel Welsh, the secretary, happened to be in the hall. 'I was roused,' he wrote, 'by a rustling sound, and on looking up I saw a spectral figure gliding gently and almost noiselessly towards the ward door. It was nearly dark. "Sister!" I said, "is it you?" "Sh!" she said and glided through the doorway into the ward. In a short time she returned, and I said, "Sister, you are ill. What are you doing here?" "It's true I've been ill", she said, "but I heard them talk about amputating that poor fellow's leg and I wanted to see if there was any possibility of saving it. I believe there is. Knowing that, I feel better." And so saying, she glided out of the hall as noiselessly as she had entered.'[31]

From that evening Sister Dora went back to work as though nothing had happened. She ordered a cab and drove out through the rain to visit a railway pointsman, who was ill at home with a poisoned foot. 'She came in so quiet and pale, I thought it must be her ghost,' said the patient. 'But she folded back the bedclothes off my foot and dressed it, and it began to feel easier. Then I knew it was her all right.' It was six months before the hospital staff found out where she had gone that day, and she laughed at them. 'What a long time it took you to find out!' she said.

Until the day of her death she never took more than a few days' sick leave again. Dr Burton was completely baffled by this case, and many pious friends were convinced the cure was miraculous. Not so Mr R. C. Lucas of Guy's Hospital, who, reading the case-history some years later, pronounced 'the termination or cure was as sudden and characteristic as the onset . . . I put it to the professors whether any actual synovitis ever terminated abruptly in this manner. The knee affection was from first to last a neurosis, viewed in connection with her highly strained temperament.' He suggested that the case of Sister Dora would form an illustration to a lecture on 'an hysterical knee-joint'.[32] As corroborative evidence, he pointed to her 'endurance and her desire to die a martyr, with all the mental strain involved'. Considering that he knew nothing of Sister Dora's family history or early life, this seems a notably shrewd diagnosis.

Despite his gloomy fears, old Dr Burton might have recalled the lecture on Local Nervous Affections given by Sir Benjamin Brodie thirty years before, in 1837,[33] which describes something remarkably like Sister Dora's case. Brodie noted that 'a particular joint was affected with pain and a great degree of morbid sensibility, attended occasionally with some degree of tumefaction although

. . . the usual consequences of abscess and destruction of the joint did not ensue'. He went so far as to say that 'four fifths of female patients who are commonly supposed to labour under diseases of the joints labour under hysteria and nothing else'. The precipitating causes were physical exhaustion and 'some moral cause having a depressing effect. Young women of the highest moral qualities and of the strongest understanding are not exempt from these maladies'. A striking feature was the 'belle indifference' of the patient, which Sister Dora clearly displayed.

The whole history of this illness and its ending must raise the question of Sister Dora's mental stability. Her heredity was bad and her childhood had been appalling. Fainting and paralysis form part of a recognized group of hysterical illnesses. Anna Pattison suffered from paralysis of many years' duration, and Mark Pattison's wife was a sceptical observer of her husband's collapses. 'The fainting is always exaggerated, like everything else which can excite commiseration. I have seen him throw himself down on the landing with great ease in similar attacks,' she wrote. From a clinical point of view, Sister Dora's religious faith might be considered a symptom of neurosis, since, as William James pointed out, the 'acute fever of religion' involves a discordant inner life, obsessions, melancholy and a radical pessimism about the human condition, from which Christianity is seen as the only hope of deliverance.[34]

Certainly Sister Dora did not appear to those who saw her every day at work as a person who could be judged by normal standards. 'I never saw such a woman before,' said an experienced doctor at the hospital. 'She had the vitality of three ordinary people.' She was slender in build, with delicate hands and feet, yet her strength seemed extraordinary. For years she ran the the hospital without a porter; she was seen to lift a drunken miner weighing fifteen stone and dump him in bed like a baby. 'Her physical strength was gigantic,' said another doctor. 'Sister Dora could sit up all night and work all day and as far as I am able to judge, she was neither physically nor mentally the worse for it. I never saw such a woman.'[35] Her devotion to work became compulsive. As Edith Simcox shrewdly observed, she attempted 'to lose herself' in physical exhaustion. She was up earliest in the morning and last to bed at night; from 1868 she had the casualty bell beside the front door connected to her own bed-head and seldom had a night's unbroken sleep. 'She always took the heaviest and roughest part of any employment on herself,' said the cook at the hospital. 'She never chose to ask her servants to do anything which she was not in the habit of doing herself.' Laughing with pleasure at her own strength, Sister Dora would take heavy buckets of water or hods of coal out of their protesting hands, and walk away with no alteration in her light, graceful a step.[36] From her father Sister Dora inherited intense vitality and driving will-power, from her mother a near-fanatical sense of duty and devotion. These qualities had gone to waste in the parents' tragic and futile lives; but in the daughter's they served a purpose.

It is well known that certain hysterical traits in able men and women may contribute to their achievement. It is said that such people 'excel in occupations of a strange sentimental appeal, such as those of nurse or welfare worker, nun, missionary and the activities of the public benefactor. In occupations such as these the hysteric may attain a resounding success'.[37] Universal love is perhaps less exposing for such temperaments than the close, equal companionship of marriage. In her public career Sister Dora became one of the heroic figures of mid-Victorian England. This was only achieved at great personal cost, for the conflicts and passions which had assailed Dorothy Pattison continued to rack Sister Dora to the very end of her life.

As soon as she was fully recovered and able to work, Sister Dora turned to a clergyman for advice.[38] She said her strong will, the pride of life, had been a source of grief and suffering for herself and others. Could she not surrender it entirely into the keeping of higher authority? The mild discipline of Coatham had failed to protect her from her own passionate temperament. Should she not enter the strictest religious order she could find? It seems likely that she was thinking of the Society of the Most Holy Trinity at Osnaburgh Street, London, an order run by its Abbess Miss Sellon, a naval officer's daughter, with positively sea-going discipline.[39] In fact the reputed severities of the Society were the source of much of the gossip about Anglican Communities for women. Sister Dora's advisor replied that he believed she was called to 'active service of mind and body'. At Walsall she could do the nursing work for which she was so well fitted;

if she left she might be turning her back on it.[40] His advice was to seek her own salvation in care for other people. Sister Dora was convinced by this, and, as she said 'resolved to stay where she was'. She plunged into such incessant work that the other Sisters were alarmed. She had one aim in life, she said, to become a good surgical nurse. 'Nobody could possibly be more ignorant than I was,' she said. 'I had everything to learn.' She admitted later that this time in her life had been 'a tolerably severe apprenticeship'. Even more severe was the next shock to assail her.

On 3rd March 1867 Redfern Davies died at his father's house and was buried in a family vault at Edgbaston Old Church. Post mortem examination revealed a false aneurism of the descending thoracic aorta, caused, it was believed, by the injury when he was thrown from his horse. 'Very few surgeons', wrote *The Lancet*, 'have displayed in their early years a more thorough appreciation of scientific surgery. . . . To his friends, apart from his abilities, he was especially endeared by the independence of his character, and the truthfulness of everything that he did.' He had met pain and the approach of death with 'unflinching fortitude'.[41] On her visit to Rachel, Sister Dora heard news of another death as well; her girlhood's love, Purchas Stirk, had died at his farm near Hauxwell, at the age of thirty-one. Everyone she encountered seemed to suffer for it. 'At this particular time,' it was noticed, 'regret and remorse seemed to have taken away from her, for a time, all desire for life.'[42] Her remorse was supposed to be for the death of her father, described by one who did not know him as 'a genial and open-handed old country Rector'. It seems far more likely to have been for the early deaths of two men who had loved her, and who had both died unmarried.

A few months after Redfern Davies died, the first of several epidemics of smallpox broke out in the overcrowded courts and alleys of Walsall, where it lingered with continual fresh outbreaks through the long, sultry summer of 1868. There was no fever hospital in the town, and the Committee determined, successfully, to keep the wards of the accident hospital entirely free from fevers. Nothing was done for the smallpox victims; they lay in their stifling little rooms until they either died or recovered. The death rate in Walsall from March to October 1868 was thirty-nine per thousand, higher than that of any town of comparable size in the United Kingdom.[43] This was the opportunity Sister Dora longed for. Close observers recorded her 'scarcely veiled longing for some hope forlorn enough to throw away her life upon'. Later she admitted how strongly she had hoped to catch a fever and die.

She confided in no one, but went out to search for patients in their own homes. The other Sisters attempted to remonstrate with her, but Sister Dora had not grown less self-willed with the years. She argued that she would not neglect her hospital duties; she would 'make half an hour', by getting through her rounds with extra speed, or cutting a meal. As for infection, she said, 'we are all exposed to that already from out-patients, who may come up to have their wounds dressed with the smallpox already upon them'. Sister Dora, with her black cloak and black nurse's bag, went down into the slums of the lower town, a wilderness of sooty slate roofs, broken only by noisome tunnels, narrow and black as a coalmine. Behind lay more houses, facing on to stifling yards, with one central water-pump, where rusty pipes, fowl pens and old iron bedsteads jostled privies and middens.[44] The whole was seen through a blear of coal dust. Inside, the houses were identical, a door from the street into the single living room, the dark kitchen beyond, the stair to the two stifling rooms above, where her patients lay indescribably crowded by their children, their animals and their inevitable lodger, usually one of the five thousand Irish labourers at work in the town. These hastily and heartlessly built dwellings were described by a local clergyman as 'brick graves where the poor are buried alive'.

There was little to be done for the patients, some of whom were dying of the terrifying confluent smallpox known as 'black pox'. Sister Dora sometimes found them at the point of death, alone in houses from which all their relations had fled in terror. She took them bottles of clean drinking water, washed them, made beds and calmed them by promising 'not to leave them while they lived'. At night she sat by the dying in the light of guttering candle ends. Once at least she stayed on in darkness, till in the early dawn she groped her way to the door to let in the light which confirmed that her patient was indeed dead.[45] Obsessed with the desire to help and the longing to die herself, she forgot rest or food.

Yet she did not die. She had reckoned without her own intense vitality and love of living. What happened in these desperate months was that the love, which in a normal life would have been given to family, husband and children, fastened itself upon the poor and suffering of this harsh town. They returned it with the generosity of the humble. This was, for Sister Dora, life's bargain, and she did not think it a bad one. Walsall was her home, and its working people 'my own people', as her family had long ceased to be. 'I came here,' she said, 'and here I hope to stay to the end. The more work I have to do the stronger and happier I feel. I *never* want to leave.'[46] She had come through a major conflict and had made her choice.

NOTES

1. Lonsdale, 76 ff. dates it before the retirement of old John Burton, i.e. before 1868. Her account contains several contradictions, and appears to confuse two different relationships.
2. F. Burleigh, *Sister Dora*, 17.
3. Pattison, 66, f. 424–5.
4. *Provincial Medical Directory*, 1865–1870.
5. W.C.H. MS.
6. *Medical Times and Gazette*, 1858. 'Radical Cure of Inguinal Hernia with Modification of Instrument.'
7. *The Lancet*, 9th April 1864 and *The British Medical Journal*, 23rd May 1863.
8. *Medical Times and Gazette*, 1864.
9. Lonsdale, 93, 203.
10. *The Lancet*, 6th June 1863, and *The British Medical Journal*, 23rd May 1863.
11. Lonsdale, 76.
12. J. Morrison, *History of the Birmingham Medical School*, 126.
13. Lonsdale, 77.
14. Pattison, 56, f. 307.
15. Ibid., 56, f. 424–5.
16. Lonsdale, 77
17. J. Manton, *Elizabeth Garrett Anderson*, 213.
18. Lonsdale, 77.
19. W.C.H. MS. and W.C.H.A.R., 1866.
20. Ridsdale, 57.

21. Lonsdale, 78, describes this illness, but gives no date, except that it preceded the retirement of old Dr Burton, in 1868. It seems to correspond with the mysterious illness of November-December 1866, described in Pattison, 56, ff. 345–91.
22. Pattison, 56, f. 355.
23. Ibid., 56, ff. 357–8.
24. Ibid., 56, f. 355.
25. Lonsdale, 78.
26. Pattison, 56, ff. 389–91.
27. Ibid., 56, ff. 424–5.
28. Ibid., 57, ff. 59–61.
29. Ibid., 19.
31. Ibid., 56, f. 389–91.
31. S. Welsh, *General Baptist Magazine*, 1889, 271–2.
32. *British Medical Journal*, 11th December 1880.
33. Hunter and Macalpine, *Three hundred years of psychiatry*, 860–64.
34. W. James, *Varieties of Religious Experience*, 144–5.
35. Lonsdale, 107.
36. Ibid., 100–101.
37. Mayer-Gross, Slater and Roth, *Clinical Psychiatry*, 136.
38. It is not clear whether this was her old friend, Edward Wyvill, or her new friend, Richard Twigg.
39. Miss Sellon also suffered from a mysterious and disabling paralysis and was carried around on a mattress.
40. Lonsdale, 43.
41. *The Lancet*, 16th March, 1867.
42. Lonsdale, 53.
43. W.C.H.A.R., 1868.
44. The last of these yards has now been demolished, but they existed within living memory.
45. Lonsdale, 52.
46. Ridsdale, 32.

CHAPTER THIRTEEN

Sister-in-Charge
1868–1870

In the autumn of 1867 a miner named Thomas Hall was admitted
to the crowded little house in Bridge Street for amputation of a
leg smashed in the pit. After he had spent eight weeks as an in-
patient the stump was still inflamed and an angry red rash spread
over the surface of his body. Dr Burton diagnosed 'the fatal
erysipelas' and hastily sent him home, where Sister Dora visited
him every day for the next seven weeks to change the dressings.
To her immense relief he did not die, and no further cases
developed, so that Dr Burton was able to say emphatically in his
report that 'no amputation has terminated fatally and *no contagious
surgical malady* has ever existed in the hospital'. The emphasis
reflected what they all knew; they had had a narrow escape.[1]

Erysipelas was one of a recognized group of 'hospital diseases'.
The others most commonly met were pyaemia, in which septic
clots formed in the veins, to be carried by the circulation to distant
parts of the body, septicaemia, or generalized blood poisoning
and 'hospital gangrene' in which the wound area, sometimes a
whole limb, mortified and sloughed away. All were highly contagious and together they were the principal cause of hospital
mortality.[2] Florence Nightingale observed the restlessness, lan-
guor and feverishness of patients crowded together in a hospital
ward. 'All operations' the nurse was told, 'are attended by the
same after-risk of erysipelas or blood-poisoning and a nurse must
never forget how quickly a very slight wound may progress to
a fatal termination'. She was warned to watch for the signs of
'surgical fever', raised pulse and temperature, restlessness, headache and malaise, disturbed sleep, later delirium and finally coma

leading to death.[3] This was the central problem of Sister Dora's work as a nurse of accident cases.

No theory had ever been brought forward to offer a rational explanation of the hospital diseases; until the publication of Pasteur's work and its application by Lister to surgery their nature and cause remained a total mystery. They were often assumed to be the product of polluted 'miasma'; ex-medical students were heard to speak nostalgically of 'the good old surgical stink' of the wards in their teaching hospitals. Florence Nightingale, writing in 1863, refused to accept the possibility of contagion, which 'pre-supposes the existence of certain *germs*', and insisted that 'abundance of pure air will prevent infection. All my hospital experience supports this conclusion'. She pinned her faith to open windows day and night. Others, including Sir James Simpson, believed the infection to lie in the fabric of the buildings themselves, and that the only remedy was hutted hospitals, demolished at regular intervals. Among substances applied in the hope of combating infection were Friar's Balsam, myrrh, glycerine and zinc. Other suggestions included wire mesh at the windows to exclude flying particles of 'malignancy', and heavy bandages, which effectively prevented the drainage of already infected wounds. Surgeons were in the position of a man looking for a dropped pin in a dark room, and their nurses were equally baffled. Sister Dora did not understand the cause of wound infection until almost the end of her career; but meanwhile she was to achieve surprisingly good results by the simple, though laborious method learnt from Redfern Davies, 'the utmost possible cleanliness in nursing'.

Although the cause of Thomas Hall's erysipelas was unknown, doctors and committee agreed that the hospital must move from its makeshift quarters in Bridge Street without delay, as 'the wards were evidently impregnated with malignant air to a hopeless extent'.[4] They had been collecting a building fund since 1864 and now they began house-hunting in earnest. Various schemes fell through for financial or legal reasons, until they found the ideal site. Old paintings of Walsall show, on the edge of the town, a sharp ridge crowned by a bleak redbrick villa called 'The Mount'. A large garden, with blackened trees and grass, sloped down to the Wednesbury Road. Opposite, in 1868, lay an open space, trampled bare by generations of Walsall boys playing football, and beyond that the town's racecourse. So much open space offered hope of escape from 'malignant miasma'. At first the owner, Miss Harriet Richmond, proprietor of Walsall's one genteel girls' school, recoiled in horror from the idea. 'A hospital!' she cried. 'I could not even think of such a thing!' but the chairman's blandishments and an offer of ready money prevailed. The four-square, windswept building was solid and plain, with high, well-lit rooms opening off a central hall; it had gas and water though no drainage.[5] The main rooms formed three wards, with a total of twenty-four beds; a coach-house, down a steep and highly inconvenient flight of steps, became an out patient surgery, and the mortuary was established in a distant gardener's shed. The cost of conversion was £742, to which Sister Louisa contributed £5 and Sister Dora £10.

The foundation stone of the new hospital was laid on Easter Monday 1868, and by 23rd April Sister Dora applied for the Committee's permission to entertain all her old patients to a house-warming tea in the Bradford Ward.[7] Just as the date for moving approached, Sister Louisa caught measles; infectious diseases were a recognized hazard for adults from sheltered backgrounds who came to work among the poor. She was not young and she took it badly. The entire move and the arrangements for the new hospital passed automatically into Dora's hands. By 13th May she was called in to the Committee meeting; from this time she became in name and in fact 'head of the nursing department'. In this building she was to do for industrial workers what Florence Nightingale had done for army casualties in the Crimea. Their working situations were in some ways similar; society had grown used to the idea that workmen were the cannon fodder of industry. Though Florence Nightingale had friends in high places, and worked in a blaze of publicity, while Sister Dora was a provincial, unknown outside her own region, factual reports and statistics show her to have been equally revolutionary.

Everything conspired to give her an unexpectedly free hand. The move to the new hospital was accompanied by changes in the Sisterhood, which profoundly affected her future. Briefly, the Chaplain, John Postlethwaite, intended to go to South America as a missionary, and therefore resigned his parish at Coatham.

His new appointment fell through, but Mother Theresa had already nominated the Rev. R. L. Page to Christ Church living and the Chaplaincy of the convent. The work was therefore divided between the two clergymen, 'which naturally severs the House at Coatham and the Walsall Hospital from the North Ormesby one', wrote Sister Frances. 'One cannot help being sorry for it, but it must be so.' The Sisters at Walsall were left in some doubt where their obedience lay; 'it is for all those engaged in the hospitals to decide which side has justice'. Frances wanted to discuss it with Dora, but felt 'she was afraid I might talk too much about the alteration that has taken place'.[8]

Sister Frances and two of the Sisters at Walsall chose to remain under the direction of the main community at Middlesbrough. Thereafter Dora and Frances, though they were fond of each other, were seldom able to meet. Young Father Page was only in his middle twenties, but already a very different proposition from Mr Postlethwaite. As befitted a future Oxford Superior of the Cowley Fathers, he had a clearly defined ideal of the religious life, and a sharp eye for constitutional anomalies. In 1867 the Sisterhood was reconstituted under the name it now bears, the Community of the Holy Rood, and work began on the re-drafting of the rule in accordance with canon law. Predictably, differences of opinion arose, including, as a tactful arbitrator wrote in 1869, 'a mutual distrust between the Mother and Chaplain, each heartily respecting the other personally, but entirely distrusting each other's fitness for the particular office each holds'.[9] To the credit of both, the distrust was conquered, a Chapter held, and a proper constitution drawn up.[10] In 1871 Sister Frances, with Mother Theresa, took final vows in the Chapel of the Cowley Fathers at Oxford. There was a period of trial and error, with some withdrawals, but in 1876 the Convent of the Holy Rood was established at Middlesbrough, where succeeding generations of Sisters have ever since been held in affection and respect. Mother Theresa had the joy, after years of struggle, of seeing her community grow and thrive, and of knowing that Sister Frances would succeed her as Mother Superior. Their lives were lived in a great tradition, but theirs was a calling Dora did not share.

Sister Dora, given the choice in 1867, elected to remain at Walsall under the direction of Mr Postlethwaite and the Coatham

Homes. She did not, in the words of the *Dictionary of National Biography* 'leave the Sisterhood', but the work of the hospital was hived off from the main community; thereafter 'the connection of the Sisterhood with the charities at Coatham and Walsall consisted merely in name'.[11] Mr Postlethwaite seems to have had a good heart and a muddled head, both reflected in the curious hybrid ecclesiastical title he now adopted, 'Pastor of the Homes of the Good Samaritan'.[12] Sister Dora called him 'the formidable Pastor', but in reality she could make rings round him. His administration was well-meaning, but amateur. Sisters were sent out and recalled on a bewildering variety of good works; first Sister Louisa was withdrawn, a few months later Sister Phoebe, and at least six others came and went in the years 1866–9. Old Dr Burton complained that the hospital was 'seriously under-nursed'.[13] Dora hated the waste and inefficiency involved. Tactfully she persuaded the Chaplain to leave her alone at Walsall to settle patients in the new building. By his weak and vacillating direction, she was left in an extraordinarily exposed position for a woman of her time, with neither husband, family nor religious vows to protect her. Her innate dignity and independence were her shield, but, given the current conventions and her own temperament, Rachel's fears for her sister's reputation and character were far from groundless.

Nor did Mr Postlethwaite understand or share Sister Dora's commitment to her work. Later he was to admit candidly when charged that 'his chief object in establishing hospitals was the extension of his own religious views. He would not give his time and labour merely for repairing broken bodies'.[14] Since this was Dora's vocation, they were bound to clash eventually. For the moment however the medical and lay committee members of Walsall Cottage Hospital, always thrown into consternation at the prospect of losing Sister Dora, breathed again. From now on she was undisputed Sister-in-Charge. Loneliness honed the cutting-edge of ambition. She worked single-handed and for five years could not even take a summer holiday. The Committee recorded the fact by printing her name for the first time in their annual report. The entry, in the financial statement, was modest. 'Balance in hands of Sister Dora,' it read, '£6:5:5½'.[15]

Changes on the medical side too, concentrated responsibility in her hands. Old Dr Burton, who had been in practice for some forty years, decided in 1868 to retire as acting surgeon, a position he had held since the sudden resignation of Redfern Davies in 1866. The medical committee voted that he should not be replaced, but that they would share his duties in monthly rotation. The doctor whose turn it was to be on duty had to be traced, a messenger sent after him with a note, and his coming awaited, sometimes, if he were out in his carriage, for several hours. This was too much for young John Burton, who foresaw that responsibility would fall on his shoulders as acting unpaid house-surgeon. He had already begun to leave notes saying 'Sister Dora, do as you like in this case'. Now, politely, 'offering you my congratulations on the increasing usefulness of your institution', he handed his resignation to the Committee,[16] and left Walsall to become a regimental surgeon to the Staffordshire Rifle Volunteers. The scheme, as he had the sense to see, proved unworkable and a permanent surgeon was appointed after a few months; but meanwhile, the only person immediately available in any crisis was the Sister-in-Charge. Hospital practice a hundred years ago made heavy demands on courage and character. There was no clinical team with specialized skills to share responsibility, no X-rays, no pathological laboratory, no mechanical resources. At Walsall in 1868 the hospital consisted of a roof, four walls and a subsistence budget, within which the staff had to improvise to meet bloody emergencies, usually without warning. Dora's bold, imaginative mind served her better in these conditions than a more formal training might have done; her spirits rose to meet difficulties which would have overwhelmed a timid or conventional character. She was forced to rely on first-hand observation and experience, to do the best she could in the moment of decision and thereafter have the courage to live with what she had done. No sight was too terrible for her to face, no case too hopeless. Her lion-like courage sustained patients and staff through the worst hours. This single-handed struggle against death and disaster excited her dramatic temperament; she never worked better than in a crisis. Moreover she had brains as well as character and she was learning all the time. The work never allowed her to grow stale, never ceased to challenge her intelligence. 'We are absolutely full of the most interesting cases. I am never weary of it,' she wrote in one of her rare letters to her sisters. After years of empty frustration or ravaging emotional conflict, she was living to some purpose at last. She found it deeply satisfying.

In these circumstances the management committee came to rely on Sister Dora implicitly. There is not the slightest evidence that she 'considered it her duty to influence them'[17] or condescended to them socially, and no reason why she should have done. They were a cross-section of society, including clergymen, a lawyer, a gentleman farmer, a schoolmaster, a journalist, a mineowner, a bank manager and several manufacturers. The chairman, Samuel Cox, whose portrait in bas-relief appears on Sister Dora's memorial, was a fellow Yorkshireman and a personal friend, and the secretary, Samuel Welsh, a clever Scotsman of radical sympathies. They had created a much-needed hospital by their own efforts, without receiving or demanding a penny from public funds, and she admired their independence. She had been frugally brought up and showed her loyalty in the most practical manner, saving the committee money in every way which did not affect the patients' welfare. Everyone who worked at the Walsall Hospital sooner or later heard Sister Dora say, 'Mind you don't waste *a thing*!' It became statistically the most economically-run small hospital in Great Britain, with a cost per patient in 1870 of 15s. 6d a week. At another time the cost was reduced further to £34 per bed per annum. The committee members were happy to leave practical questions in Dora's exceedingly capable hands. From the time she became Sister-in-Charge items which had caused long and vexatious discussion – could the hospital cook be a Nonconformist? – would a Roman Catholic housemaid be a cause of scandal? – quietly vanished from their agenda.[18] Sometimes they could not agree on a point and a member wrote this account of what used to happen. 'Ask Sister Dora! Had we not better send for Sister Dora? some member would exclaim out of the fog of contention. Thereupon she would appear; calmly self-possessed she would stand, never sit, with her hand on the back of the chair which had been placed for her, every eye directed to her; nor was ever many moments before she had grasped the whole question and given her opinion, clearly and simply. Nor was she ever wrong.'[19] She was gone, with a soft rustle of her long skirts, even before they had time to thank her.

With all the force of her indomitable will, she put aside the griefs of the last two years and concentrated on the work in hand. She welcomed the challenge of immediate practical problems, which demanded all her energies of body and mind. During the early months in the new hospital most of the suggestions for improvement, all sooner or later adopted, came from her side, as the committee's manuscript minutes reveal. From the beginning she set a standard of comfort and care for patients far higher than anyone else concerned had begun to imagine. She had four years' observation of nursing in somewhat primitive conditions to draw on, and it seems likely that she was influenced by Redfern Davies, easily the most distinguished surgeon under whom she worked. It is striking that from the first she began exactly as she meant to go on. The committee, prepared for a vaguely imagined angel of mercy, were confronted by a professional woman of practical outlook.

Her first move was to find good domestic staff, treat them well and make them stay. As cook she engaged a childhood friend, Sarah Watts, whose aproned lap had been her refuge in the kitchen at Hauxwell. Sarah loved Dora with the single-minded devotion of an old-fashioned family servant; she was a good cook and an excellent manager.[20] Nineteenth-century institutions were in general believers in the benefits of low diet; hospital food tended to arrowroot, cornflour and sago, with watered milk and 'broth' made from sheep or ox-head. Where bulk was permitted it was supplied by bread, potatoes and suet pudding; cases of scurvy in hospital wards were not unknown. Under Sarah's direction, joints of meat were roasted in the Walsall kitchens; Sister Dora carved herself and carefully supervised each plate. She continually requested and acknowledged gifts of fresh fruit and vegetables, while Sarah made jam and bottled their own garden produce for the winter. Patients and staff always ate the same food. In the long illnesses of those days, much depended on keeping the patients' strength up. It is impossible to say how many were cured largely by Sarah's cooking.

Florence Nightingale, whose *Sanitary Condition of Hospitals* Dora read, recommended 'all the scrubbing, and cleaning and polishing and scouring which used to go on in old-fashioned country households'.[21] This was what Dora had been brought up to, and she trained her two housemaids with Yorkshire thoroughness. Black Country dirt had one great psychological advantage; it was visible, even palpable in its gritty density, and presented an irresistible challenge to any woman of spirit. A cylinder beside the kitchen range, and huge iron kettles on the hob of every ward fire provided an inexhaustible supply of hot water, which Sister Dora insisted must be *'very* hot'. Carpets, curtains and hangings were ruthlessly discarded. The bare surfaces, floors, walls, doors and ledges were sealed with lacquer, which was then polished to a hard gloss twice a week and dusted every day with clean cloths wrung in hot water. This method was successfully followed in the Birmingham teaching hospitals; Sister Dora possibly learnt it from Redfern Davies, who had written that it significantly reduced infection. It would be interesting to know how hot the 'very hot water' in fact was, but there is no record of this. Every year she instituted a full-scale north-country spring cleaning. Bedsteads were dragged into the open air and turned upside down for the springs to be washed, paintwork renewed, every item of equipment cleaned, checked and tested.[22] The cleaners learnt to dread Sister Dora's inspection, her quiet frown at a skimped job. 'I would infinitely rather do it myself.' Everyone valued her highest term of praise, which was 'exquisite cleanliness'.

After the first spring cleaning Dora presented, at her own expense, matching blankets throughout the hospital and the immaculate wards were opened to the public for a day. A local lawyer was so impressed that he presented furniture for an entire new ward when it should be needed, and in due course the Edward Barnett Ward was opened and named after him. Other visitors, impressed with the comfort and happiness of the patients, gave donations towards the debt on the building fund. Sister Dora appealed for old, clean linen, which she stored in a work room, where wives and mothers of patients came in voluntarily to sew. The best linen was repaired for use on the beds, the worse cut into swabs and bandages. She also instituted a 'bank' of used clothing in good condition. Often, she explained, she had to cut away the clothes of injured patients and their working clothes were all they possessed. This service was a great help to hard-pressed families.

Sister Dora made the beds herself every morning and evening, and insisted on a supply of clean bedclothes. The hospital washing had formerly been sent out; she now gave one month's notice to the washerwoman and proposed to the committee that an outbuilding should be converted to a well-equipped wash-house and the work done at home by women engaged for the purpose.[23] In August 1868 the committee resolved 'that Sister Dora be authorised to provide appliances for washing to be done at the hospital'. The result was that washing and night-nursing which together cost the hospital £35 9s 4d in 1867, were done in 1870 at a cost of £7 1s 0d. Night-nursing had been done by a series of untrained 'watchers', engaged more or less at random in the town. Sister Dora dismissed all but one or two of these, whom she trained herself and applied to the committee for permission to install a system of night bells at a cost of £4 10s 0d. These connected her own bedroom with the wards, and an emergency bell on the front door;[24] she said she could be dressed and downstairs in three minutes to cope with any crisis.

She persuaded a carpenter, who was a patient in the hospital, to fit large castors to an old arm-chair, which she used to wheel helpless patients to an improvised bathroom, where they enjoyed or endured what was often the first bath of their lives. Next the drinking water supply claimed her attention. She handed round the committee table a horrific trophy of her own selection. It must have changed hands at high speed, for it was 'a glass of water containing numerous organic impurities visible to the naked eye'; the committee made a rule that all drinking water should be filtered before use.[25] A year later she was demanding 'the purchase of a self-registering clinical thermometer' and a year after that the services of a dispenser, whom she was empowered to appoint herself.[26]

The committee had hardly time to draw breath after these changes, when their Sister-in-Charge was back, this time demanding an 'outdoor porter'. After one or two unsatisfactory appointments, she had a candidate waiting, an ex-patient, 'my faithful friend Murray'. The committee meekly agreed 'the man found by Sister Dora is most suitable', and promised to build him a lodge in the grounds. Murray, at a combined wage of £53 10s 0d doubled the duties of gardener and handyman. He was a firm ally of Sister

Dora. She was afterwards quoted as authority that 'a man is indispensable' for the drying, renewing and emptying of the system of earth-closets which provided the only drainage at Walsall Cottage Hospital.[27] An efficient earth-closet demands a supply of dry earth, and Dora ensured this by having a glass passage constructed between the main buildings and the out-patient department, where earth could be dried in trays. She also used it to raise plants and it was romantically known as 'Sister's conservatory', by those who liked to fancy her arranging flowers by each sufferer's bedside, and preferred to close their minds to the less romantic side of hospital life. Not so Sister Dora. One of her strict rules was that every chamber pot must be removed and cleaned instantly, not, as was then the custom even in upper-class households, once a day. She quoted Florence Nightingale, 'Don't turn your sick room into a sewer! If a nurse declines to do these kind of things, I should say nursing was not her calling.' A patient was distressed that she should wait on him in this intimate way. 'Now don't you mind me,' she said cheerfully, 'because I assure you, I really don't mind at all.' The same patient remembered how she would never leave him until she was sure that he was really comfortable in bed. 'Aye,' he said, 'her was a grand tucker-up.'[28] These homely but rigorous standards of cleanliness seem to have been effective. In 1868, for the first time there were no deaths in the hospital from January to October.

The coach house converted to out-patients' department was already proving too small for the numbers passing through it. In 1869 it received 71 fractures, 104 burns and scalds and 290 flesh wounds; by 1870 the total number of out-patients was 2318. Most of the patients, both in and out, were men in the prime of life, in excellent health at the time of their injuries, while the smallness of the hospital reduced the risk of cross-infection. Nevertheless, the success of their treatment, set against a death rate in the town of 39 per 1000 during the same period, represents a real achievement. Whether Sister Dora's passion for cleanliness is attributed to a Puritan upbringing, suppressed sexual guilt or simple Yorkshire thoroughness, its results were striking. Soon they began to be noticed by medical men outside the immediate neighbourhood of Walsall. Lawson Tait recalled in 1890 how, when he came to Birmingham as a young man twenty years before, serious accident cases had been jolted in from miles around to the General and Queen's Hospitals. But, he added, 'old John Burton of Walsall, aided by Sister Dora, had just begun to show what a cottage hospital could do. . . . These local hospitals are a credit to any community; cases are treated quite as well and far more safely in cottage hospitals near the place of accident'.[29]

The most urgent need, which became obvious after six months in the new hospital, was for a permanent surgeon who should be available every day. In the autumn of 1868, after nine months with no deaths, a series of accident cases arrived which caused Sister Dora the deepest anxiety. Among them were a railwayman who had fractured his spine, a quarry worker in whose face a charge of gunpowder had exploded, and a labourer who had lain undiscovered with a broken thigh in a clay pit full of icy water. All three of these, and one more, died before the year was out. Sister Dora petitioned the medical and lay committee, and a special meeting of the General Committee was summoned on 15th September at 7.30 in the evening 'for the purpose of consulting on the propriety of the appointment of a House Surgeon'.[30]

The discussion was long, gloomy and inconclusive. Clearly they badly needed a house surgeon. Equally clearly they had no money to pay him. Then something happened extremely fortunate for Walsall and for Sister Dora. A square-built, sandy-haired, youngish man stood up in the Hospital hall and said, with a marked Scots accent, that he would be prepared to undertake the duties of acting surgeon, in return for an occasional honorarium.[31] On October 16th he confirmed the offer in writing from 30 Bridge Street, Walsall, 'I beg to offer my services as Surgeon to Walsall Cottage Hospital.'[32] He would attend the hospital every morning to see in-patients, and cases referred by Sister Dora from amongst out-patients. He was willing to operate on two afternoons every week, with a volunteer anaesthetist and Sister Dora to assist. The meeting, as one man, accepted this offer. So came into being a working partnership which was to last ten years, and to be broken only by Sister Dora's death.

The new acting surgeon, James MacLachlan, came from Glasgow. He had been a medical student there during Lister's years as Professor of Surgery, one of the large and enthusiastic class which banged on the desks to applaud each morning as the

Professor entered the lecture theatre. It was probably the largest, certainly the most appreciative medical class in Europe. Young MacLachlan admired his Professor enough to adopt Lister's style of hair and side-whiskers, which he wore for the rest of his life. By chance we know one of the questions he had to answer in Lister's class examinations, set in March 1862. 'Explain the principles on which simple incised wounds ought to be treated.' Marks were given for mentioning avoidance of inflammation, which had direct bearing on MacLachlan's work in the Walsall casualty department. From the revered figure of Lister, young MacLachlan learnt a high ideal of duty, which was to sustain him through twenty years of work at Walsall as medical officer to the workhouse and the borough, police-surgeon and acting surgeon to the hospital.[33] He qualified M.D. in Glasgow in 1863 and Ch.M. or Master of Surgery in 1865. At the time of his appointment he must have been about twenty-eight or thirty years old, though his square-cut features appeared older.

In every way MacLachlan and Dora were opposites, which is perhaps why they made such an effective team. Where she was dashing, impulsive and imaginative, he was steady, firm and unemotional. He had a dry sense of humour, which pulled her wilder flights of fancy sharply back to earth. He was a realist, disillusioned, with a not unkindly cynicism about human nature. He had been brought up as a Roman Catholic, and indeed his only brother became the Catholic Bishop of Galloway, but he regarded religious feelings with tolerant amusement. It was a rare occasion when he admitted to Sister Dora that her prayers for the patients were 'the real thing and no humbug', and his praise pleased her far more than the adulation she was accustomed to receiving from visiting ladies and clergy. He was equally blunt about Dora's looks; the shining eyes, delicate skin and slender waist most people admired, were, he told her symptomatic; she had had pleurisy twice and would be a fool to run risks with her health, though here she had the pleasure of proving him wrong. There was nothing remotely romantic or sentimental in their relationship. MacLachlan, a comfortable bachelor, seemed as indifferent to women as he was to worldly success, or indeed to most things outside his work. Here he showed himself not brilliant but painstaking and very thorough; his colleagues were right when they said 'his valuable services gratuitously rendered to the Hospital for many years contributed materially to its success'.[34] Every morning for years he made a round of every bed of the hospital with Sister Dora, and gave her clear directions for the day. Every evening she went round the wards alone, but if she was anxious about a patient, she sent the porter to fetch Dr MacLachlan, who not only came, but came promptly and efficiently, whatever the hour. Sister Dora became very fond of this uncompromising character, who took the place in some ways of the brother she no longer saw. The hospital secretary who saw them at work together said, 'There was no one who more fully enjoyed her confidence; to him, more than to the clergy or individual members of the committee she opened her mind and was in every way frank and friendly.'[35] He was to be a true friend.

By the end of 1868 the new hospital was well established and Dora began to plan a Christmas party with a tree and presents for every child who had been a patient during the year. There was hardly time to clear up after this before she began preparations for the adults' party, to which as many ex-patients as could squeeze into the large ward were welcomed on New Year's Eve. Rachel sent a pair of turkeys or geese from the farm at Bellerby, which Sarah Watts roasted in the hospital kitchen, and all sat down to supper at which Sister Dora carved. Afterwards, there was singing, some kind of entertainment, and conversation. Old patients were often surprised by how much Sister Dora seemed to know about them. 'I *never* forget a patient!' she used to boast. She insisted that patients would not recover fully unless they were happy. It was useless to treat them like well-cared-for farm animals and neglect their human needs. 'What a one-sided nurse I should be,' she wrote, 'if I only looked after their bodies and could not give any refreshment to their minds or souls.' A visiting nurse, objecting to the 'low songs and jokes' of the workmen in the accident ward, got little sympathy. 'You can't hope to keep men out of mischief', said Sister Dora frankly, 'unless you keep them amused.' She appealed for games, chess, draughts, backgammon, for books, pictures, magazines and toys for the children, whom she taught to play hide-and-seek among the haycocks. Local iron works, whose men she had nursed, presented garden seats, and a wrought-iron archway supporting a lantern over the garden gate.

She begged gifts of shrubs and plants and got the committee's permission to lay out a pleasure garden for the patients in summer.[36] At the foot of the slope ran the railway, with a ceaseless clanking of goods trains carrying coal and iron ore. The noise did not appear to disturb Sister Dora; railways to her generation were an unqualified blessing, and a view over a railroad had inspired Neale's famous sermon, in which the signal 'stretches out its arms, and by the sign of the cross directs the passing train'. To the patients, especially the railwaymen among them, the passing trains were a free entertainment. Each engine and driver had its distinctive whistle, which they recognized, and the ward echoed with shouts of 'Hullo, that's our Bill' or 'There goes Jack!' Sister Dora nursed many railwaymen, and always expressed admiration for the masculine mysteries of gauges, boilers, signals, plates and shunting. Drivers and firemen were among her favourite patients.

On dull days she made time to read aloud in the evenings, not from improving literature, but from adventure stories, which she enjoyed as much as the men did. Once she chose a love-story, which to the delight of the other patients reduced a large and sentimental Irishman to tears. 'He was driven to wiping his eyes on the sheet,' she said triumphantly, 'and we all laughed and cried together.' The boys were always trying to catch her for a game of chess or draughts. She seldom had time to sit and finish a game, but would glance at the pieces and make her moves swiftly with one hand, as she passed up and down the ward at her work, while her slower-witted opponents sat puzzling over the board. She took as much pleasure as they did in her own skill, and entered into the game as whole-heartedly as a child. Again and again, patients remembering their stay in hospital, starting with pain, shock and anxiety, remembered the following days and weeks as the happiest in their lives.

This building formed Sister Dora's world. Her home, to which she climbed in the evening, when she had, as she said, 'put everyone straight for the night', was one large plain, comfortable room on the top floor. The windows were always open in summer, with spotless curtains billowing in the wind. It overlooked Walsall Race Course, and to Dora's delight she could actually see, from the upstairs windows, the horses running. The minister of the

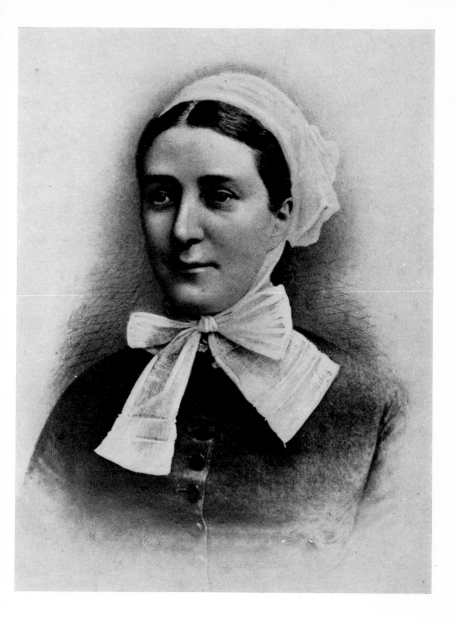

13. Sister Dora wearing the nurse's cap to which she gave her name

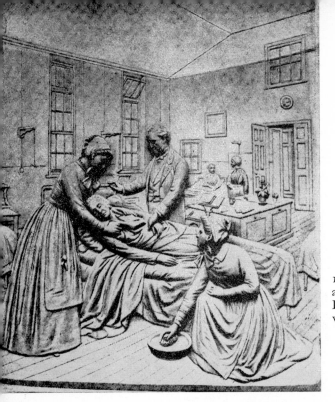

14. Dr James MacLachlan, a student nurse and Sister Dora in the men's accident ward. The portraits are from life

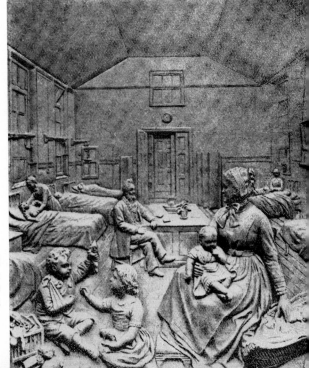

15. Samuel Cox, the Hospital Chairman, and Sister Dora in the children's ward. Note the children's toys for which Sister Dora had appealed

Congregational Church next door called one day, and was astonished to find himself swept upstairs into her sitting-room to watch, as he cautiously said, 'the only horse-race of his life'. One of the jockeys was thrown, and the people who carried him on a stretcher to the hospital were mystified to find Sister Dora ready and waiting, with everything set out to give him first aid.[37]

Visitors to the hospital prepared themselves, with characteristic Victorian relish, to meet 'the three terrors of human life, pain, disease and death in their most ghastly forms'. They were relieved, or perhaps disappointed according to temperament, to find themselves in an atmosphere of confidence and cheerfulness. A visitor to Walsall hurried to the hospital to see 'the celebrated Sister Dora', and wrote in some surprise, 'She is a tall, black-haired, handsome woman, brimming over with energy and fun. She picks out the humorous side of everything she tells one and laughs over it, though the next minute she had brought tears into my eyes. Her sense of humour must be the greatest blessing and help to her in her work. Such things she told us! pouring them out one after another as if it were a treat to have friends to chatter to.' Sister Dora used to say, 'My dears, if I could not laugh over the things that happen here I really do not know how I could go on.' The same visitor noticed her air of easy mastery, 'taking an evident pride in her own good management, which she is much too transparent and open-hearted to hide.'[38]

News of her excellent and economical management began to spread through the voluntary hospital world, far beyond the confines of Walsall. Many applications came for Sisters to act as trained nurses to private patients, which had to be refused, as all the other nursing Sisters had been recalled by Mr Postlethwaite to Coatham. Still more alarming to the Walsall committee were attempts by other hospitals to lure Sister Dora away from them. 'Applications have been received', said the secretary, 'from the largest hospitals in the kingdom and offers have been made to induce the Sister at Walsall to undertake the nursing in these institutions.'[39]

Fortunately for the Committee, Dora was far too busy to listen to these blandishments. The Franco-Prussian war in 1870 marked the peak of the Black Country iron trade. The number of blast furnaces increased in the next three years from 1700 to 2158; the saddlery trades all worked overtime,[40] with a proportionate increase in accidents. Sister Dora longed to go to France and nurse the wounded, but, as she said, 'my work was cut out for me in Walsall, so I made up my mind I ought not to let anything, however exciting, take me away from it.'[41] She and Dr Mac-Lachlan shared the labour and satisfaction of cases like the miner Henry Bond, who had fallen down a pit-shaft at Darlaston and fractured both thighs. A few years earlier he would have been a helpless cripple, but on 12th October 1870, after thirty weeks as an in-patient, he left the hospital on his own feet. Doctors from all the industrial towns north of Birmingham were beginning to send their serious surgical and accident cases to be nursed at the Cottage Hospital. In 1870 she had 139 in-patients, and the following year 177 serious cases, of whom only 17 died, chiefly railway-men run over by trains or miners crushed by falls underground. She began, under MacLachlan's direction to keep a summary of cases treated which, though less detailed than later reports, shows the weight of her nursing responsibilities.[42] Every day she worked her way through a crowded out-patient department, seeing personally more than two thousand patients each year. 'Fractures, burns, scalds, ulcers, abscesses, 15 dog bites and 257 teeth extracted,' she noted laconically.[43] The hospital was winning the confidence and support of all classes in the community, and it showed in one unmistakable way. Income from subscriptions and collections rose during two years from £798 5s 10d to £1188 16s 2d. All sorts of people contributed, from the Labourers Accident and Burial Society of the Cyclops Iron Works, to a little girl of ten who 'got up a Christmas tree' and proudly brought 15s in pennies and halfpennies. The committee, while thanking them, and the medical staff for 'efficient and gratuitous services', were in no doubt who was really to be thanked. 'The success', they wrote, in their Annual Report for 1871, 'has been chiefly promoted by the unwearied devotion of the Sister-in-Charge, whose services have been beyond all praise.'

Dora had achieved, at least for the present, what she had struggled so long for. She was living as if she had no wishes, no future, nothing but present duty. She could not have said herself where the boundaries of the spiritual and the practical lay, for charity was woven into her daily work. She had given up the struggle to make something of herself by conscious effort of will; she lived unreservedly in the problems, successes and failures of each day, finding no contradiction between her beliefs and her growing knowledge and skill. She had little time to think, less time to write, and her letters were hasty scrawls, written at her table in the ward, with continuous interruptions. There is, though, one brief note to her old friend Miss Finch at Woolston, which reveals something of what she felt. It was written in the spring of 1870, four years after her father's death, the breaking up of her old home, the breaking of her own engagement, and three years after the death of Redfern Davies. Evidently nothing had changed at sleepy Woolston, and they still missed her there, but for herself, she felt, everything had changed.

'And so,' she wrote, 'you wish me still at Woolston! I could wish myself back, to do differently. I think I could do so much better now than I did then. I wish I could come and see you for an hour and tell you of my happy life here. It is a busy one, but *very* happy; everybody is so good and kind to me, I am only afraid I shall get spoilt. But I have learnt more, and I think (I say this in all humility) I have learnt to love God more. Eternity has become real.'[44]

NOTES

1. Lonsdale, 48, describes an epidemic of erysipelas at Bridge Street, but the report specifically denies this.
2. F. Nightingale, *Sanitary Condition of Hospitals*, 3.
3. R. Williams and I. Fisher, *Hints for Hospital Nurses*, 127–38.
4. W.C.H. MS., 1867.
5. It survives as the administrative block of Walsall General Hospital.
6. W.C.H.A.R., 1868.
7. W.C.H. MS., 1868.
8. Pattison, 56, f. 369.
9. H.R.C. Correspondence on revised constitution.
10. Ibid., Constitution as finally printed.
11. Ibid., Chapter Minutes, 1873.
12. *The Guardian*, 28th July 1886.
13. W.C.H. MS., 1868.
14. *Walsall Observer*, 26th July 1879.

15. W.C.H.A.R., 1870.
16. W.C.H. MS., 1868.
17. Lonsdale, 73.
18. W.C.H. MS., 1863–7.
19. The writer was Edward Fitzgerald, see p. 267 below.
20. Lonsdale, 53, identifies her only as 'Mrs. H. —'; she was the source of many of Miss Lonsdale's more emotional passages.
21. F. Nightingale, *Notes on Nursing*, 139.
22. W.C.H.A.R., 1869–71.
23. W.C.H. MS., 1868.
24. W.C.H.A.R., 1870.
25. W.C.H. MS., 1870.
26. Ibid., 1871–72.
27. H. C. Burdett, *Cottage Hospitals*, 154.
28. F. Burleigh, *Sister Dora*, 23.
29. Lawson Tait, *Address in Surgery to B.M.A.*, 1890.
30. The blue printed slips summoning members still exist.
31. It was some years before the committee was able to offer him a regular £50, less than the wages of Murray the porter. In the middle 1870s he received £60 a year.
32. W.C.H. MS., 1868.
33. *Walsall Observer*, 15th December 1888.
34. W.C.H.A.R., 1888.
35. *Reprints*, 26. A portrait of James MacLachlan from life, working with Sister Dora and a student nurse in the men's ward, appears on her memorial.
36. W.C.H. MS., 1870–1.
37. Lonsdale, 254.
38. Ibid., 113, quotes this letter verbatim.
39. W.C.H.A.R., 1868.
40. G. C. Allen, *Industrial Development of Birmingham and the Black Country*, 200–1.
41. Lonsdale, 93.
42. Appendix, A. Case Summary for 1872.
43. W.C.H.A.R., 1870–71.
44. Lonsdale, 29, quotes this letter.

CHAPTER FOURTEEN

The Patients
1870–1872

In the autumn of 1870 Dr MacLachlan came to Sister Dora with a piece of advice which greatly surprised her. He urged her strongly to leave Walsall, go to Edinburgh as a student and qualify in medicine and surgery, when she would be free to practise wherever she chose. Clearly James MacLachlan was a reader of the medical press, which was currently devoting columns to the vexed, and to medical men vexing, question of 'lady doctors'. In June of the same year Miss Elizabeth Garrett, after passing a series of vivas and submitting a thesis in French, had qualified as M.D. Paris to the cheers of students at the Sorbonne. Even the somewhat dour *British Medical Journal* admired 'the indomitable perseverance and pluck' of Britain's first woman doctor.[1] In October Sophia Jex-Blake led the group of seven young women who, as medical students in the Edinburgh Extra-Mural School, were seeking admission to the wards of the Royal Edinburgh Infirmary. It was this gallant band, called, from the terms of their petition, the *Septem contra Edinam*, that MacLachlan wished Dora to join. He had worked with her for two years; he knew her character and capabilities, and he believed her natural quick wit would make up for her erratic education. Very much to his surprise, she refused. He did everything in his power to persuade her. In November the Edinburgh Seven faced the jeers and shouts of the riots at the Surgeons Hall, when hostile students pushed a sheep into the examination room with the woman candidates. 'It has more sense,' remarked a professor drily, 'than those who sent it here.'[2] The newspaper reports were sensational, and Sister Dora said she 'shrank from the publicity of such proceedings'. As she never, in her whole life, shrank from anything, however risky, which she really wanted to do, this must be regarded as a conventional excuse. The truth was something which she could not easily explain to him; she found in nursing a different and deeper satisfaction than the intellectual interest of medicine could offer.[3]

James MacLachlan was firmly on the liberal side in the question of women doctors; he was also the last person on earth to be influenced by convention in any important practical matter. The cottage hospital badly needed a resident house-surgeon; there was no prospect that it could afford one in the nearly future.[4] He decided, in defiance of all medical etiquette, that he himself would train Sister Dora in the duties of the post. In a large teaching hospital or city infirmary this might have provoked a scandal; at Walsall no one seems to have questioned his decision.

The first essential was to teach her some anatomy. He lent her books, dictated notes, set her to trace diagrams, all of which she mastered with ease. He summoned her to dissect privately in the out-house which served as hospital mortuary, and asked her to attend all post-mortem examinations. He later confessed that he had been anxious to know what her attitude would be. Not that he expected a vulgar prudery; he knew her too well for that, but he feared Sister Dora's religious beliefs might be hostile to scientific study. The famous confrontation between Wilberforce and Huxley at the British Association meeting at Oxford in 1860 had left prejudice on both sides. Churchmen complained that scientists offered a purely mechanistic theory of the universe, 'the reduction of all spiritual states to physiological causes', while scientists counter-claimed that religion had no right to impose limits on genuine intellectual inquiry. Dr MacLachlan was quite unprepared for the determination with which his pupil reconciled these conflicting views. She said she found God not only in mysterious unknown problems but in proven facts. This seemed to her the true relationship between religion and scientific knowledge, though it was to take more than half a century for most scientists to arrive at her view. Here, as so often, unconsciously, she was ahead of her times. The study of anatomy filled her with a mixture of wonder and delight; she exclaimed over the articulation of bones and muscles with the same spontaneous pleasure that she gave to the trees and the grass on her rare excursions into the countryside. The existence of life and breath which most people took for granted, seemed to her a miracle to be approached with the deepest reverence.

This reverence for life was accompanied by a respect for the fact of death, which use and custom could not weaken, and here master and pupil fell out. Post-mortems at Walsall were attended by visiting students from Birmingham, who smoked cigars and worked in their shirt-sleeves, laughing and joking with the comfortable familiarity of long habit. The first time Sister Dora heard some of their broader jokes she said nothing from a sense of professional courtesy, but MacLachlan, seeing her sharp glance and heightened colour, guessed she was offended. Next morning, when he called for his rounds, she asked him with icy politeness to step into her small office. James MacLachlan, who had a dry sense of humour, delighted to tell the story against himself. 'Her wrath, which she had apparently been nursing all night, burst upon my head.' The magnificent creature strode up and down the little room like a tigress, eyes flashing with anger. 'She did not object to the discourtesy towards a woman, she said, but he should at least not encourage the disrespect shown in the presence of death.' All attempts to defend himself were in vain; his feeble excuses were swept away in a torrent of angry words. They went round the hospital in silence, and the doctor retreated as best he might. Two hours later, a messenger brought a note to his house. 'I completely lost my temper', wrote Sister Dora, 'and I am penitent. Can you forgive me?'[5] He wrote at once, apologizing and promising that in future the young men would behave better. This clash of two strong characters cemented their friendship as nothing else could have done.

In 1873, MacLachlan was officially appointed senior surgeon to the hospital 'with responsibility for all operations performed in the in-patient department'. The following year, with a glowing testimonial from the Committee, he was appointed Medical Officer to the Walsall Union.[6] He never made any pretence of suffering fools gladly, and in middle age grew increasingly a martinet. Junior doctors complained of his 'tyranny' and he forced the resignation of one colleague; but Sister Dora, though she deferred to him professionally, always stood up to him personally, and he valued her skill at its true worth. Under him, she served effectually as casualty officer.

Redfern Davies had always stressed the importance of treating eye injuries promptly, and it may be remembered that he had equipped the hospital with a set of ophthalmic instruments. Sister Dora had a particular interest in eyes; very few weeks went by without a workman stumbling into her surgery with a fragment of metal or hot cinder embedded in his eyeball, since protective goggles were never worn at work. She accordingly applied to the Eye Infirmary, Steelhouse Lane, Birmingham, for permission to attend dissections and see their cases. Though women medical students were meeting with hostility or blank refusal at hospitals all over the kingdom,[7] here Sister Dora was made welcome at once; neither she, nor anyone else, seems to have recognized how unusual this was. She became an expert at removing foreign bodies, varying from a small speck of grit or coal dust to a splash of molten metal, from the eye. She would evert the lids over a probe and delicately pluck out the particle. Where metal was embedded in the cornea she would place the patient against the light to detect it, and neatly dig it out with the small spud made for the purpose. Patients were willing to trust her with this most delicate of operations, and thanks to her prompt treatment of emergencies, cases of ulceration or infection seem to have been rare.[8]

Dora was finally capable of carrying out all the duties of house surgeons and dressers, as set out in the standard text book, Heath's *Manual of Minor Surgery*.[9] MacLachlan, a most conscientious man, entrusted her with an increasing amount of surgical work. In fact she carried out the duties of de facto house surgeon. These included the emergency treatment of 'machinery accidents', first arresting the haemorrhage, if necessary by pressure on a main artery, cleansing, suturing and splinting. Dora's experience bore out Heath's opinion that 'it is extraordinary how well even severe machinery accidents turn out owing to the previous good health of the patients'. She became skilful at recognizing all types of fractures, by no means easy where the patients often had existing deformities from old injuries at work. She kept padded splints and sandbags at hand for 'putting up' broken arms and legs, which was done without anaesthetic; her firm bandaging over the top of the head to support a broken jaw was particularly admired by a visiting Professor of Surgery from Birmingham. When the broken jaw was the result of a fight, she might also have to reduce the opponent's fractured metacarpal bones, by flexing his fingers over a ball of material placed in his palm. She persevered in dressing and re-dressing broken fingers to save the patient a useful hand, but if necessary she could also amputate a finger or thumb cleanly through the joint and stitch the flap.[10] Her success rate, even in compound fractures, was high, except with fractures of the pelvis, which, if accompanied by crushing injuries to the bladder or viscera, meant in those days that there was no hope for the patient.

She could perform a tracheotomy in an emergency and Dr MacLachlan left to her, as a routine matter, the opening of abscesses and whitlows in the out-patient department. More serious was the dressing of dog-bites, potentially very dangerous because of the possibility of rabies. She kept the patient, and if possible the dog, under surveillance for several weeks. The danger was so real that this woman of lion-like courage confessed to a terror of dogs, 'even the smallest cur that bares its teeth at me in the gutter'. She was careful to hide this fear from her patients, whose fierce Staffordshire terriers, ready to fight to the death, were a source of deep pride to them. There was no effective treatment for rabies, which was later to be almost eliminated by the strict quarantine of imported dogs. Nor was there a satis-factory treatment for burns and scalds. Pasteur's studies in fermentation, published in the years 1860–5, had already put the germ theory upon a scientific footing, while Lister's first papers on antisepsis in surgery had followed shortly after, in 1867.[11] Yet very few people related these discoveries to the severe illness, marked by fever, wasting and pus, which so often proved fatal in burns cases. Nor did they know that patients with burns over more than fifteen per cent of the body surface, or less in children, were liable to develop shock from loss of plasma, and to die even before infection set in. These deaths, particularly of children, were heart-breaking to Sister Dora, but remained completely mysterious. Today the hazards can be opposed by aseptic methods, by intravenous fluid replacement and by skin-grafting, but for Dr MacLachlan and his nursing sister, the only possible treatment was to cover the burn with lint soaked in carron oil, and hope that natural healing would follow. Even small burns took weeks to heal, and demanded the utmost patience and ingenuity in nursing.

It is not recorded when Sister Dora began the practice, which she insisted was absolutely essential, of isolating any serious case of burns in a small ward reserved strictly for the purpose. Whenever possible she preferred to dress burns or scalds in the patient's own home. Serious burns could remain months in hospital, and, observed a doctor, 'are by no means favourite cases with nurses or dressers'. Sister Dora did, however, secure the healing of smaller burns, and, to everyone's surprise, showed that by massage and exercise she could prevent the contractions which often crippled burns patients.

Sister Dora's final duty as house surgeon was to assist Dr MacLachlan at operations. After making all the preparations which formed the normal work of a nurse, she scrubbed her hands and took her place opposite him, ready to sponge, hold back flaps, and tie ligatures on the blood vessels as he took them up. She practised tying ligatures in private, and developed exceptional manual dexterity. Her experience was wide. In this small cottage hospital, with makeshift equipment, major operations were performed every year. One year's report mentions fourteen amputations of crushed limbs, four excisions of joints, three strangulated hernias, and fourteen removals of tumours, including the still rare and dangerous operation of ovariotomy. The death rate after operation in this particular year was one per cent. It is not mentioned that Sister Dora gave anaesthetics; house surgeons were particularly warned never to let a nurse do this, but in an emergency she would probably have been capable of it.

James MacLachlan was naturally proud of his pupil. 'She can set any fracture better than most general practitioners,' he claimed, and patients often heard him say, when she reported a new case, 'Do what you think best, Sister. You'll most probably deal with it better than I should.'[12]

By the end of 1870 he told the Committee that he conscientiously felt he need no longer attend every out-patient session. He would call once or twice a week to see selected patients, but Sister Dora could deal on her own initiative with all cases not referred to him.[13] He was generous in giving her credit for the hospital's success. On 5th March 1873 he wrote a special report 'to call the attention of the Committee to the great amount of good being effected through the Out-Patient Department. In other hospitals it is the practice merely to prescribe for the out patients and leave them to carry out the instructions in their own homes, with the result that not infrequently they are never carried out. . . . In this hospital wounds are dressed, daily if necessary, by the Sister and wounds which under ordinary hospital treatment would be months in healing are cured in an incredibly short time.'[14] Her bandaging was so skilful that he invited a Professor and a class of dressers from Queen's Hospital for her to give a demonstration, and told everybody afterwards the Professor had said, 'Your Sister Dora could pass a first-class examination in surgery.' For his own part he came to rely on her implicitly. Patients and the public believed that she worked by some super-natural 'womanly instinct', but he described it as a combination of minute observation and great practical experience. One night, after an amputation, she said she felt 'convinced that something was wrong in the ward', and hurried to the patient's bedside to find a secondary haemorrhage from a slipped ligature. She stopped the bleeding by pressure on the main artery while a messenger ran for James MacLachlan, who said she had undoubtedly saved his patient's life. Another time she said, 'I am sure that patient will develop tetanus.' 'I asked how she knew for he showed no symptoms,' said Dr MacLachlan. 'She said she could not tell how, but she felt convinced. She was right, the patient died.'[15]

He was too honest to pretend that he agreed with Dora in her decision not to qualify. Glad as he was to have such good nursing for his patients he considered she was wasting her abilities and that she needed the corrective of working with people as intelligent as herself. His verdict on her character is interesting because it is so much more balanced than the sentimental raptures she normally inspired. 'Apart from her excellence as a nurse and manager, there was something fascinating in the charm of her manner, so playful and winning in all her ways. No one who has ever seen Sister Dora could possibly forget her.' Yet he added a serious qualification to his praise. 'Her glorious nature, physical and mental, was marred by undisciplined impulse. Her character would have been best formed by marrying a man who would have dominated her, and she would have shone subdued.'[16] Perhaps he was thinking of Redfern Davies, whom he had known and admired. Events were to prove his judgment sound, for Dora's impulsive emotions brought her tragic unhappiness, literally to her dying day.

For the present she felt completely fulfilled. She did not want to leave Walsall because the hospital was her home, the Committee a sort of composite husband to be served or cajoled, and the patients above all her children. 'My dearest children,' she actually wrote to them, when called away, and her love for them poured out in a passion of protective devotion. The out-patients, sometimes over a hundred at a surgery, crowded the dingy little waiting room on three afternoons a week. After 1874 she saw them every day except Sunday and their numbers rose in one year from 2809 to 9940.[17] They wore a uniform of poverty and toil, women in shoddy skirts with check shawls wrapped round head and shoulders, men with sweat rags and trousers still greasy with coal-dust. Both sexes showed hands scarred and calloused, often mutilated by their work. Sister Dora claimed that by looking at a man's hands she could tell his trade. This seemed to the patients wonderful. 'Sure isn't Sister Dora like the blessed Saints?' said an impressionable Irish bricklayer. 'One look and she told me I was a builder!' 'His clothes were full of dust, he smelled of mortar and I had just taken a piece of brick out of his eye,' said Sister Dora, dryly, 'so it was hardly remarkable!'

Endlessly they passed before her, poisoned fingers, crushed hands, cut heads of boys, scalded bare feet of children, workmen with sparks or fragments of metal in their eyes, women with varicose veins, raging ache of decayed teeth, all the occupational ills of hardship and neglect. Their courage was miraculous; she could never admire them enough.

No one in all her life knew Sister Dora as her in-patients knew her. She would arrive at the bedside of a total stranger who, for the duration of his illness, became closer to her than her oldest friends or her own family. Joseph Clare, a mayor of Walsall, could remember the exact day he had entered hospital as a young currier's labourer, trapped in the machinery twenty-seven years before. 'I'm bound to say what no other Mayor of Walsall can,' he said at a public meeting. 'I've been an in-patient of this hospital for two months. During that time I spent many sleepless nights and anxious days, for my accident was such as few get over, but thanks to Dr MacLachlan and Sister Dora I recovered, and the hospital became a home to me. No man is prouder of Sister Dora than I am and none has greater cause to be so. Never in my life have I known a woman like her, and I remember her as if it was yesterday.'[18] A young man of 22 named William Chell, a stoker on the railway, was run over in the dark by an engine and tender, during the night of 17th April 1872. He described how he was carried into the hospital on a rough stretcher in the middle of the night, with one leg crushed beyond repair.[19] It was amputated at once, and he remembered nothing of the confusion of darkness, pain and shock, except 'that Sister was always there, and when I came to after the chloroform she was on her knees beside me, with her arm supporting my head, speaking to me, and through all the pain and trouble I had afterwards, I never forgot Sister's voice.' He was seventeen weeks in the hospital and had to face another operation before his leg healed, but Sister Dora would not let him despair. Because of the strange hours railwaymen work, she allowed his mates to visit him at any time, however inconvenient to herself. Slowly he grew stronger and became a leader at the evening singing; he declared he could 'sing till he was hoarse' with Sister Dora. He tried to describe the quality in her which had drawn him back from the edge of death, but it was beyond him. 'I could not tell you all her goodness to me,' he said simply. 'Words would fail me if I tried.' Another favourite patient was a young man wanted by the police on a criminal charge. He had cut his sweetheart's throat, fortunately not fatally, and then his own, and had been brought in by the police for dead. He was laid on the floor in the hall, when Dora, passing by, heard him breathe with a sudden gasp. She moved him into a bed, with head raised to close the wound, and nursed him devotedly, with stern warnings to other patients not to gossip and not to let him see any newspapers which might distress him. She confessed she would have liked to help him escape, but this was not possible because a policeman sat by his bed day and night. She had to content herself by visiting the police superintendent and demanding indignantly, 'If you must send your men, send them in plain clothes to spare my patient's feelings, and please do not send again the one you sent yesterday, as he was not very civil to him'. After this visit, as Dr MacLachlan remarked with amusement, 'There is quite a competition among the policemen for the hospital post'. The young man was discharged to prison, where Sister Dora wrote to him regularly and helped him to find a job after the end of his sentence.[20]

Sister Dora and the police came to know one another well, for they had many cases in common. Dr MacLachlan, as Police Surgeon, regularly gave evidence in cases of violent injury which had found their way to the hospital. These included attempted suicides, like the young man with the cut throat, gang fights and wife murder. What particularly distressed Sister Dora were assaults on children, infanticide and back-street abortions.[21] Fortuately the police cases also had their lighter side. One of these was represented by Betsy who lived in a common lodging house in a back court, and, like the overwhelming majority of women patients, suffered from varicose ulcers, always described as 'bad leg'. From long practice Dora developed great skill in the firm bandaging of these legs and would persevere with them for months on end, visiting the patients at home, to save a hospital bed. One evening she arrived at the lodging house to find no Betsy, but ironical remarks of 'Betsy's gone away on a visit'. She understood at once the meaning of the expression and set off with her surgical bag to the lock-up. Betsy, finding her leg better, had taken a walk down the street and been unable to resist a pair of trousers conveniently hanging outside a slop-shop. 'You thought no one could see you, Betsy,' said Dora, 'but if you'd thought to look up as well as sideways, you wouldn't have taken those trousers.' She set to work briskly and visited the gaol regularly for the length of Betsy's sentence, in order to complete her treatment.

Many patients came to her with stab wounds as a direct result of drunken fighting with knives, belt buckles and broken bottles. On the testimony of the police she was capable of breaking up a fight herself. One night, returning home from a patient she was passing the end of Marsh Lane, a street near the Walsall Canal, when she heard the shrieks and yells of an 'Irish fight', a bloody, pitched battle with sticks and stones between rival gangs. She turned down the street and climbed a high doorstep, to see over the heads of the crowd, the two leaders, both old patients whom she knew by name. She yelled at them above the din to stop, and saw them stand, for a moment or two as she said, 'like two furious bulldogs with their tails between their legs'. They then rushed upon one another again like wild animals, till she jumped down from the doorstep and flung herself between them, holding them apart. 'Either of them could have broken my arm as easily as he could have snapped his tobacco pipe,' she said, 'but they let me win the day and the fight was at an end.'[22] The police, who had been twirling their nightsticks uneasily on the edge of the crowd, stood respectfully aside to let her pass.

The Irish immigrants bore the blame for many of the troubles of the Black Country which were not of their making, poverty, over-crowding, sordid housing and disease. They were among Sister Dora's favourite patients; she appreciated their family feeling and admired their loyalty to their church. Not even Dr Mac-Lachlan was allowed to ridicule their superstitions, 'How can you scoff at the poor people's childlike faith?' she said. 'Think what their lives are like, and ask yourself, have you anything better to give them in exchange?'[23] At the same time, she admitted their fondness for strong tobacco and stronger drink raised problems in hospital. One night, when she was in bed, she smelt the unmistakable reek of burning shag from the ward below. She put on a shawl and went down to find a patient called Pat hastily hiding a clay-pipe, still alight, under the bedclothes. 'What have you got there?' she demanded sternly, 'Let me see! Oh Patrick, you might have set fire to the hospital!' Sadly, he surrendered it, saying, 'Sure, 'tis nobody can deceive you, Sister, and 'tis myself that will never try again!' She worked for weeks over a young man who had received a compound fracture in a drunken fight, and who went out promising loudly 'never to touch a drop again'. That night he was brought back, cut, bleeding and fighting drunk. The other patients felt as lost as children when they saw the indomitable Sister Dora lay down her head on the little table in the ward and cry bitterly.

No account of Sister Dora's patients would be complete without a special mention of those who really were children. There were always children running about the hospital corridors or playing in the garden, most of whom seem to have suffered from tuberculosis of bones or joints, the product of bad food and bad housing. They had to stay in hospital for many months, but Dora insisted they should have as normal a life as possible, with plenty of games, indoors and out. The children's ward was filled with toys, picture books and games of which she could never have too many.[24] She could still tell stories and sing songs with the same skill which had held the village children at Little Woolston spellbound in her teaching days. Dr MacLachlan commented on her 'dextrous management of children of all ages'. At the same time he noticed with approval she did not coddle. 'She could love without spoiling them. She was as healthy as the breath of morn.' At times she could be a notable disciplinarian and nothing roused her quick temper so fast as sneaking or bullying. One day she was talking with the doctor at the window of her little office, when she saw a schoolboy pushing the head of a howling baby through the railings outside. 'Out rushed Sister Dora into the streets like a flash of lightning,' said MacLachlan. 'She seized the young gentleman by the collar, and delivered a shower of boxes, first on one ear, then on the other. She laid it on hard; they must have been no joke at all. In fact,' he added with simple pride, 'they were positively masterly boxes on the ear, just like everything else she did.' By contrast, to sick children she was unfailingly gentle. It took a long time to treat these children; in fact one ten-year-old boy named Sam stayed so long in the hospital that he could help with the daily routine and the other patients nicknamed him 'The Doctor'. Fresh air and Sarah's cooking usually cured them in the end. It was one of Dora's great pleasures to see their 'old un-childlike faces' revert to normal childhood.

By contrast, her greatest anxiety was the small children, burned or scalded in overcrowded workshops and kitchens, of whom she sometimes had three together in the children's ward. The wailing of a hurt or frightened child was something she could not bear. 'It goes to my heart to hear it,' she said. 'I never allow them to feel or be unhappy if I can possibly help it.' By day she would wrap a baby in a shawl and carry it around the house on her arm; by night she would move its cot into her own bedroom. Not all these children could be saved, and she maintained from experience that all but the youngest understood enough to be terrified by the exhaustion of approaching death. She would leave all her other work to sit by a dying child, if necessary for hours, to reassure and comfort it. 'While they are in hospital, they are my children,' she said. 'It is not right, if they are in danger, to shift the responsibility on to others' shoulders.' The deaths of these children were among her greatest griefs.[25]

A number of the hospital's industrial accident cases were in fact children. Children had always been employed in Black Country industries. Early in the nineteenth century no boys were left in Walsall Union Workhouse, for all were used in the narrow seams of the mines. In 1863 a Royal Commission reported on children in a number of industries including the metal trades of the Birmingham district. Mr J. E. White, the inquiring commissioner for the Black Country towns was startled and disturbed by his discoveries.[26] Over thirty of the children had never heard either of Jesus Christ or Queen Victoria. Their world was limited to their own grimy street and the workshop. 'A violet is a pretty bird'; lilac 'is a bird'; 'believe I would know a primrose, it's a red rose like'; 'don't know if a robin redbreast is a bird'. A picture of a cow bing milked was shown; 'he's a lion'. Girls almost grown up were unable to tell the time by the clock. White investigated the whole range of trades in which children were employed, from steel pens and buttons or glass-moulding, to loading kilns in the brick-yards, where a girl of twelve shifted the equivalent of thirty-six tons in an ordinary working day. The risks to child metal workers emerge very clearly from a nailer's account. 'They get a bit of red hot iron in their shoe and that of course will burn alarming. Four years ago my boy, then betwixt ten and eleven, got two pieces of iron in at the top of his trousers and before they could be got out they dropped and catched his leg burning two wounds each as big as the face of my hammer and the scars are there now and always will be.' The same nailer reported that children 'fret more with the learning and sweat more – fret wonderfully the little ones do'.

The Commission's report shocked the public and in 1864 the Factory Acts Extension Act protected more than seventeen thousand of the younger children. The Education Act of 1870 made boy assistants harder to find and their wages rose from four shillings per week in 1860 to ten shillings per week in 1875.[27] Yet regulations remained difficult to enforce, since owners left the job of engaging assistants to butties or over-hands. All through her life at Walsall Sister Dora continued to treat boys and girls of twelve to fifteen maimed by accidents or injury at work. One of them, a motherless boy of fourteen later wrote his account of his time in hospital.

'I ENOCH SIMPSON Working in the Iron Works Pelsall Met with an accident on the eighth of May 1869[28] I was then about fourteen years Old there was little or no delay in conveying me to the Hospital but when I arrived there every bed was full, but Sister Dora looked at me and when she saw I was badly hurt she instantly made up a bed on the floor. The while I was taken in and laid on a large table, then she took of my clothes and washed me, then laid me in the bed she had prepared for me, I lay their a few days until another bed was vacant she then moved me to it, on this second bed I lay for three months attended to in all my wants by Sister Dora, from six in the morning until ten at night and often later than that and at any hour in the night she would come to me, and why Sister attended to me so early was to wash me and clear away the corruption that dis-charged from my leg so that I may be clean, this was the start of the day for the first three months of my Hospital life. But I had not been there above a week when Sister Dora found me a little bell as there was not one to my bed and she said "Enoch you must ring this when you want Sister". This little bell did not have much rest for whenever I heard her step or the tinkle of her keys in the hall I used to ring my bell and she would call "I'm coming Enoch" which she did and would ask "what do you want?" I often used to say "I don't know, Sister", not really knowing what I did want. She'd say "do you want your pillows shaken up or down or do you want moving a little?" which she'd do, then she'd start to go into the other ward, but very often before she could get through the door I'd call her back and say my pillow wasn't quite right or my leg wanted moving and she'd come and do it again, then she'd go about her work but at the next sound of her step my bell would ring. Some of the other patients remarked I would wear the bell out or Sister but she'd say "Never mind for I like to hear it and its never too often" and it rang so often that we heard Sister say that she often dreamt she heard my little bell and started up in a hurry to find it was only a dream. That lasted for three months during which Sister Dora and Dr. MacLachlan tried all in their power to cure my leg but it was no use for it had to be taken off or else it would have taken me off. She came and sat by my bed and talked to me for a long time and explained to me how near I was to death, and though afraid of losing my limb ought to consent as the only means of saving my life, and by her persuasions I did consent and on the same day my leg was amputated. Until the end of those three months I was gradually getting weaker, but from the time my leg was taken off I began to get better. I trusted her, for through Sister's love and care to her patients they all placed the same confidence in her. I was in the Hospital eight months in which time I learned to love Sister Dora as a mother, for having none myself. She used to say she was my mother, but she used to say that to all of us, and those patients who were the most trouble she seemed fondest of.'[29]

The fame of Sister Dora spread, not only among former patients, but their families and their friends. Dr MacLachlan related with a grin a conversation he overheard in the train between Walsall and Birmingham. Two women in the railway carriage with him were discussing the Sister-in-Charge. 'Ah, her's got no nerves!' said one. 'Hasn't her!' said the other. 'Why, her'm as tender as a baby.' 'What!' said the first, 'stand by and see a man's leg cut off?' 'Ah,' said Sister Dora's supporter, 'that's just because her's used to it. Mark my words, her'm real soft-hearted and no mistake.' By 1872 it seems that everyone in Walsall had come round to this opinion; Sister Dora had finally overcome the traditional local mistrust of the 'jubous'. The Committee noted thankfully that suspicion of the hospital was at last at an end, and that 'nothing has tended more to the excellent arrangements in the domestic department and the skilful, systematic management of the nursing, to secure the confidence and support of all classes. We owe no small debt of gratitude to the Sister-in-Charge'.[30]

Happily the patients found a more imaginative way than a formal vote of thanks to show their gratitude. One afternoon in June 1873 Sister Dora was summoned to the front steps of the hospital. There she found a dozen of her ex-patients, all railwaymen from the South Staffordshire line, resplendent in their best off-duty suits, with flowers in their button-holes. In front of them the porter held a pretty, glossy little bay pony, with a rosette in its head-band. The pony was harnessed to a small open carriage, in which, they said, 'they hoped Sister Dora would take the air'. The railwaymen from their own wages had subscribed £50 for this present. Dora, who had been such a good rider in her young days, had never owned a horse of her own. She was enchanted with the pony, which became the pampered darling of the hospital. Two members of the executive undertook responsibility for its grooming, and the maintenance of the little carriage; both, in a town of harness-makers, were always immaculate. The Committee built a stable and coach house for it, at a cost of nearly £70, then a considerable sum.

At first she feared she would never have time to drive the carriage, which was used mainly to pull the garden roller and take delighted convalescent children for rides. In 1874 the Committee voted unanimously 'that the cost of keeping Sister Dora's pony be defrayed out of the hospital funds, as it is used for the benefit of patients'. At first she was too proud and independent to accept this, but the Vicar of Walsall called on her and persuaded her to agree, on the grounds that it would give them genuine pleasure.[31] Gradually she found she could save time by taking the carriage when she went out on her rounds, and the Walsall boys discovered a new diversion, fighting one another for the privilege of 'holding Sister's pony', while she attended her cases.[32] When her patients were far afield and the nights cold, the porter or an ex-patient, would drive the pony-carriage, so that she could keep her hands warm and supple for her work. Murray, the porter, looked back on these drives under the cold starlight as 'some of the jolliest hours of my life. She never stopped talking to me, telling me stories, and many's the time I wish I could recollect her way of putting things. We had patients all about, and drove as many as eleven or twelve miles of a night. Once we drove to Lichfield and back, to a midnight service in the cathedral. It took us a good part of the night, but Sister Dora, why, she never seemed to feel the cold, nor to be a bit tired the next day.'[33]

Dora's character, and her supposedly miraculous powers, made her in the Black Country a legend like Florence Nightingale. A cult grew around her, as round a local saint in the Middle Ages. Her relics, a cup, a glove, a letter, a nurse's belt or scissors were treasured for years by their owners. Her picture hung in the place of honour in countless Walsall homes. Even the children shared in this feeling; a schoolmaster was amused and touched to see 'how little ragged dirty urchins playing in the streets would run up as she walked along, pulling at her gown to attract her attention and not satisfied till she had bent down from her majestic height to kiss their grimy faces, which they held up to her with utter confidence'. She could not have been so loved if all her powers had been devoted, as Mark Pattison claimed, to self-glorification. Was she really the remote, aristocratic figure of her legend, 'with whom none could ever venture to take a liberty, who worked without in the least descending from her social position'?[34] Some people painted a different picture even in her lifetime. 'The secret of Sister Dora's popularity', said the Secretary of the hospital, who saw her every day, 'was her goodness of heart, her genuine, frank open manner, which won her the confidence of everyone and endeared her to all, but especially to the poor. No inducement such as the offer of the management of larger institutions could induce her to leave; she worked for love of the people of Walsall'.[35] Fortunately Black Country memories are long and their loyalties deep-rooted. In 1963, when the hospital was celebrating its centenary, some people were still found who could claim with pride to have been 'Sister Dora's patients'. An old gentleman at Bloxwich was still showing his grandchildren 'Sister Dora's thumb'. One bonfire night, more than eighty years before, he had held a firework which had exploded in his right hand, shattering the thumb. He was rushed to the hospital, with splinters of bone hanging through the skin. Dora told him the top of the thumb 'must come off', and amputated it herself, with a swift, clean cut through the first joint. He was a brave boy; the stump healed, was usable and became a source of life-long pride to its owner.[36] Another surviving patient, Mr William Page, was ninety when he was asked if he remembered Sister Dora as a remote figure. He could still describe her kindess to him when he had gone into hospital as a frightened small boy of four who had caught his hand in the mangle rollers in 1876. His father was a railwayman, one of the subscribers to the pony and trap. A family friend, another railwayman, on coming out of hospital, had thanked the Sister by taking her for a row on the lake in Walsall's Arboretum. 'It would be quite out of keeping,' declared Mr Page, 'to think of her as high-handed or snobbish with anyone'.[37] The final comment comes from an anonymous patient, who was evidently a man of few, but very well chosen words. When asked his opinion of Sister Dora, he said, 'Well, I have a leg more than I would have had, if it hadn't been for her.' After a pause for thought he added, 'Her was the best woman that ever cut a loaf.'[38] It would be simple but too shallow to say that these people loved Dora because she was an attractive and amusing person, or that they realized the rarity of her skill. Extreme suffering sweeps away the common, surface standards of judgment; anyone who has ever known great pain or fear can recall the anguish of isolation they impose, the rigid despair which stares out from concentration camp photographs. Sister Dora, from some depths of her nature, drew the power to enter this desolation. When she was there, patients, even those at the point of death, no longer felt themselves alone, face to face with the enemy. Her power was love, which the patients tested in matters of life and death, and always found steadfast. They were inarticulate people, but they could feel, with Othello:

> *She loved me for the dangers I had passed;*
> *And I loved her that she did pity them.*

NOTES

1. J. Manton, *Elizabeth Garrett Anderson*, 186–92.
2. E. Moberly Bell, *Storming the Citadel*, 77.
3. E. Lutzker, *Actes du XIe Congres International d'Histoire des Sciences*, notes that one of the Edinburgh seven, Edith Pechey, held an appointment in 1875 at the Birmingham and Midland Hospital for Women. Sister Dora seems neither to have met nor mentioned her.

4. In fact no house-surgeon was appointed until 1891.
5. Lonsdale, 107 and 177.
6. W.C.H. MS., 1873–4.
7. J. Manton, *Elizabeth Garrett Anderson.*
8. *Reprints.* The general public, with a fixed and sentimental pre-
   conception of nursing, refused to believe in Sister Dora's study
   of practical anatomy, but it is well attested.
9. C. Heath, F.R.C.S. *A Manual of Minor Surgery and Bandaging for the
   Use of House Surgeons and Dressers,* first published in 1861, ran
   through many editions in the next three decades.
10. One, at least, of these cases was still alive to show her handiwork
    in the 1950s.
11. *Lancet,* 1867, i, 326, 351, 387, 507; ii, 95.
12. Lonsdale, 108.
13. W.C.H. MS., 1870.
14. W.C.H. MS., 1873.
15. S. Welsh, *General Baptist Magazine,* 1880.
16. S. Baring-Gould, *Virgin Saints and Martyrs,* 384.
    Dr MacLachlan was not identified by name in this passage, but
    the description of the speaker strongly suggests him.
15. S. Welsh, *General Baptist Magazine,* 1880.
17. W.C.H.A.R., 1874.
18. Ibid., 1898.
19. W.C.H. MS., 1872.
20. Lonsdale, 111–14.
21. The weekly police-court news in the *Walsall Observer* reveal how
    common crimes of violence were.
22. Lonsdale, 177.
23. Ibid., 249.
24. The children's ward is portrayed from life on the memorial. The
    bearded figure sitting at the table is the Chairman, Samuel Cox.
25. Lonsdale, 86.
26. E. Royston Pike. *Human Documents of the Victorian Golden Age,*
    124–32.
27. G. C. Allen, *Economic Development of Birmingham and the Black
    Country,* 206.
28. According to the minutes, he was re-admitted three times in the
    next few years, and so came to know Sister Dora exceptionally
    well.
29. Lonsdale, 85–90. The most valuable work Margaret Lonsdale did
    was to collect these first-hand accounts of Sister Dora, though
    she often received less credit than she deserved.

30. W.C.H.A.R., 1872.
31. W.C.H. MS., 1873–4.
32. One of these boys, Sidney Boyd, survived to broadcast about her in 1957.
33. Lonsdale, 206.
34. Ibid., 67.
35. S. Welsh, *General Baptist Magazine*, 1887, 228.
36. *Centenary History*, 26.
37 and 38. *Sunday Mercury*, 6th October, 1963.

CHAPTER FIFTEEN

The Nurses
1872–1874

❊

The news that the nursing at Walsall Cottage Hospital was excellent spread by word of mouth among the doctors of the Midlands. Dora continually received requests, none of which she could fulfil, to send nurses to private cases. One of these, however, was difficult to refuse. It was a telegram from Canon Lonsdale, son of a much loved Bishop of Lichfield who had died two years before of a stroke 'occasioned' it was said 'by excessive letter writing after a trying diocesan meeting'. Canon Lonsdale urgently needed a nurse for his daughters' governess, who was dangerously ill with pleurisy in his own house.

Late that night, the Lonsdale family, waiting anxiously, heard the station bus pull up outside their quiet house in the Close. One of the schoolgirl daughters, Margaret, ran to the window to look out. She saw a slender black-clad figure leap lightly down from the bus and offer a sixpenny fare. 'What! Take sixpence from you, Sister! Blowed if I do!' said the conductor. Dora looked, said Margaret, 'very merry, like a boy escaped from school'. 'I couldn't find you a nurse,' she announced, 'so I've come myself. Where is my patient?' She vanished into the sickroom, for the rest of the night, and the girls had to wait impatiently for the morning to see her. She came down to breakfast cheerfully fresher than those who had spent the night in bed. They were enchanted by her looks, speech and manners; at luncheon and dinner 'she kept the family in fits of laughter', but vanished swiftly as soon as the meal was over, to her patient's bedside. That night they wanted her to rest, but she would have none of it. 'Oh, I'm used to night nursing,' she said. 'I always find I can stay up seven nights if I go to bed on the eighth.'

The three weeks that followed were tantalizing to the young girls. Their life was exceedingly quiet; the family lived in the same house for more than fifty years, while their father spent much time in the study, at work on his translations of Horace and Virgil. They longed for the company of this fascinating stranger, who dispelled dullness but was only interested in her patient's crisis and recovery. At last, as the governess began to recover, they found a way to get her to themselves, by taking her out for drives in the carriage. The first time Dora saw the country-side she clapped her hands and exclaimed with delight at the most ordinary things. 'Look at the trees and the grass! I had forgotten how *green* they were! It is so long since I saw them.' As they drove through the country lanes beyond Lichfield she laughed out loud like a child at the sight of the flowers in the hedgerows. In the early mornings they saw her slip out to gaze up at the sandstone pinnacles of the Cathedral darkened by the drifting smoke of the Black Country, ten miles away. The governess recovered. Sister Dora packed to escort her to her home in the south. Soon she would be gone out of their lives, perhaps for ever. Greatly daring, young Margaret Lonsdale approached her. 'Would you allow me to train as a nurse with you at Walsall?' she begged. Sister Dora laughed. 'No, certainly not,' she said lightly. 'You're *much* too dainty a creature'.[1]

She had learnt to be cool, even ruthless, in holding admiration at arm's length. She suffered, like everyone else in the medical profession, from ladies with a morbid interest in her work. 'They are disappointed,' wrote a doctor disgustedly, 'or they want something with which to kill ennui, or they have religious convictions on the subject.'[2] Dora endured many trying visitors, like the lady whom she took round the hospital in 1872, showing her wards, operating theatre and kitchens, in hopes of a useful donation. The visitor was deeply impressed, and wrote afterwards, 'I think I'll do some texts for a new ward they have just opened, by way of expressing my feelings.' Sometimes, if really pressed, she frankly got rid of them, as when she said to a young girl, 'What a pity you have come all this way, for I am going to be busy with my out-patients and have no time for talking. No, I do not care to be photographed or written about or anything of that sort. Good-bye!' The poor girl was left gazing after 'the tall stately figure in her long, black garments, her face beautiful with the light of holiness',[3] as Sister Dora vanished swiftly down the path. Such treatment was brutal, but there was some excuse for it. Sometimes visitors fainted. Others addressed the patients with a lachrymose and whining sympathy which set Dora's teeth on edge, and must have caused some ribald amusement in the wards, once they had been safely seen into their carriages. Yet, however much she disliked the idea, there was an undoubted demand for nursing training, and the work at Walsall was now expanding too fast for her to do it alone. 1872 was the heaviest year's work she had yet known. There were more than two thousand out-patients and two hundred in-patients, no longer purely local people. Cases were sent from Birmingham, Coventry, Gloucester, Glasgow, Liverpool, Sheffield and even London. During the year seventeen men died, most of them within a few days of admission; they had been run over by trains in shunting yards, crushed in the mines or scalded in blast furnaces. In the autumn of 1872 Dora recognized the need for more staff, and with very mixed feelings proposed to the Committee that she should train 'lady-pupils'. These were not to be paid probationers, but educated women who could afford to maintain themselves and pay a premium for their training; she proposed to charge them twelve pounds a year. She pointed out that for nursing experience Walsall could offer 'peculiar and special advantages not possessed even by London hospitals' in accident work.[4] She would also undertake to send 'trained and efficient nurses for private cases'.[5] This would help the perpetually struggling hospital; once she had got the scheme running, income rose in one year from £798 to £1188.[6] The Committee advertised that 'Ladies desirous of being trained would do well to communicate with the Sister-in-Charge'. All terms and conditions were handed over to Sister Dora, who converted a female ward into a rather bleak dormitory for the ladies, and drew up the regulations which they had to accept. From this time onwards there were always two or three of them at work in the wards.[7]

In spite of the hard conditions there was never any shortage of applicants, who often came from a distance. Among those who became Matrons or Superintendents of Nursing were Ellen Ravenhill of Gloucester, Alice Hunt of Derby, Louisa Lawson of Ilminster and Hannah Tomline of Ryde, Isle of Wight.

They did not have an easy life, but at least they were never bored. Sister Dora herself was not what was conventionally called 'a trained nurse'. She had been thoroughly drilled in housekeeping at Coatham, and well grounded in minor surgery by Dr Mac-Lachlan, but she had never passed through any recognized training school. She described her nursing education frankly to her new pupils, 'I do assure you, my dears, I unlearn every year what I learnt the last!' It is clear, from quotation that she herself read both Florence Nightingale's *Notes on Nursing* and C. V. Cullingworth's *Nurse's Companion*. This, and their own reminiscences, makes it possible to reconstruct much of the training she gave her young pupils.

The first stage was to teach them housekeeping and ward management to her own standard. The students despaired of attaining the speed with which Dora could skim round a ward, as 'with deft hands she straightened a coverlet that did not hang quite square, lifted the lid of a boiling kettle or pushed a bed that was a little out of line close up to the wall. Nothing escaped her eye.'[8] Next they learnt the regular routine of bathing, moving, changing and feeding helpless patients, taking pulses and temperatures, measuring and testing of urine. Sister Dora particularly stressed the importance of turning helpless patients regularly to prevent bed-sores; she would pull out a bed from the wall, stand behind the head-rail and lift, apparently without effort, a miner or puddler weighing sixteen stone. She would never allow the young nurses to go through their routine work with mechanical efficiency; they must use it as an opportunity to observe the patient, every change in his face, voice or attitude. They should not need to ask him how he felt, for they should understand his feelings. 'I try to put myself in the place of these poor men,' she said, 'to see with their eyes and to feel their wants and difficulties as if they were my own.'[9] Only then could the nurse give an intelligent and truthful account to the physician or surgeon. 'If you cannot observe you had better give up being a nurse for it is not your calling, however kind or anxious you may be.'

She taught the nursing of sick children as a special art. 'Much patience and unselfishness is needed,' she said, 'and, above all, *imagination* is absolutely necessary. We must learn to put ourselves in the place of a child.' She showed what she meant by points of apparently minor, but really essential, detail. A thirsty child must be allowed to drink freely. 'It is very irritating to have a tumbler of water held to your lips and then withdrawn just as you are beginning to enjoy it. You would not like it yourselves!' She made them imagine the terror of a child who had never been bathed in its life, when confronted with this strange experience. 'Few things frighten a little child so much as being seized by a stranger, undressed among clouds of steam and violently plunged in. Coax the child in gently, feet first and splash warm water over it by degrees with your free hand. Use all your tact with children.' She would never allow them to leave a frightened or unhappy child to cry itself to sleep. 'Soothe it and amuse it very gently and quietly at the same time,' she said. 'When it is calm it will fall asleep of its own accord and sleep well.' To convince worried mothers of the truth of this, she invited them freely into the children's ward, an unheard-of practice at that date. She taught the young nurses to trust the marvellous natural resilience of child patients. 'They have so much life in them and such power of recovery, that with God's blessing they seem able to survive in a miraculous manner. Never give up hope of the life of a child.'[10]

The next stage in the nurse's training was to assist Dora with the daily dressings which, since the hospital took only surgical cases, occupied a large part of each working day. Dr MacLachlan had taught Dora, what he himself had learnt from Lister's pre-antiseptic teaching, that one must expect the formation of pus.[11] Part of the wound was always left open for drainage, and dry dressings applied, which, as they became encrusted with pus, had to be changed at least every two days. Sister Dora's method was to soak off the old dressings, by squeezing warm water over them from a special dressing sponge to a basin, which the student held beneath the wound. She then removed the old dressing inch by inch with forceps. When suppuration persisted, she applied lint poultices of bread or linseed oil to 'draw' the wound, binding them on with home-made bandages of old, clean linen. The nurse had to change poultices regularly to maintain the heat.

The whole process of dressing, constantly repeated, was at best tedious, at worst agonizing and exhausting for the patient. Skill, speed, a light firm touch and a gentle but confident manner were essential. 'Never touch a wounded limb as though you were afraid of it,' advised Sister Dora. 'It gives unnecessary pain and inspires no confidence. Handle it very gently, but quite firmly.' Her own touch and manner were said to be perfect.

She tried to teach her nurses the same confidence in meeting an accident or emergency. 'Whatever happens, never show you are afraid,' she said. The secret was to be prepared. She kept an accident bed, with mackintosh, cradle, sand-bags, blocks and fracture boards, always made up, and the pupils were taught to have ice-packs and hot water bottles ready. She taught them how to undress an injured patient, cutting clothes along the seams and drawing them away from the injury, and how to clean men brought in with the grime of their work still on them. On several points she was clearly in advance of her time. One of these was in the recognition and prevention of shock, where Dr Mac-Lachlan came to agree that her own method, founded, as she said, 'mainly upon common sense' was more effective than his own. Particularly when casualties were burnt or scalded, she did not attempt to touch the wounds, but wrapped the patient in blankets and cotton wool, with ice to the head and hot bottles to the feet. She left him to rest, later offered sips of milk and brandy, and after a few hours was usually able to dress the wounds without further shock or distress.[12] Even more revolutionary in the 1870s was her mouth-to-mouth method of artificial respiration. The students watched in amazement as she put her lips to the mouth of a patient in a state of collapse, and breathed into his lungs until his own breathing began.[13] This method was so successful that she used it habitually, though when Margaret Lonsdale described it, an indignant correspondent to the *British Medical Journal* described it as impossible to believe.

The last duty Sister Dora taught her nurses was to assist Dr MacLachlan at operations, which occurred on two afternoons a week. They had to scrub down a deal table, cover it with mackintosh sheeting and sprinkle fresh sawdust thickly on the floor. It was their duty to set out basins, jugs of hot and cold water, soap, towels, swabs, a clean side-table or tray and the instruments.

These she washed with very hot water and soda, dried and placed on a clean towel. The patient, and everyone assisting, washed well with soap and hot water before every operation, and the wound was dressed with old, clean linen from the hospital's store. A standard manual of surgery advised that 'Sponges should be scrupulously clean; they must never be used for any other purpose and particularly should not be employed to wipe blood from the floor',[14] which suggests that standards of cleanliness at Walsall were unusually high. Nothing of course was sterilized, but Dr MacLachlan's patients seem usually to have done well and Sister Dora's pupils were always in demand as surgical nurses. One became superintendent of military nursing to the Prussian army.

Efficiency was not enough. Sister Dora demanded from her nursing students nothing less than total dedication to their calling. 'Tell her', was her message to an intending applicant, 'that this is not an ordinary house, or even hospital. I want her to understand that all who serve here, in whatever capacity, ought to have one rule, love for God, and then I need not say love for their work. I wish we could use and really mean the name Maison Dieu.'[15] This idea must have been in her mind since childhood, for *Maison Dieu* is the Norman name of a street in Richmond, where the medieval hospice of the town once stood.[16] She demanded from these unschooled women total self-possession and calmness at any time, nor did she attempt to shield them from agonizing sights and sounds. Some confessed they could not bear it, and to those she repeated the advice of old Sister Mary in her own early days. 'Look upon your work as a privilege. Do not look upon nursing as an art or a science, but as work done for Christ. As you touch each patient, think it is Christ himself, and then virtue will come out of the touch. I have often felt that myself.'[17]

Yet, to the surprise of many of the nurses, Sister Dora did not encourage displays of piety or affected sympathy in the wards. 'You may be sure they will judge you by what you do, not by what you say,' she would say. 'Don't come into the wards unless you can come with a smiling face.' Ladylike condescension irritated her above all; she would find the luckless nurse some particularly unpalatable domestic chore, watching her out of the corner of her dark eyes with undisguised amusement. Sometimes she was frankly impatient with tiresome pupils. 'I could have *beaten* that silly goose!' she was once heard to say. These girls from ultra-respectable homes soon found that, in any conventional sense, Sister Dora was quite unshockable. If they complained of a woman who arrived covered with cuts and bruises after a fight with her husband, and disturbed the out-patients by shouts and curses, Dora looked thoughtful. 'D'you know,' she said, confidentially, 'if I had been her, and had a husband like that, I should have been a *fiend*!' Another morning, she was called by a pupil to see a dog-bite, which had been covered with a horrifying home-made plaster incorporating dog's hairs. 'Well,' she said interestedly, 'we often heard of a hair of the dog that bit you, but I've never actually seen one before.' She emphasized that they were there to nurse the patients, not to reform their manners and morals, though that might follow if they won love and trust. When an Irish labourer refused to drink anything but stout for his breakfast, Sister Dora saw that he got it. She would not allow the patients to be surrounded by an 'invalidish atmosphere' which depressed them. The usual practice throughout the nineteenth century was to keep the patient in bed, for days or weeks at a time, until the muscles grew weak from lack of use. Dora used to say, 'Let him walk; it will help him.' She enrolled two men, each with one injured arm, as 'an extra pair of hands', and when she was away sent one of them the message, 'Mr. Baker I hope is attentive to his duties and has broken *no more pink cups.*'

It is clear that all this, so remote from their sentimental imagining of the nurse's calling, was a great shock to many of Sister Dora's pupils. Among these, after a few years, came, at her own entreaty, Margaret Lonsdale of Lichfield.[18] This young woman had led a sheltered, indeed a blinkered, existence. She had woven her dreams around the remembered figure of Sister Dora, whom she called 'a real princess', whose friend and confidante she hoped to become, 'always with her, working under her, learning from her'. The realities of the black and gritty town, the crowded hospital, the practical duties which filled every minute of Sister Dora's day were a bitter disappointment to her. She was determined to prove herself, and she worked hard and well, but some-

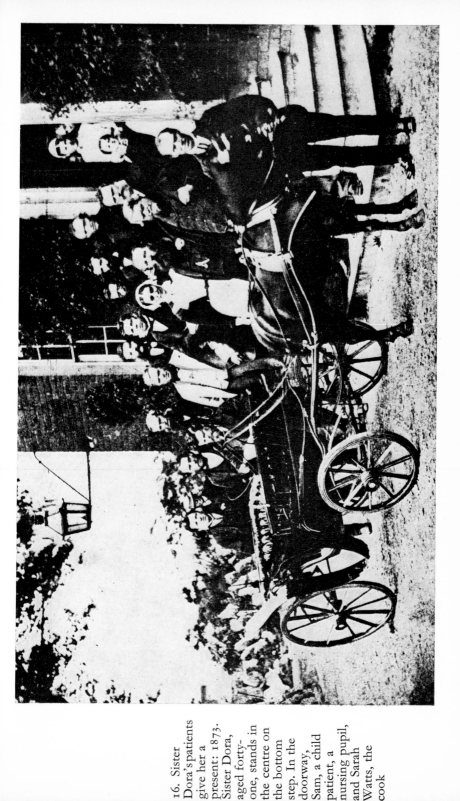

16. Sister Dora's patients give her a present: 1873. Sister Dora, aged forty-one, stands in the centre on the bottom step. In the doorway, Sam, a child patient, a nursing pupil, and Sarah Watts, the cook

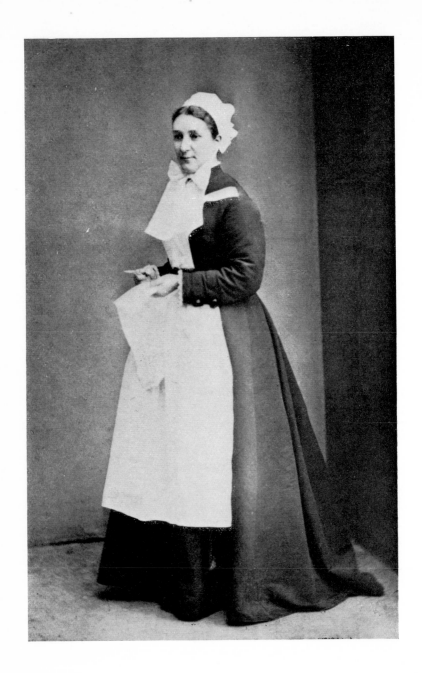

17. Sister Dora cutting a bandage

thing of her chagrin shows in her account of Walsall and her training there. These months, when the lonely, frustrated girl brooded over a relationship which only existed in her dreams, were the germ of what Mark Pattison, in one of his inimitably disagreeable phrases, called 'Miss Lonsdale's romance, *Sister Dora*'. The town seemed 'begrimed with dirt', the people 'half civilized savages', the committee members 'engaged in trade', the clergy 'hardly men of congenial spirit'. Sister Dora, according to her, 'found no one in Walsall of her own social position and lived, of her own choice, a solitary life, devoted to study, meditation and prayer'. The young nurse's relations with the Sister-in-Charge, were not at all what she had hoped for. Much of her time was spent in routine work in the women's ward, for Sister Dora 'did not care to nurse the women, unless there were some very engaging children in their ward and preferred leaving them in the charge of her lady-pupils'. She complained of Dora's 'strong, almost violent prejudices', her intolerance of slowness or clumsiness in others, which was a terror to nervous probationers, her favouritism among pupils, and her jealousy of any nurse 'who showed signs of ability to fill her place'.[19] This is a formidable list of faults, and although it was denied by many people when Margaret Lonsdale's book came out, it cannot have been wholly imaginary. Dora did love her patients with a primitive, maternal passion, which left little time for the young nurses in her care.

Yet she could, when in the mood, be an excellent teacher, with an inborn gift for the vivid phrase or lively demonstration which stays in the memory. She instilled observation, perseverance, method. Her manner was crisp and concise; she never wasted words and expected to be understood the first time. She knew that she was impatient with clumsy beginners and confessed it with disarming repentance. 'I was anything but forbearing, dear, I was overbearing,' she wrote to a former pupil, 'and I am truly sorry for it now.' Even after a grinding day in the hospital, the nurses' supper, at which she presided, was a hilarious meal, and when she went away she wrote most affectionately to her young students, 'Don't forget your prayers, do get all you want for your meals, and don't have any troubles that you do not tell me.'[20]

The best proof of Sister Dora's ability as a teacher was the career of her favourite pupil, Louise MacLaughlin.[21] This girl came from the social class which nursing reformers hoped to attract to the profession. Her seven brothers included clergy, army officers and an Indian magistrate. She was the daughter of a Shropshire clergyman and granddaughter of an Earl. Yet nothing could have been more down-to-earth than her attitude to work. She completed her training at Walsall, and in 1876, with a devoted female friend, set out as a Red Cross nurse in the Serbo-Turkish war. These two redoubtable ladies, armed with green-lined parasols and a crate of permanganate of potash crystals, arrived in August at a Balkan village of mud-huts, dust and flies. They found rows of wounded lying on the straw-strewn floor of a Turkish cafe, where Louise put her Walsall training into practice. 'We turned out all the furniture,' she wrote, 'we rubbed and scrubbed and splashed about carbolic and water until we felt clean, and the rooms smelt so. We washed mattress cases, blankets and linen in neat permanganate of potash, and made up beds on trestles and planks. This is a much cleaner plan than laying them on the floor; there is a free draught of air under them, and it is easy to sweep and scrub beneath. The windows were always kept open, the floors washed, every used dressing thrown into proper receptacles and taken away.' She treated the Serbian peasants as though they had been Walsall iron-workers. 'The secret to keep men in a cheerful, hopeful, helpful state is to make them do as much as possible for themselves, avoiding invalid ways and occupying their minds. It is much better to adopt as many of their own habits as possible.' This account reproduces both the letter and the spirit of Sister Dora's teaching, and the result was all she could have wished. '*Not one death occurred*,' wrote Louise in November. 'All our "hopeless" cases are alive and walking about.'[22] She invited Sister Dora to join her in the Balkans, though for various reasons this was impossible. Dora was unselfishly delighted and proud when her old pupil received the Cross of Honour of the Red Cross. Louise MacLaughlin was to be a very good friend to her in the last months of her life.

Another favourite pupil, unnamed, left a full account of Sister Dora's working day at the hospital. This makes clear why she regarded marriage as irreconcilable with her work, for every waking minute was devoted to the patients. Her day began before dawn, when the mournful hooters of pits and iron-works sounded through the darkness.

'Sister Dora,' wrote the nurse, 'used to come down into the wards at half-past-six in the morning, make the beds of all the patients and give them their breakfasts, until half-past seven, when it was time for her own breakfast. She was skilful and rapid in her work, a great matter where invalids are concerned. . . . After her own breakfast, she read prayers, on the staircase so that all the patients in the three wards could hear and join. Then came the daily ward work, the washing of patients and dressing of wounds. At half-past ten there were usually old out-patients who called regularly to have their wounds poulticed or lanced. The doctor appeared at eleven and went his rounds with Sister Dora. At twelve came the patients' dinner, at which she attended minutely to every detail and always carved herself. Then she read prayers in the nurses' little general sitting room. Then followed dinner for the nurses, a very movable feast as far as Sister Dora herself was concerned. . . . Out-patients began to arrive at two o'clock. . . . The doctors got through their part of the work quickly for they passed on to her the minor operations entrusted to experienced dressers in large hospitals. The setting of fractures and drawing of teeth were common operations to her; her bandaging was so good that a surgeon from Birmingham called upon all his students to admire and study her handiwork. The treatment of out-patients took between two and three hours, so the in-patients' tea at five o'clock had sometimes to be prepared by the servants. About six the nurses had their own tea, but it was rarely Sister Dora got a quiet meal for either someone would come tapping at the door saying she was wanted, or the surgery bell would ring, as indeed it did all day long. After tea she went into the wards again and this was the time to which patients looked forward all day. She would go and talk to them individually, or they would sing while she washed up the tea-things, or play at games in which she occasionally took part. . . . By eight o'clock wounds had been dressed for the night and the patients' supper was served. Sister Dora read prayers. Just before bed time came her own supper, when she was often very merry, and would relate her experiences with intense drollery. This was the time to which we lady-pupils looked forward. She was the first to be up and the last to go to rest; how she managed to get through such constant hard work was a marvel.'[23]

In 1874 the number of serious accidents was reduced by a long-drawn miners' strike, which in turn threw the iron-workers and railwaymen out of work. The winter was bitterly cold, and the women and children suffered from the effects of hunger. Some-times, looking round the crowd of patients waiting in the street for the gates to the out-patients hall to be unlocked, Sister Dora would murmur to one of the nurses, 'What would have become of all these poor people, if there had been no hospital?'[24]

By autumn 1874, the first pupil nurses had completed their training. Two, or possibly three, of them were capable of taking charge for a short time while Dora went away. For some years she had been worried about her discharged patients, specially the children, who needed good food and air but were forced to return to back alleys. She would have liked to keep them longer, to run wild in the hospital grounds, but her beds were always needed for urgent cases. In September she took six boys who had undergone surgical operations for a day's picnicking among the larches and heather of Sutton Park. 'Her joy,' said their host, 'at the sight of the children's pleasure, was boundless.'[25] The success of this day decided her to take a party to the seaside. With the help of funds provided by the pupil nurses, she set off in October 1874 for Rhyl, where she had booked cheap out-of-season lodgings. The landlady was completely won over. 'Instead of disliking us,' reported Dora to the givers of the money, 'she is so good to the patients, and takes trouble with the cooking.' It was her first holiday for years and she was happy in their pleasure. 'I do not know when I have enjoyed anything so much!' she wrote. 'Our family ranges from two years old to a grey-haired man of sixty. Only one of them had seen the sea before; their remarks are so amusing; it is fun for me. They are never tired of the shore, are out in the morning at seven and never come in before eight at night. I take the little child out and let it run without shoes or stockings. One boy who limped when we came was running races today! I took them all out in a boat. I am only grieved that

I did not have them weighed when we came.' Every afternoon she left them on the beach, and went to church for the unaccustomed luxury of daily Evensong. Looking back over the six years since 1868, when she had taken charge of the hospital, she found much to give thanks for.

To the Committee, the doctors, the patients and the nurses Sister Dora had become an institution; they could not imagine that she might have problems of her own, or could ever leave the hospital. In fact she was more than once in difficulties with the authorities at Coatham. Mr Postlethwaite, as Chaplain and administrator of the Homes, was continually harassed by shortage of nurses.[26] He wrote long-windedly and rather plaintively to the Walsall Committee on 6th September 1872 that because of the distance 'the supply of nursing aid was consequently attended with considerable inconvenience'. He added, 'Whenever Sister Dora should be *removed* from the charge at Walsall I should prefer not to send another Sister.' This dark hint caused 'considerable excitement', and they wrote asking what he meant by this expression, since they 'sincerely trusted the date of her removal might be far distant'. He replied that 'if Sisters tarry long at Walsall (and your Committee does not like changes) excepting in name they become almost separated from us, and I cannot fulfil my duties to them at such a distance'. He revealed that he had conducted 'a prolonged correspondence on this and another matter with Sister Dora'.[27] The Committee members were thrown into consternation and confusion. As always in a crisis they sent for Sister Dora to attend their next meeting.

'You have been in charge for upwards of seven years,' said the chairman. In fact it was six, but he had lost count. 'How *should* we manage without you?'

Sister Dora replied with the utmost composure that she did not consider she had received notice to leave Walsall. 'For the past four years I have been unaided by Sisters from the North, and I trust the nursing of the hospital has been carried on in a satisfactory manner?'

'You mean,' said the chairman, evidently clutching at straws, 'you would still consent to remain in charge and carry on the work in future?' Sister Dora, smoothing her cuffs, as always when pleased, 'kindly consented'.

'Then there will be no inconvenience or difficulty!' exclaimed a member. 'The work of the Hospital will be carried on just as before!'[28] On 27th November Mr Postlethwaite reluctantly gave his consent 'to reappoint Sister Dora, without further reference to me.'

In fact, this was a serious step for Sister Dora, tantamount to defying an order from her superior officer. The nurses were curious as to her reasons; probably they had heard some of the old gossip and were curious for details of cruel discipline at Coatham or scandalous Ritualistic practices. Finally one of them plucked up courage to ask Sister Dora why she had not returned to the north when requested to do so. Whatever she expected, she must have been surprised by the reply.

'Because,' said Sister Dora crisply, 'I am a woman and not a piece of furniture.' No explanation could be more convincing, or more in keeping with her character.

She was believed and believed herself to be hostile to the movement for women's social freedom. Until the age of thirty she had been brought up, like her sisters, with 'a profound sense of her own inferiority in mind and body' because she was a woman. In 1873, when her work was becoming well known, a woman correspondent wrote asking her about nursing as a career, and was disconcerted to get the reply, 'I feel pretty much like Balaam of old, as if I should give quite the contrary advice to what you want of me. You would like me to urge women working in hospitals. I feel more inclined to harangue about women doing their work at *home*, being the helpmeet for man which God ordained and not doing man's work.'[29] Queen Victoria herself could hardly have said more. Sister Dora was quoted to over-adventurous girls as an example of submission. Friends denied that she 'would not submit to the quiet domestic life of an ordinary woman'.[30] 'There are plenty of so-called female apostles in the present day,' wrote an editor, 'of whom Sister Dora never was one, ready enough to prate about women's rights. They might be better employed in trying to learn the noble lesson she has bequeathed to them, of the reality of woman's work.'[31] This was the lesson associated with the Sister Dora legend; the reality of her professional position was different. As Sister-in-Charge of an accident hospital she proved that women were capable of hard work, responsibility and judgment. She could always manage what she called in all sincerity, the stronger sex. The patients, helpless in their splints, or neatly tucked under their red blankets, trustingly accepted her authority. A surgeon marvelling at her effortless control of the wards, called her 'a woman born to command'. Clergy of any church or chapel were welcome visitors, but a minister who had the misfortune to get in the way at a crisis never recovered his nerve after the 'concentrated sharpness' with which Sister Dora told him to '*Shut that door!*' She resisted any attempt by clergy to enforce religious observances on the patients. Even towards the physicians and surgeons her attitude was more independent than perhaps she or they realized. In the public view nursing was the feminine profession par excellence, in which 'the quick eye, the soft hand, the light step and the ready ear second the wisdom of the physician and execute his commands'.[32] In real life, things might be very different. The 'lady nurse' was sometimes more experienced than the newly qualified house-surgeon, and often of higher social position. Sometimes, as in Sister Dora's case, she was working voluntarily, for charity, where the hard-pressed surgeon or dresser needed his fees.[32] 'Contact between them,' wrote a surgeon, with the wariness of experience, 'is difficult and precarious.'

Sometimes, it must be said, the pioneer trained-nurses were high-handed as well as high-minded. Poor Margaret Lonsdale, who seemed fated to trouble, went on from Walsall to Guy's as a 'lady pupil'. Here she wrote an article which for three months roused the medical press to uproar. She maintained that medical men resented 'Sisters in the proper sense of the word', who were ladies by birth and education, for sinister reasons of their own. The old 'scrubber' nurse, whose recreation was taken 'too often, alas, in the nearest public house', had permitted 'practices and experiments' upon helpless patients, which a trained sister would never allow. Nor would she tolerate 'the low tone of morality for which the wards were remarkable. The presence of a refined lady puts an end to any undue familiarity between doctors and nurses, and *imposes a moral restraint* on the words and ways of medical students, who are as a class universally acknowledged to be uncouth'.[33] Doctors responded in various ways to this genteel dressing-down. One protested that he had never witnessed the least impropriety; another, evidently a realist, wrote that one

Sister Dora

might as well complain because students and nurses are men and women.[34] A surgeon wrote wryly that, 'with whatever natural shrinking from near contact with refinement' most doctors valued good nursing for their patients.[35] The general tone, however, was much more hostile than this. It is clear that the new lady nurses, starched sticklers for propriety, for rigid routines, for spit and polish, in whose presence, as Florence Nightingale insisted, it must 'seem impossible to the most unchaste to utter an immodest jest', were far from popular. Many a doctor and patient sighed for the comfortable old days, before 'this fashionable mania for nursing'.

Yet the medical committee at Walsall seemed to have been quite happy to entrust to Sister Dora duties far beyond those normally given to a nurse. It is not difficult to see how this came about. The voluntary cottage hospital was small, poor and hard-pressed; it would never in her lifetime afford the services of a resident house-physician or surgeon. Many of its cases were emergencies where prompt treatment was a matter of recovery or mutilation, sometimes of life and death. The relationship between Dr MacLachlan and Sister Dora was one of exceptional friendship and trust. The medical and lay committees both knew they would never find anyone else to take on the amount of work she tackled single-handed for no pay. Her tact and charm made her position acceptable to men who would have resisted a woman of aggressive or masculine personality. 'Her feminine devices were endless,' wrote an appreciative colleague, and naturally they gave her a free hand. Sister Dora sincerely believed herself to be an anti-feminist, yet she effectively showed the world what could be achieved by a woman of skill and character.

NOTES

1. Lonsdale, 79–81.
2. *The British Medical Journal*, 17th March 1880.
3. Ridsdale, 4–5.
4. *Walsall Observer*, 1st February 1873.
5. W.C.H.A.R., 1872.
6. Ibid., 1873.

264

7. W.C.H. MS., 1871 and 1879. One is shown with Dr MacLachlan and Sister Dora, on the memorial.

8. Ridsdale, xiii.

9. Lonsdale, 120.

10. M. Lonsdale, *Care and Nursing of Children*, passim, recorded several of these sayings, which, she said, 'I learnt from Sister Dora.'

11. R. Godlee, *Lord Lister*, 149.

12. Lonsdale, 83.

13. Ibid., 159.

14. C. Heath, *A Manual of Minor Surgery*, 1st edn., 91–6.

15. Lonsdale, 102.

16. Personal observation.

17. Lonsdale, 223.

18. Ibid., 2nd edition 1887, 6.

19. Ibid., 68.

20. Ibid., 144.

21. No relation of Dr MacLachlan.

22. E. Pearson and L. MacLaughlin, *Service in Serbia under the Red Cross*, 170–84.

23. Lonsdale, 93–9.

24. W.C.H.A.R., 1874.

25. Lonsdale, 126.

26. He could no longer call on the Sisters of the Community of the Holy Rood, who were already over-worked in their hospital and orphanage at Middlesbrough.

27. W.C.H. MS., 1872. He did not reveal what the other matter was but there are hints of a question of conscience which continued to trouble her.

28. W.C.H.A.R., 1874, and W.C.H. MS., 1872–4.

29. Quoted Lonsdale, 110.

30. Ridsdale, vi.

31. *The Saturday Review*, 1st May 1880.

32. *St. Paul's Magazine*, August 1871.

32. O. Sturges in *The Nineteenth Century*, June 1880. A relative of my own, gold medallist at the Middlesex Hospital in 1893, used till his ninetieth year the old-fashioned expression 'lady nurses'. He remembered the drop in dressers' fees when trained sisters took charge of the dressings, and how many budgets were unbalanced by the change.

33. M. Lonsdale, *The Nineteenth Century*, April 1880.

34. *The British Medical Journal* and *The Lancet*, May and June 1880.

35. *The Nineteenth Century*, June 1880.

CHAPTER SIXTEEN

Sister of Charity
1870–1874

❊

As a nurse, Sister Dora was unwilling to compromise her professional judgment by religious vows. Yet the ideal of the dedicated life never lost its hold upon her. It seems probable that she, like her married sister Sarah, remained an Associate Sister of the Community. No letter or minute recording her resignation or dismissal exists anywhere among the papers of the Convent of the Holy Rood. She visited the Convent in the last few months of her life. 'Sister Dora', she said, 'is the only name by which I am known or ever will be known.' She signed all letters and documents, including her own will, as 'Sister Dora', and described herself in 1876 as 'belonging to a Sisterhood'.[1] She accepted an Associate Sister, Phoebe Milligan of Saltburn, as a nursing student, and, when seeking a successor to herself as Sister-in-Charge, chose another Associate Sister, Ellen Coleman.[2] She still wore the familiar black dress, with crisp white ruffles at neck and wrist. Her black cross on its neck chain and her jet buckled belt are still preserved at Walsall. The only change in her habit, as may be seen from photographs, was practical. The novices' cap, with its muslin frills, demanded much starching and goffering. Dora felt time could be better spent. She made herself up a new cap, still tied with a butterfly bow and streamers under the chin but folded smoothly back over her dark hair. It was to be known to generations of nurses as 'a Sister Dora'.

Whatever her position in canon law, there is no doubt that Sister Dora had a strong spiritual influence on patients and friends. There is an eye-witness account of her at the age of forty by a young parish priest. She had always chosen to worship not in the great Gothic parish church crowning the hill, but in the Chapel of St Paul, jerry-built in 1826, in a rather meagre classical style, to serve the needs of the working population of Walsall Wood.[3] In 1872 this Chapel became an independent parish church. Sister Dora presented an engraved alms-dish, still in use, and befriended the new vicar, Edward Fitzgerald, a young Cambridge man of twenty-six, who had previously served in the parish as curate and who was also classical master at Walsall's ancient grammar school.[4] His first thought when he saw Sister Dora was that she reminded him of a Greek goddess. Like herself, he was a worker. Despite the difference in their ages they understood one another well; Fitzgerald was one of the few people to whom Sister Dora gave a personal memento during her last illness. At her invitation he held services in the hospital, where he was able to observe her closely.

'When the services were over,' he wrote, 'I used to stay and talk with the patients and thus had many opportunities of seeing Sister Dora at work. Never did she attempt that impossible feat of "cramming religion down people's throats". She always used much tact in dealing with them. She knew they were scanning her conduct and would judge of Christianity by the way she presented it to them in her actions. But never did she seem to forget that men's souls are worth infinitely more than their bodies.' He saw an example of her influence with a difficult patient, who grumbled incessantly, whatever was done for him and crackled his newspaper noisily throughout prayers. This man became very ill and for several nights Sister Dora hardly left his bedside, taking endless pains to make him comfortable. One night, in the darkened ward, he suddenly said, 'I hope they pay you well for this.' 'Yes,' she said, 'very well.' 'What do they give you, then?' he said. 'I want to know.' 'So I told him', related Sister Dora, 'how I believed I was paid.' Next morning, to Fitzgerald's astonishment, the patient was actually heard to say 'Amen'; not, as Dora explained, that he agreed with religion, 'but I suppose he thought it would please me, and that was kind of him'. Fitzgerald gave as another example an iron-worker called Powell, who was dangerously injured. 'He woke one night and found Sister Dora kneeling by his bedside, praying quietly, but in spoken words. He made

Sister Dora

no sign but lay and listened and heard her pray most fervently for his soul. It impressed him deeply. He had never thought his soul of much value before, I imagine, and he was touched by such an evidence of her deep care for him.'⁵

Fitzgerald was so impressed with Sister Dora's power of reaching people who ridiculed conventional religion that he enlisted her in a project very near to his heart. He wanted to hold a mission to his poor and neglected parish, and in particular to its numerous alcoholics. The habit of steady, hard spirit-drinking was wide-spread in the district. 'I remember one Saturday night walking five miles into the Black Country,' wrote Cormell Price, the friend of William Morris. 'In the last three miles I counted more than thirty people lying dead drunk on the ground, more than half of them women.' Sister Dora was not, in the accepted sense, a temperance reformer. She would drink a glass of wine herself on any social occasion, and it was said 'nobody ever heard her urge upon working men the duty of never touching a drop of drink'. If she had, they would certainly not have listened; but she did grieve over men injured in drunken fights or households brought to poverty by drinking, especially where the mother of a family was an alcoholic. So, rather reluctantly, and insisting that she would on no account speak, she agreed to attend a meeting for work-people. The scene which followed became a story to tell against herself. Tea was being poured from the parish urn by charitable ladies, when she noticed that most of the company was provided with little bottles of gin to fortify it. A former patient rose to his feet rather unsteadily and welcomed the guest. 'When I was in hospital,' he declared, with a hiccup, 'Sister gave me strong porter! Sure her never denied me a drop.' This speech was greeted with loud applause. Suddenly Sister Dora lost her temper. She stood up with flashing eyes and berated them until, as she said, 'every head sank and every heart quailed.'⁶ She did not, though, alter her firm opinion that to preach against drinking was a waste of time, unless society offered working people sports, entertainment, good company, and a place, other than the gin shop where they could be, as she said, 'sure of spending a merry half-hour and having a good laugh'. For this reason she always invited former patients to come back for Sunday evening parties at the hospital. If ex-patients, men or women, were locked up as

268

drunk and disorderly, she would go down to the Police cells to give them a personal invitation.

Three years after the first parish mission at St Paul's another was held, and in this Sister Dora played a key part. She proposed to Edward Fitzgerald that they should make a special effort to reach some of the town's prostitutes. Full-time professional prostitution was rare in the Black Country, but occasional prostitution, to supplement the miserable wages of working women or to provide for their children when they were out of work, was a commonplace. Girls would go into public bars, drink with the colliers or canal bargemen, then lead them away to dark alleys or backyards. Sometimes wives would go in search of their husbands, and savage fights between the women would follow.[7] Work among prostitutes was known to be difficult, and the results often disappointing, but certain Church of England communities, notably the Clewer Sisters, had undertaken it successfully. Sister Dora had nursed many individual prostitutes and grown fond of them; moreover, as she said, 'life had given her the opportunity of studying human nature and now she could put it to use'. If the clergy would hold a special midnight service for these women, every night for a week she undertook to find a congregation for them. 'There's hardly a poor man or woman in Walsall whom I do not know personally,' she said, 'I could go up to anyone in the street and ask them in.'[8]

So they took possession of a dingy, ramshackle little building, at the corner of a rookery of courts and alleys called Town End Bank, soon to be demolished. It had been a cholera hospital during the great epidemics of the 1830's. Here Sister Dora set lamps in the windows, and left the door open. Then she went up and down the alleyways, knocking at each house and saying, 'Open the door – it's only Sister. I want to speak to you.' Once inside, she asked, 'I want you to come with me into a room we have got hard by, and listen to something some friends of mine have to say to you.' By two's and three's women slipped into the improvised hall, where Sister Dora met them at the door and greeted each one by name, asking, 'How are you now?' or 'Is your arm better since I did it up for you?' Eventually, about thirty-five people joined in hymns and prayers and listened to a short address. It was the strangest service the young clergyman ever remembered. During his speech, a man pushed his way in jostling and jeering. 'Make him be quiet, Sister, do,' implored the women, and Sister Dora turned to the newcomer. 'Now then, Jack, none of that,' she said coolly. 'Sit down here by me and behave yourself.' To Fitzgerald's amazement the man sat down meekly beside her and listened to the rest of the service. In retrospect, however, her authority, remarkable though it was, struck him less than her manner with the women. 'There was something very touching,' he wrote later, 'in her attitude towards them. No condescension, no standing apart. No saying "I am holier than thou". It seemed to me that she knew them nearly all by name and she told me she had doctored nearly all of them at different times. Many of them used to seek her only after nightfall, but she was always ready to help.'[9] Sister Dora was determined not to lose touch with these women. She felt that, as a woman, she shared responsibility for their troubles. 'I feel so ashamed and distressed for them,' she said, 'to think I have been able to do no better than that for them, with all my trying.'[10] She would go in search of a missing girl, asking fearlessly for her by name in the roughest parts of the town. Just as the problem with the men was to provide an alternative to drinking, the problem with women was to find employment which offered a living wage. 'They are so terribly hedged in,' wrote Dora to a woman friend, Mrs Ridsdale. 'They cannot get back to the narrow way. Many do not fall from sin, but from their trusting, loving nature. I have visited them individually and heard their stories.'[11] Two of the women were arrested for robbery, and these she visited in the cells. For a few she managed to find work. 'Like her Master,' wrote Fitzgerald, 'she seemed never to despair of a human soul.' Her acts of charity she kept hidden. After her death, her solicitor, James Slater, revealed that she had used her private income largely to help old patients, whom she considered her special responsibility. She had given or lent money to convalescents until they were able to find work; where this proved impossible she had paid the passage money for whole families to emigrate. Sometimes a man was discharged from hospital, but was unable to work, because his tools had been pawned to buy food for his family during his uncompensated illness. Sister Dora redeemed these pledges, and, if the man could not repay her in cash, cheerfully accepted services in kind. Many small carpentry jobs about the hospital were done free as a result.[12] It was well known, and often resented, that Sister Dora seemed to have little liking for her own sex. Again, after her death, it emerged that this contempt was confined to idle women of the moneyed classes. To working women she had been a generous friend. On the evidence of a country physician at Sutton Coldfield, 'servants worn down by sickness, governesses and others dependent for their living on their own exertions, she often provided for. I was asked by her to find lodgings for them and give medical supervision and, when they left, to pay all their expenses and charge them to her.'[13] She was known to receive many letters from these women and from former patients; her executors, hoping to record her widespread charity, searched for them among her papers after her death. She had been careful to destroy them; not a single letter of thanks remained.

Her personal kindness was already well known in Walsall itself. It was revealed to the Black Country as a whole by a colliery disaster. In November 1872, flood water poured into a pit at Pelsall, cutting off twenty-two men for five days; they died of exposure and starvation, one boy having chewed his own boot-laces. During the week that the women waited at the pit-head Sister Dora lived among them, organizing an endless supply of food, hot drinks, blankets and shelter for their small children.

'Out of doors the scene is weird and awful,' wrote a correspondent; 'the intensity of the darkness is heightened by the artificial lights. Every object the most minute stands out in bold relief against the inky darkness which surrounds the landscape. On the crest of the pit-bank, policemen like sentinels are walking their rounds; the wind is howling and whistling through the trees, and the rain is hissing down in sheets. A form glides among the hovels, in the pelting rain, over the rough bank and through miry clay, now ankle deep. Her face is radiant with kindness and affection. On she glides, with a kind word to all. . . . Who is this good Samaritan? She is the Sister who for seven years has had the management of the nursing department at the Cottage Hospital at Walsall.'[14]

This is the first independent description of Sister Dora at work. Without seeking personal fame, she was becoming famous. 'We have just been to see the celebrated Sister Dora and I must tell you about her at once,' wrote a visitor to Walsall in 1872, who concluded his account, 'she is certainly as fascinating a woman as ever I came across.' She won the admiration of her bishop, the tall, rugged Selwyn of Lichfield, who had been the first missionary bishop in Melanesia. He came to have a great affection for Sister Dora, in whom he saw what he most valued, the common touch. He firmly denounced what he called 'the gentleman heresy', the social pretensions of the clergy, and insisted that he was bishop of the people. He came regularly into the Black Country to hold open-air services, and was to be seen eating his sandwiches on the cinder heaps beside the canals and waving cheerfully to passing bargemen. These journeys often included a visit to Walsall, where at Sister Dora's request, he visited the workhouse, to which she had no right of entry. She knew the paupers, young and old, sick or well, had to spend their days in a low, dark, damp hall. The bishop, having seen it for himself, insisted on improvements, although no infirmary was provided for the sick until 1896. He confessed that for him 'the simple Cottage Hospital had a special charm' and he nicknamed the indefatigable Sister Dora his 'one horse Chay', because she liked to do everything single-handed.

Her fame began to extend beyond the boundaries of the Black Country and the diocese. Frances Pattison, Mark's wife, described her remarkable sister-in-law to the Radical writer Edith Simcox. There are arguable grounds for thinking that she also described her to George Eliot, and that certain strands of Dorothy Pattison's personality are woven, through the character of Dorothea, into the complex tapestry of *Middlemarch*.[15]

This general and growing interest in Sister Dora was not because of her family background or personal life, which remained unknown except to a very few close friends. It was because of her religion. 'No topic excites the English world more than a religious topic,' wrote Mark Pattison himself in his *Memoirs*, and he did not exaggerate. Religion had the glamour in the 1870s of space-travel to the 1970s, with the same quality of being at once esoteric and universal. Everyone was curious about Sister Dora, though she did little to encourage speculation. She was reserved about religion, unusually so for an age when public displays of religious fervour formed part of ordinary social behaviour. Her public worship was simple. Every day she stood on the central landing of the hospital and read aloud Morning and Evening Prayer from the Book of Common Prayer. The double doors of the three wards were propped open so that patients could join in if they wished. In addition she read the collect and grace before the patients' lunch, and was careful this should not be neglected in the bustle of the day. 'Whatever you do, don't forget mid-day prayers!' was almost the only warning she gave to a pupil left temporarily in charge. Early every Sunday morning she was to be seen in her usual place, a corner at the back of St Paul's Church. Her well-worn prayer-book is still to be seen in the vestry at Hauxwell Church.[16] Every Sunday afternoon the wards were open to old patients, patients' families and friends. There was a short service, followed by a large, cheerful tea party and community hymn singing. Sister Dora played the piano and sang with whole-hearted pleasure, while miners, puddlers, railwaymen, their wives and children joined in lustily. Her voice remained as fresh and strong as when she had led the village choir at Hauxwell; if she attended a strange church on holiday, the most decorous Anglican congregation would turn round to see who was singing. For the enjoyment of her men she learnt the rollicking revivalist tunes of Moody and Sankey, but her own preference was for the hymns of Charles Wesley, who expressed her inmost feelings with elemental directness and simplicity. Her favourite was:

> *Then let us attend*
> *Our Heavenly Friend*
> *In his members distrest*
> *By want of affection or sickness apprest:*

> *The prisoner relieve*
> *The stranger receive*
> *Supply all their wants*
> *And spend and be spent in assisting his Saints.*

> *By word and by deed,*
> *The bodies in need,*
> *The souls to relieve,*
> *And freely as Jesus hath given, to give.*

On Sunday evenings if none of her patients were in danger she took the train to Wednesbury, for Evensong at St James's, Richard Twigg's church. These services were a source of great joy to her; there were no pew rents to exclude the poor, and no gift, however small, towards the Church's school, orphanage or old people's home was ever rejected. Sister Dora fixed her eyes on the unfamiliar altar, candles and cross; she was heard joining the singing of the choir with all her heart and soul. She listened to Richard Twigg's searching sermons which, she said, 'sent you away supremely uncomfortable about yourself'. He had started life as the youngest of a large poor family, in the West Riding mill town of Horbury. He left school early and supported himself as a clerk in Leeds, where he served as a lay worker under the great Tractarian, W. F. Hook, who helped him to take a degree at Durham and enter holy orders.[17] He knew industrial life at first hand, and was quite undaunted by the situation he found when he took charge of St James's Church and parochial schools, Wednesbury, in 1856. The parish lay in 'the lowest and most neglected part of the town', which had been devastated by the great cholera outbreak of 1849.[18] There was not a single tree or shrub over five feet high, and the church was hemmed in by industrial buildings. The population was described as 'males 2057, females 1882, Irish 565'[19] as though to emphasize the sub-human status of the immigrant.

Richard Twigg loved this parish. It was useless to tell him, as many did, that he was wasting his talents 'among the smokiest dens, and the half-civilized savages' of the Black Country. Soon St James's had lectures, classes, daily Matins and Evensong, and Holy Communion every Sunday instead of the usual once a month. The first parish missions in the Midlands, possibly in the Church of England as a whole, were held there. More than a thousand children came every week to the Sunday School. This ceaseless work was sustained by a life of intense personal devotion; Richard Twigg passes hours of the night in solitary prayer in his church. He is still remembered as 'The Apostle of the Black Country'.[20]

He understood Dora well, perhaps because they were alike in temperament. He forced her to look beyond her actions to her motives. Did she use the love and admiration which surrounded her 'to win souls', as she claimed, or to satisfy a need for power, long thwarted in her early life? It was a measure of her honesty that Sister Dora accepted this criticism as just. Dora returned his interest by nursing Mrs Twigg through her last illness, and continued to visit the family after her death. The Twigg children loved her. 'She was a lovable creature, so gay and winsome,' wrote one of the daughters to Baring-Gould. 'She used to come into our rather dull and sad home (our mother died when we were quite children) after evening service. She would nurse one of us on her lap, and the others would gather round and she would tell us stories.' The same daughter, grown up, added truthfully, 'She was a *real* woman, though, with all a woman's failings.'[21]

Sister Dora would have been the last person to deny it. She knew better than anyone the violence of the sudden impulses which often threatened to overcome her better judgment. She said she fought hard battles with herself, 'and by no means always came off victorious'. Her patients saw nothing of this inner conflict; to them she appeared as saint and guardian angel combined. Legends began to gather round her in her lifetime in the medieval tradition of dying beggars kissed and miraculous cures.[22] This cult developed after her death to fantastic lengths. Her virtues were even used as a stick to beat the people she had served. Margaret Lonsdale, determined to emphasize her heroine's spiritual qualities, said, 'She hated her life in this world', but endured it to improve those members of the working classes who 'grovel in sin and darkness, to lift and raise your souls to her own level, above sordid cares and weary drudgery, above low pleasures, brutal sports and animal passions'.[23] The patients can hardly have recognized in this admonitory figure the Sister Dora with whom they had such absorbing conversations about dogs and tumbler pigeons. She was said to object to their speech. 'Pain was often caused to her refined and Christian feeling,' said the Vicar of Walsall in a memorial sermon, 'by the oaths and language which proceeded from blasphemous tongues – what agony such conversation gave a pure soul like Sister's!'[24] She was held up to young girls as an example of vapid meekness, 'a loving, patient spirit, a sweet self-forgetfulness and devotion'. Her forthrightness, her passion and her astounding courage were all conveniently glossed over in her official image. Pious memoirs reduced her heroic figure to the insipid likeness of a plaster statuette in a church furnisher's window.

'There is a hidden life,' as F. Denison Maurice wrote of the Anglican religious orders, 'from which the outward life of charity proceeds.' This spiritual life, in Sister Dora's case, was marked by resolution and a profound reserve. It is clear that from the time of her broken engagement and illness in 1866 she adopted an increasing ascetic discipline, which may have been dictated by her abnormal temperament. It baffled and distressed her friends, who could see no meaning in it. A member of the hospital committee said he had worked with Sister Dora for fifteen years but had never seen her sitting down. 'It is better to wear out than to rust out,' she said. 'There seems so much work to be done, I grudge every moment I must spend taking care of this body.' When excited by a crisis or an interesting case she slept only four hours a night. Often she stayed up all night with a patient in danger. She loved the silent, dark hours of night duty and slept little in the day time. On many freezing nights she was woken from sleep by the clanging night-bell, which hung at the head of her bed. Dr MacLachlan used sometimes to scold, and sometimes to tease her about the drunk and disorderly casualties who woke her at night to attend to their cuts and bruises. She took the challenge seriously. 'It is hard,' she admitted, 'to see the Master in these poor degraded people, and yet, the Inasmuch holds good for them as for all men.'

Sometimes she would go to her room at the normal time, but deliberately avoid sleep by sitting on the hard floor and singing softly to herself the hymns which she called 'the dearest companions of her solitary life.' Her old servant, who slept next door, heard her praying far into the night. Food, like sleep, was a grudged necessity. Sister Dora, who herself carved in the wards and personally arranged every plate of food which was set before a patient, seldom ate a meal uninterrupted. She arrived back from visiting patients in the town too late, or had out-patients waiting, or was called away by the casualty bell. 'The diet she allowed herself,' a young nursing pupil noticed, 'was very meagre.' These girls looked forward to supper-time, when the day's work was done and Sister Dora would entertain them at table with 'intense fun and drollery', for her sense of the ridiculous was irresistible.

Yet on Fridays, or during Lent she would often look in at the door of their bare little dining-room and say, 'I don't want any supper tonight; I am going to bed. Good night.'[25] No one dared to argue.

Two acknowledged marks of mystical experience are authority and joy, both of which Sister Dora showed to the most casual observer. Colleagues and patients alike relied on her authority; visitors invariably noticed her happiness, which seemed to them so at odds with the sombre surroundings of her life. She sometimes suffered the depressions known to the mystical temperament, in which seasons of lively and difficult faith alternate, but these depressions, though sharp, were seldom lasting. Faith confirmed her passionate sense of the goodness of life; her love of God was feminine and ardent. As a young girl remarked with naïve surprise, 'Sister Dora made religion seem romantic.' In the last years of her life, by intense contemplation, she said, she 'sometimes seemed to see Jesus face to face as she went about her duties'. Like St Theresa she felt joy 'penetrating to the marrow of her bones'. Those who saw her every day felt that Sister Dora lived 'two lives inseparably blended. The outward life one of hard, unceasing toil; the inner, a constant communion with the unseen world'. Nurses grew used to the sight of Sister Dora rolling down her sleeves and buttoning her cuffs after a difficult dressing, with the words, 'Well, we must pray', which she said in the practical tone of one recommending hot fomentations or clean lint. At night when the wards were quiet, the other patients often saw her kneel at the bedside of one who was dangerously ill. If he was unconscious and unable to hear her, she said, 'That is no matter; our prayers go up for him just the same.'[26]

She never demanded religious conformity from others. The hospital committee issued each discharged patient with a printed form requesting his minister of religion to 'return thanks' publicly for his recovery. It was, in effect, a free advertisement. A Scotsman, a radical self-educated watch-maker, a reader of Voltaire and Tom Paine, indignantly refused to sign it. He said it was against his conscience. The committee, scandalized, tried to compel him. Young Mr Fitzgerald reminded him how good Sister Dora had been. 'Aye,' said the patient, 'I watched her closely, and she's a noble woman. But she'd have been that without your Christianity!' As a last resort they asked Sister Dora to coax him. To their amazement she refused, saying she had too much respect for his conscience to interfere. Her nearest neighbour at the hospital was the Roman Catholic Church of St Mary's the Mount, where she was on excellent terms with the priest. It is not easy to appreciate now how unusual this was in her day, when Agnes Jones, an educated woman, visiting the timeless beauty of Rome, could only see 'a city given over to idolatry'.[27]

The circle of friends bound together by the spell of her presence broke after Sister Dora's death into rival religious factions. Richard Twigg claimed her as a member of his Ritualist congregation, the Methodist Ridsdales were convinced she would have found her spiritual home with them, while the Roman Catholic priest revealed that she had approached him for instruction. Margaret Lonsdale believed she 'hated her life' in this world, and found her only satisfaction in mystical fulfilment, while Edith Simcox maintained that her 'very moderate Anglicanism was scarcely a part of Sister Dora's nature. . . . The secret of her passionate love of work lay in the impulse to run away from herself, the need to lose her own consciousness in the whirl of action'. A modern writer considers Sister Dora 'held firmly all her life to her own interpretation of the Evangelical creed'[28] but nothing seems further from the 'converted' state of the Evangelical churchman of the last century than her continual anxious quest for truth. Mark Pattison, imagining the rival religious groups gathered for this once-loved sister's funeral, dismissed them all, predictably. 'I shall not go to her funeral,' he wrote, 'as I should be sadly out of place among those Sisters and long-coated hypocrites.'[29] These judgments tell us more about the writers than they do about the living woman; her faith remains inexplicable in conventional terms. It is best described by the Congregational Minister, Thomas Hinsley. Sister Dora's religion, he said, 'was not dogmatic, controversial, old or new, or denominational. It is known how well she loved her Church, but no Noncomformist ever thought about the difference in the charm of her conversation. Her religion was as natural to her, and appropriate and fresh, and pleasing to all as the perfume or colour of the individual flower is. It was as impossible to describe as the charms of the flowers, but it was delightful to be within its influence.'[30]

In 1874 with two well-trained student nurses at the hospital, Sister Dora was able to leave Walsall for the first time in the five years she had been in sole charge. There were family threads, never quite broken, waiting to be picked up again. She went to Guernsey to stay at Forest Rectory with Eleanor. Her niece Nora, the child who had so delighted in the story of John Gilpin, was grown up and about to be married. Sister Dora entered into the wedding preparations, said Eleanor, 'with all the zest of a girl'. She arranged flowers, copied lists, sewed the bride's trousseau, and helped with the trying-on of the wedding dress, as though nothing more important had ever happened in her experience. Caught up in her enjoyment, the whole family felt themselves living at a higher pitch; 'it was hard', they wrote later, 'to believe that her actual life was passed in scenes of suffering and pain'. To their bitter regret, she suddenly left them a few days before the wedding, because of a crisis at Walsall. It was a sharp reminder that her life was committed to duties beyond their imaginings. 'No one in our little village', wrote Eleanor, rather wistfully, 'will forget that visit, nor her rich voice in church. Her absence seemed to us the great disappointment of that wedding day.'[31]

Dora stayed longer upon her other visit, a meeting with Rachel and her children for a shared seaside holiday at Coatham and a visit to Sister Frances at the Middlesbrough convent. There were now five Stirke daughters, Mary, whose birth she had witnessed, Jane Anna, Dora, Rachel and Philippa.[32] The sight of Rachel, after an interval of five years, was shocking; she looked ravaged and exhausted. As soon as they were alone together, while the children played upon the sands, she came straight to the point. Her heart was failing; she had been warned that she had not long to live, and she needed Dora's help. Rachel was under no illusions about her family's attitude to her marriage and she feared, with some reason, that Mark might attempt to deprive Robert of his children after her death. 'Whatever their father thinks best for the children when I am gone, let it be,' she said. 'Help him, but trust his judgment.' Dora, who had always been grateful for Robert's kindness, promised to do this. Yet Rachel was still not easy in her mind. She repeated often '*Never* let them be separated from him', and Dora, deeply moved, gave her word that she never would.[33] She loved the five girls, whom she visited without fail every year for the rest of her life. 'They are such good children,' she wrote to Mark. She grieved at the sight of Rachel's failing strength, but comforted herself with the thought that this favourite of all her sisters, 'our sweet Rachel', had married a man whom she greatly loved, and known many years of happiness.

On 8th November 1874 the scattered members of the Pattison family heard the news of Rachel's death. She was buried among her husband's people in Aysgarth churchyard, within sound of the great waterfall. Mark, who had ceased to care deeply for his other sisters, was broken by the shock. 'She is buried today at Aysgarth,' he wrote in his journal, 'my heart has been in Wensleydale since Sunday. . . . My world is half-perished in her loss!'[34] To Dora the news brought no shock or surprise; she had been expecting it for months. She clung to the memory of Rachel and Robert, their love and their last hours together. They had sat by the fire talking together, 'as only husbands and wives can', said Sister Dora to Eliza Ridsdale. A few hours later Rachel had become distressed. Robert held her in his arms to support her; she smiled at him, when he realized she had already ceased to breathe. Dora, who had watched so many death agonies, was grateful for this end. 'It was beautiful,' she said, 'to be taken right from the heart of home, husband, children – yes, beautiful!'[35]

Rachel's death left her with a problem of conscience which was not settled until the end of the year. Mark was determined that one of his sisters should take charge of the motherless girls and bring them up by Pattison standards. On 30th November he 'wrote to Fanny expressing my wish that she would go to Bellerby to mother the children'. He received in reply 'Vexatious letter from Fanny, who is insisting on going back to Middlesbrough and leaving the Bellerby children to themselves'.[36] Mark was somehow unable to believe in the reality of his sisters' professions; his next choice fell upon Sister Dora. It was her duty, he said, to leave her work and look after the orphans. Dora was alarmed. Suddenly she realized that Walsall, with its drifting smoke and roaring furnaces, was home, as the moors and streams of Yorkshire had never been. The people of the Black Country were nearest her heart, 'yes', she admitted, 'nearer than my own flesh and blood'. Above all, she loved her work. 'I cannot make up my mind,' she wrote, 'to give up all this work and go to them. I admit it is selfishness on my part which makes me hesitate. No one knows what it would cost me to give up work, home, friends and go to that barren moor.' When she spoke of leaving, James MacLachlan grew angry. The work of the hospital depended on her. She was a fool, he said bluntly, to consider leaving hundreds of patients, to keep house for a family, which any other woman could do just as well. 'And if you leave, Sister,' he said with grim humour, 'then I might as well go and lay my head under the next railway train.'[37] Yet she had written her letter of resignation, and actually laid it before an appalled committee, when Sarah Pattison's kindly husband, Dr Richard Bowes, came to the rescue. As family doctor, he would help Robert Stirke bring up the five motherless daughters. He and Sarah, who to their sorrow were childless, would help to arrange schools, holidays, outings and treats. Mark appears to have protested, but now Dora dealt firmly with him. 'As to the arrangement at Bellerby, I am content, for it is carrying out Rachel's plan. R. Bowes' considerate kindness to them all is a beautiful trait in his character.'[38] She ended the year with a prayer of thankfulness that 'everything seems to have grown dearer'. She was on the brink of her greatest work.

NOTES

1. Ridsdale, 6.
2. H.R.C. Register of Associates.
3. The building proved unsound and was replaced in 1893 by J. L. Pearsall's fine Gothic church in local sandstone.
4. *Walsall Observer*, 5th June 1875.
5. Lonsdale, 172–4.
6. Ridsdale, 30–31.
7. E. R. Pike, *Human Documents of the Industrial Revolution*, 294–5.
8. Ridsdale, 45.
9. Lonsdale, 186, quotes Fitzgerald's account of the missions.
10. Ridsdale, 32.
11. Ibid., 45.
12. W.C.H. MS., 1868.
13. Lonsdale, 127.
14. Quoted S. Baring Gould, *Virgin Saints and Martyrs*, 377. The

scene is represented, from contemporary sketches, on Sister Dora's monument.

15. This suggestion is fully developed in Appendix B, *Dorothy Pattison and George Eliot.*
16. It was presented by Eleanor's daughter, Lady de Saumarez, last survivor of the large Pattison family.
17. *Midland Advertiser*, 17th and 24th May 1879.
18. J. F. Ede, *History of Wednesbury*, 310–12.
19. Ibid.
20. F. W. Hackwood, *Religious Wednesbury*, 117–19.
21. S. Welsh, *General Baptist Magazine* (1889), 272.
22. Lonsdale, 52.
23. Ibid., 2nd edn., 1887, 5.
24. W. Allen, *Three Sermons*, 1879.
25. Lonsdale, 197.
26. W. James, *Varieties of Religious Experience*, lists Sister Dora among the undoubted Saints.
27. Jones, *Memorial of Agnes Jones*, Diary for 1862.
28. M. Price, *Inasmuch as*, 15.
29. Pattison, 131, f. 57.
30. Lonsdale, 255.
31. Ibid., 125, quotes this letter to herself from Eleanor Mann.
32. P.C.C., 1879, f. 38. The spelling Stirke had been adopted by this date.
33. Pattison, 57, f. 71.
34. Ibid., 130, f. 90.
35. Ridsdale, 8–11.
36. Pattison, 130, ff. 93, 97.
37. Lonsdale, 130.
38. Pattison, 57, ff. 69–71.

CHAPTER SEVENTEEN

Disaster Area
1875

❋

No one in a position to know doubted the dangers of a serious epidemic in Walsall. They had been steadily impressed on Sister Dora by a succession of people. Old John Burton had never forgotten his experiences as a young man in the cholera outbreak at Haddington. Redfern Davies's family had played a leading part in establishing the first Fever Hospital at Bath Row, Birmingham, where father and son donated their services as physicians. The Poor Law Medical Officer of Walsall, Dr Drewry, described his alarm at the condition of sick paupers in the workhouse. There were no nurses, no sick wards, and paupers suffering from infectious diseases were isolated in unheated outbuildings, including a woodcutter's shed. Drewry was so disturbed that he had threatened to report the Guardians for negligence to the Local Government Board.[1] All agreed that the town needed a fever hospital. If Sister Dora had any doubts about this, they were swept away by her experiences in the relatively minor smallpox epidemic of 1868. She threw all her personal influence and powers of persuasion into the campaign to make the Borough build an isolation hospital. A site was bought on the outskirts of the town in Deadman's Lane, an unpropitious address hastily changed by municipal bye-law to Hospital Street. Building went on in 1872, but too slowly. It was overtaken by the world-wide smallpox epidemic of 1872–3. *The Lancet* reported that in June of 1872 there had been 127 deaths in Walsall from smallpox alone.[2]

The summer was unhealthily damp; while the fever hospital slowly rose, sporadic outbreaks of infectious diseases, especially smallpox, occurred all over the town. Sister Dora, as in 1868, went out to nurse them in their own homes; she herself suffered a few days' sharp illness, described as 'some unknown fever caught from a patient'. She had to send home two patients who developed smallpox and a little boy of six with measles, and this distressed her. Dr Drewry noted 'various local causes which favour the spread of any epidemic and which are particularly bad at Walsall – to wit defective sewerage in overcrowded courts, which are ill supplied with water. The special causes seem to have been even worse at Walsall than elsewhere, such as the enormous number of unvaccinated children, the overcrowding and the difficulties in the way of isolating cases of infectious disease'.[3] Another local doctor wrote of Walsall's 'large area of squalid buildings, peopled by a degraded and outcast race',[4] as a danger to the whole district, since the town stood on a main railway line, and formed a centre for workman from other places. Everyone hoped that Walsall's problems would be solved when in August 1872 the Epidemic Hospital opened at last. There was room for fifty patients, twenty in four acute wards and thirty in male and female convalescent wards. Outside stood a wash-house, a mortuary, a disinfecting oven, and a shed for the horse-ambulance. The wards were entirely bare, cold and lofty. None of the windows would open, for they were closely barred with iron to prevent the escape of infectious patients. Ventilation was by cowls set at intervals in the iron roof. The whole had cost £2000 and was the pride of the Medical Officer, who maintained that 'There is every possibility of the hospital being extensively used'.[5]

The next three years proved him wrong. The working people of Walsall regarded this grim, prison-like building with loathing and dread. It was administered by the Board of Guardians as an annexe to the workhouse. There were no nurses; the only attendants were able-bodied paupers from the workhouse, with an ugly reputation for pilfering, drunkenness and brutality. During the years 1872–5 the patients consisted mainly of children from the workhouse, where there was a serious outbreak of scarlet fever, and the waifs and strays of the streets. Not surprisingly, a high proportion of patients died. Walsall mothers refused to let their sick children be locked up in 'the Epidemic', and no one would enter it voluntarily who had relatives or neighbours to care for him, however roughly, outside. In February 1875 the year's first cases of smallpox were notified at Walsall.[6] At once it spread in the crowded courts and alleys with terrifying speed. Smallpox spreads by direct and mediate contagion, and by air; whole epidemics may start with a single case coming from afar. As usual the Irish were blamed. 'Wherever these abject and deplorably ignorant creatures colonize,' it was said, 'dirt, disease and misery are sure to follow.' In fact the most potent cause was overcrowding; the disease spread street by street through contact with bodies, living or dead, bedding, or the communal rags in which whole families were clothed. Of all diseases smallpox evoked especial horror and terror; its potential victims awaited hideous disfigurement, blindness or death, with the apathy of despair. The duties of Medical Officer in an outbreak were large but vague. He was ordered to 'give such warning or instruction to the persons affected as may be calculated to induce them to have recourse to medical treatment'.[7] In other words, he had no powers of compulsion. Dr MacLachlan, who had succeeded Dr Drewry as M.O.H., did his best to persuade patients to enter the Epidemic Hospital. He always met the same reply. 'Leave us alone; we would rather die at home.' Nothing seemed to convince the poor of the danger they were in. A landlord was fined for letting a house where a whole family had died without disinfecting it, and a woman for selling the clothes of her dead son to various buyers, all of whom were attacked by smallpox.[8] The appearance of the smallpox ambulance with its sinister black hood in any street, was the signal for doors to be slammed and shutters bolted. Patients with streaming pustules were hidden in upstairs rooms to infect every member of a household crammed from cellar to attic with helpless humanity. By February 1875 reports spoke of smallpox as 'rife' in Walsall, and the County Asylum refused to accept any patients from the town.[9]

Meanwhile at the Walsall Cottage Hospital the wards were quiet, and there were three student nurses, two of them reasonably experienced. This was the situation one morning at the end of February when Sister Dora came to the Secretary, as he was dealing with correspondence in the Hospital's little office. They talked about the urgent need to isolate new cases if the smallpox epidemic was to be contained.

'Do you know,' said Dora, 'I've an idea that if there were some one at the Epidemic Hospital whom people could trust, they would send their families to be nursed. After all, no one is afraid to send their relatives here.'

'Yes,' said Welsh rather gloomily, 'but who is there whom people trust, who would be willing to nurse there?'

'I would go,' said Dora.

He was completely taken by surprise and tried to talk her out of it; but she had an answer to all his objections. What would happen to the Cottage Hospital in her absence? 'Oh, plenty of people would come here,' she said, 'but who wants to go to a smallpox hospital? Besides, it would only be for a short time.'

'But what if you should catch the disease and die?'

'Then,' she said cheerfully, 'I should have died in the course of duty and no one can die better than that.'[10]

She went off, laughing at his glum expression. That afternoon she approached Dr MacLachlan and next morning the Mayor. To the young nurses, she simply said, 'You must divide the work between you, and try to do your best till I come back.' By the afternoon of the next day Saturday 27th February, she set out.

The site of the old Walsall Epidemic Hospital is now a slum clearance area, where tall engine houses look out over acres of rubble. Margaret Lonsdale, who visited it during 1875, described vividly how it used to be.

You drive down the hill on which the Cottage Hospital stands and go on, seemingly for ever, through dirty, dreary streets and lanes. Then you leave even these signs of habitation behind you and pass along a road with heaps of slag from the iron furnaces on either side. You arrive at last at the Epidemic Hospital. It seems the end of the earth and you look back on smoky Walsall with the crowning church steeple and teeming inhabitants as from a desert land. The hospital is a long, low building, of one storey forming two sides of a square, with entrance in the angle. In front about a quarter of an acre of ground is planted with cabbages for the use of the patients and these dismal-looking rows of blackened vegetables seem to add to the desolation of the scene.[11]

James MacLachlan drove Sister Dora down this road on a raw February afternoon, as the winter dusk was closing in. All around them giant slag heaps shut out the sky. The only living creatures to be seen were the rag-pickers, crawling over the mounds of foul garbage on the dumps, in search of saleable clothing or scrap iron. Not a tree, not a bush showed on the skyline. As Sister Dora stood on the doorstep and looked around here, she shivered with an instinctive, primitive dread. She said it was the first and only time in her life that she felt the loneliness of her long struggle against suffering and distress. Her courage failed; she clutched MacLachlan's arm and exclaimed, 'Take me back! Oh please take me back! I cannot bear this dreadful place! I know I said I would come here, but I did not know it would be like this!' Dr Mac-Lachlan knew Sister Dora and how to deal with her. He was never a man to waste words. He simply unlocked the door and said, 'Come in.'

Inside lay more than twenty-five patients, men, women and children of all ages, all in the acute stages of smallpox. From the moment they opened the door the air was heavy with the greasy foetid smell typical of the disease. 'It smells of the pox,' said Dr MacLachlan. In front of the fire, airing some sheets, sat a very old, very dirty Irishwoman who was the workhouse 'nurse'. Dora described her as 'a regular old Sairey Gamp and Grimes combined, who shouts at the patients and is filthy.' She made up her mind to get rid of her as soon as possible. On a quick round of the beds she made another discovery. 'All these patients are *alive*'! 'That is generally the case,' said MacLachlan unemotionally, 'with smallpox and dirty people.' His last sight that afternoon was of Sister Dora rolling up her sleeves in the kitchen and putting on water to heat for washing the patients. Next morning Samuel Welsh knocked at the Epidemic Hospital door. Sister Dora opened it. 'What are you doing here?' she said. 'What are *you* doing here?' 'I have come to take care of the patients.' 'Then,' he replied, 'I have come to take care of you.' She let him in, watching him with covert amusement. 'He kept a respectful distance from me and the patients,' she wrote to the young nurses at the Cottage Hospital, 'but do not tell him I said so!' She was grateful, though, and sent him off to the Town Hall with a list of her demands, disinfectant, flea-powder, bars of soap, scrubbing brushes and flannel for children's nightgowns. The babies had been wrapped in old newspapers and bundles of rags, until the flannel arrived, when she reported, 'I made garments for all my urchins today.'

By the end of the first week she was writing as if she felt completely at home. 'I have made everything as respectable as I can. My room is between the wards with little windows peeping into both. There is just room for my bed in one corner, chest of drawers and slip for my washbasin, so I shall do very well.'[12] What cheered her most was a visit from one of her policeman friends, who declared that everyone on his beat was saying they would not mind coming to the smallpox hospital now, with 'Sister' to nurse them. On her second day, seven new cases arrived, by 10th March another nine. In all, according to Dr MacLachlan's report, twenty-five cases were admitted in February and fifteen new cases between 27th February and 15th April, of whom six suffered from confluent smallpox. Thanks to Sister Dora's care, only one patient died, though five had died in the Workhouse before being transferred to Hospital. Some of them were very ill; the worst case, a boy of eighteen was delirious and got out of bed to stagger round the hospital until she isolated him in an empty ward. One man was threatened with blindness, and a woman struggled so violently that it took two people to hold her down. There were two babies, one a year old and one even younger, who wailed day and night. 'They are so cross, poor things,' said Sister Dora, who finally found she could soothe them by holding them in a bath of warm water. By the end of the first fortnight she reported, 'They are getting quite fond of me.' It was harder to know what to do for the adult patients; all she could attempt was continual cool sponging to relieve their discomfort, until the fever began to subside and the pustules to dry up. She persevered with cold compresses, continually changed, which she hoped might reduce the disfiguring scars. The worst problem was the public's superstitious dread of the disease, which made it impossible to get help. 'I have my hands full,' wrote Dora on 1st March, 'for I cannot get a decent woman to come, although we pay well. I have two "critturs" from the workhouse; one is so hopeless I have to do the work for her; the other sits up at night, so can do no more.' Dr MacLachlan found two old women to do what even Sister Dora admitted was 'the loathsome washing' of clothes and bedding. Her chief helper on weekdays was the porter. On Saturdays he went off all night 'on the drink'

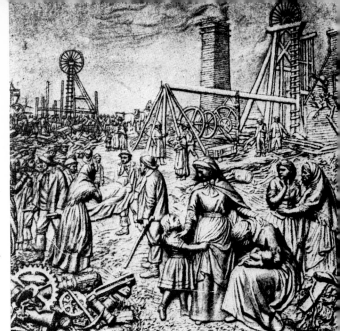

18. Sister Dora comforts women and children at the Pelsall Colliery disaster of 1872

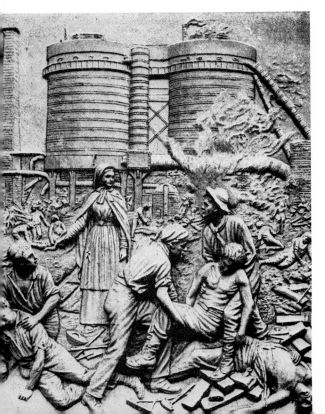

19. Sister Dora after the blast furnace explosion at Walsall in 1875

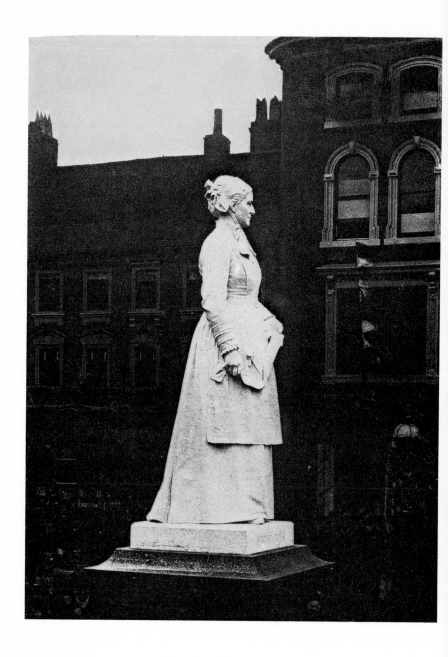

20. The original Sister Dora statue

as he frankly explained, and returned on Sunday evenings having
spent his week's wages. Dora overlooked this for the sake of his
kindness and his practical help. 'The fellow is an old soldier and
very good to me,' she wrote, 'always lights the kitchen fire and
does the range; he even scrubbed the kitchen floor early this
morning to save me.'

As March passed she established a regular rhythm of life. Dr
MacLachlan visited every day. Fitzgerald visited and found Sister
Dora entirely herself in these gruesome surroundings. 'She was
very cheerful indeed,' he wrote, 'and I remember she admitted
that she did hope, if she got the smallpox it would not make her
too hideous!'[13] As he was a classical scholar, this led to an ani-
mated conversation about Pompey's handsome soldiers, quite in
her usual style. Samuel Welsh brought books, flowers, fruit for
the patients. She made the well-scrubbed wards, she said, 'gay
with flowers and sweet with violets' for Easter Sunday. She even
found time to read aloud to the patients in the evenings. Privately,
she admitted that she missed the interest and the continual change
of surgical nursing. Above all she missed her old patients, and she
wrote them a letter, asking the nurses to read it aloud and 'tell
me everything they say'. It contained affectionate messages for
each of them by name, and an apology for leaving them so
suddenly.

My dear children,

What did you say to your mother running away? I dared
not tell you, and could not trust myself to come and wish you
good-bye, for I felt it too much. You know how I love you all
and care for you and it is for this very love that I have left you.
The smallpox was spreading in the town and might have spread
to your wives and families. Patients would not come to this
hospital until they heard I would nurse them. Now they are all
willing to come and there is not one come in who does not
know me. . . . All have been out-patients or had someone at
the hospital belonging to them. We are like old friends.

This boast, made with such ingenuous frankness, was true. The
crisis of confidence was over. By 27th March, when she had been
working in the Epidemic Hospital for a month without, as she
said, even putting her bonnet on or walking as far as the gate, the

new cases were getting fewer. The disease lingered for months, but the danger of a total disaster was past, and it was her presence which had averted it.[14]

Spiritually the weeks spent so much alone were a period of strange contentment. On 4th March the text for the day was 'I will allure her, and bring her into the wilderness and speak comfortably to her'. Its beauty seemed to sum up her situation, and continued to haunt her for weeks afterwards. She wrote to Richard Twigg on 10th March, 'I think I may almost say it is a closer walk with God. With the pestilence all round, you cannot help living every day as if it were your last.' A month later she wrote in almost the same terms to her brother Mark. He had broken a silence of nine years to send her a letter about a legacy, evidently in his most freezing style. 'I was glad to get any kind of letter from you,' she replied, 'though I cannot say it was "a nice letter". I think if you knew all my thoughts you would believe that I *do* take an interest in you. Never anything issued from your pen but I get it, so that I may know something of you. Goodbye, dear Mark, I say goodbye lest this should be the last letter you receive from me.'[15] She even wrote to her solicitor, asking him kindly to pay all her bills immediately 'for I wish to set my house in order'. As the number of new cases dwindled, the danger grew less, and she began to turn her mind to the future. On the last day of April she wrote, 'I thank God daily for my life here. I believe he sent me, and has blest it, and I hope from henceforth I shall serve him better.'

Many times during the summer Dr MacLachlan and Sister Dora believed the epidemic was over, but the variable incubation period for smallpox meant that single unexpected cases kept appearing. She went out to search for new patients in the little smallpox ambulance, no longer an object of dread, now that she was seen, as an onlooker said, 'with her jolly face laughing and smiling out at the window'. In early May she wrote, 'I am still a prisoner here, surrounded by my lepers, but I do feel thankful that I came for no one hesitates to come here, now they know I will nurse them.' The cases grew milder as the epidemic waned, though they persisted through May and June. In July James MacLachlan took Sister Dora for drives in his open carriage to enjoy the air, which seemed like a miracle of freshness after her weeks of imprisonment. She confessed she had sometimes felt ill, 'breathing the poison so much'. From June onwards she began to return three times a week to the Cottage Hospital, with the precaution of a bath and a complete change of clothes each time. There she attended out-patients, assisted MacLachlan with operations and dealt firmly with the young nurses who had quarrelled among themselves and with Sarah Watts, in her absence.[16] With so few patients at the Epidemic Hospital, she had leisure in the evenings, and begged Samuel Welsh to lend her what he rather primly called 'sensational railway fiction', the yellow-backed shockers sold on station bookstalls. Sister Dora adored a thriller; she sat up night after night devouring them. When, in August 1875, she at last closed the Epidemic Hospital, she was forced by the risk of infection to burn them. 'Oh dear,' she was heard to say, as they curled in the flames, 'I did enjoy those stories!'

Sister Dora received official recognition from the Mayor and Corporation, which reported to her employers on the Cottage Hospital Committee, 'there can be no doubt that the efficient manner in which she discharged her self-imposed duties tended in great measure to stay the ravages of the disease.'[17] 'We were in a great fix,' said the Mayor frankly. 'We had no nurse, but she came, like the good Samaritan she always was, and thanks to her, the plague which threatened has left us.' He proposed a vote of thanks to loud applause.[18] Dr MacLachlan, in his report as M.O.H., said that only the opening of the Epidemic Hospital under Sister Dora had kept the epidemic in check. For good measure she had spring-cleaned and whitewashed the building, discovered a damp wall in the kitchen, and demanded new floorboards from the startled Board of Guardians. The *Dictionary of National Biography* erroneously states that she 'resigned her connection with the Cottage Hospital to take charge of the Epidemic Hospital'; but there was no question of this. Nominally she was in charge of both hospitals and she went with the full support of the Committee. The same however could not be said of the Sisterhood.

These months at the Smallpox Hospital had a result which neither Sister Dora nor anyone else had expected. They led directly to the breaking of her connection with the Coatham Homes. For the last four years she had in practice been making her own decisions, but she had remained nominally under the direction of the Reverend John Postlethwaite and his nursing Sisterhood. In taking charge of the Epidemic Hospital without asking or even telling him, she had gone too far at last. Mr Postlethwaite wrote with unwonted sharpness to the Hospital Secretary. 'Her going without even consulting me was not only contrary to the rules, but leads me to fear a repetition, which might involve me in responsibilities for which I am not prepared. I knew nothing of her intentions and was not aware she was going to the Epidemic Hospital until I heard she was there, and I am therefore not prepared to assume responsibility or fill her place, if she absents herself again. May I also point out that had Sister Dora died, the consequences might have been very serious?'[19] As his attitude to religious vows, and the hiding of his real motive for opening the Cottage Hospital had already shown, he was nervous of public opinion. In fact the popular picture in the early memoirs of gentle Sister Dora browbeaten by a harsh fanatic is a ludicrous reversal of their roles. Mild, timid, conventional, Mr Postlethwaite must have spent some anxious hours wondering what his headstrong Sister would involve him in next. This time, he had really had enough. His attitude was so unexpected, said the hospital Secretary 'that the members of the Committee were quite disconcerted, but Sister Dora soon put them at their ease, for she announced her intention to sever her connection with the Sisterhood'.[20] Her resignation passed without ill feeling on either side; it was no more than a recognition of fact. She was loyal to the Home, always praising its excellent work and the kindness of the Sisters.[21] She always spoke with affection of her time at Coatham, and the Chaplain remained to his dying day extremely proud of her. Perhaps time softened the remembrance of how impossible it had been to keep her in order.

Sister Dora resigned in the summer, and found one unexpected freedom as a result. For more than ten years she had worn the habit of a nursing Sister. Now, if she went on holiday, she could wear what she pleased and pass unnoticed. 'Look out,' she wrote to young Eliza Ridsdale who was arranging to meet her, 'for a plainly dressed, ordinary lady. On holiday I lay aside my Sister's dress so that I can enjoy myself freely in recreations like swimming, or skating in winter – two of my favourites. But I have quite forgotten how to dress in any but Sister's fashion!'[22] When met by the Ridsdales she was wearing a black dress and jacket, and a black straw bonnet trimmed with blue ribbons. She who had been vain about her gloves, was disconcerted to find her small shapely hands had grown a size larger, from hard work. 'I cannot wear sevens any longer!' she exclaimed. She went to Yorkshire for a short summer visit to Rachel's girls. Robert Stirk had taken a new farm named Grazing Nook, near Fingall, in the country which Dorothy had hunted as a girl. Kind as ever, he offered to mount her if she cared to ride again, but it was too long since she had been in the saddle. She accepted the loan of a sturdy cob in the dog cart, and drove for miles over the moorland lanes, returning happy and excited, with glowing cheeks. The holiday must have been short because she was back in her surgical wards early in September. The hardest work of the year still lay ahead of her.

On a Friday afternoon, 15th October 1875, the worst accident ever known in Walsall took place at the works of the Walsall Iron Company in Green Lane, the Birchills. At about half past four molten metal from the blast furnace was being tapped into the prepared moulds for pig iron. Nearly the whole of the molten iron had been run out when the tuyère at the base of the furnace burst.[23] A number of men were standing round when a thick cloud of red hot ashes and a torrent of molten metal was blown over them. The owners at their desks in the works office opposite, thirty yards away, saw a cloud of flame burst from the boiler and had just time to throw themselves on the floor out of reach of flying cinders; a storekeeper and his mates were knocked to the ground by the blast, and not a pane of glass was left in the windows. The noise brought men running from all over the foundry, and though many of them had seen pit disasters, they all declared they had never seen such an appalling sight in their lives. Fourteen men, one of whom could not even be identified, and a young boy 'holder-up' were writhing where they had been flung on the ground. Three in their terror and agony ran to the canal which ran by the works and jumped into the water. A workmate jumped in to rescue them and found to his horror that when he grasped a burnt arm large portions of flesh came away in his hands. All the men had their clothes burnt from them and large areas of tissue destroyed.[24]

The owners of the iron works, two brothers called James and Kenyon Jones, kept their heads in this nightmare. They sent one messenger to warn the Cottage Hospital and call Sister Dora, and the other to fetch blankets, oil and cabs from the station. Sister Dora arrived to direct the lifting of the men, whose screams, said an onlooker, could be heard from far off. They moved the burnt men by saturating them with oil, rolling them on to blankets, and lifting the blankets by the corners on to the seats of waiting cabs.[25] By the time they had climbed the long hill to the Mount, Sister Dora was back at the Hospital waiting for them, having made arrangements 'with intelligent promptitude'.

Not a bed in the hospital was free when the news came. She sent all the patients in Barnett Ward home, with the exception of a little girl who was too ill to move, and whose cot she wheeled into her own bedroom. There was just time to scrub and disinfect the ward before the first patients arrived, still carried in their blankets. The bearers set them down on the hall floor, where Margaret Lonsdale, passing on her way to duty in a ward, saw with horror that they looked 'more like charred logs of wood than human beings'. They were all in a state of shock, cold, clammy and tortured by thirst. Sister Dora, before attempting any other first aid, knelt beside each in turn, speaking to him by name and dextrously slipping spoonfuls of brandy between the pale dry lips. Only when the danger of total collapse was past would she allow them to be moved. One by one she had the survivors carried in and with infinite difficulty cut their scorched clothes away from them, for the surgeons to dress their burns. Their groans and cries for water rang through the building, to the horror of the other patients. A general call was sent out to all members of the medical committee, and four of them worked with Dr MacLachlan until three o'clock the following morning.

Sister Dora, calm in the chaos, concentrated on practical matters. The first step was somehow to get rid of the crowd of well-meaning visitors, the Mayor, the Chamber of Commerce, the lady volunteers, who crowded the hospital, only to faint at the sight, sound and smell of the burnt men. 'You had very much better go home,' said Sister Dora, with concentrated sharpness, to an unfortunate clergyman, who had sunk under a wave of nausea on the stairs. This was no work for amateurs. Two, or possibly three of the men were already dead, and the bodies were carried straight to the outhouse which served as mortuary. Another five or six had small burns from splashes of molten metal; these she dispersed among the wards for her pupils to nurse. The patients whose beds they took were put on mattresses in the passage until they were fit to be sent home. The homely, familiar small hospital took on the air of a beleaguered camp or a refugee centre after some great natural disaster. Sarah, in the kitchen, produced extra meals and an unending supply of hot drinks day and night, for the rescue workers. The remainder, ten men burnt deeply on face, neck and arms, some on their legs and one all over the body, Dora laid in rows in one ward where she attended them herself. Three were men in their late fifties, three others only twenty. She must have known from the start that all were beyond hope.

The peculiar difficulties of treating burns had been recognized, though they could not be accounted for, throughout medical history. As early as 1607 Fabricus wrote of an 'ulcus profundum et putridum' after the separation of a burn slough. The great French surgeon Dupuytren, writing in the nineteenth century, recorded suppuration, fever, wasting and death in patients with deep burns, even where these were not extensive.[26] Within a few hours every burn was colonized by a variety of the bacteria which abounded in hospital, presenting an extreme example of cross infection, the 'hospital disease' which was the dread of every nineteenth-century surgeon and nurse. In 1875, in a small provincial hospital, the nature of bacterial contamination was barely guessed at. None of the resources now considered essential for the treatment of large burns, laboratory tests, air-conditioning, blood and plasma transfusions, chemotherapy or skin grafting,[27] were available to Sister Dora and the surgeons at Walsall. All she could do was to keep the badly burnt men in rigid isolation, for the sake of the other patients, and to protect their burns as far as possible by ample dressings. She knew from experience that, because of natural recuperative powers, this sometimes allowed smaller burns to heal. She abandoned all her other work and shut herself up in the ward with her men, allowing no one else to attend them. She asked the clergy of every church and chapel in the town to appeal in their Sunday sermons, for all the old clean

linen which Walsall households could spare. During the following
days, literally hundreds of bundles of old linen were brought to
the hospital from all over the town. She also asked for mineral
water which, with brandy, was all the men could swallow. Later
she begged for fresh eggs, and fed them with spoonfuls of egg-
flip. The owners of the iron-works, James and Kenyon Jones,
devoted themselves to their injured workmen, and scoured the
countryside for eggs and fruit. The poorest in the town brought
Sister Dora small coins from their savings 'to cheer her heart' as
they said.[28]

During the first night the man whose whole body was burnt
died. He knew he was dying and his agony was so intense that he
welcomed death. Hearing his mates call for help from all sides, he
said simply, 'They wants you worse; go to them first.' His name
was Phillips and Sister Dora said she would always honour his
memory. Next day, Sunday, a second man died; the remainder
lingered, some for as long as ten days. No one at that date could
fully understand the cause of their illness, but all showed the same
symptoms, fever, wasting, apathy or confusion and raging thirst
from loss of plasma. Sister Dora scarcely left them; she moved
continually from bed to bed, feeding them with spoonfuls of fruit
juice, or brandy in mineral water. The smell of dead and decaying
flesh in the ward was so appalling that even the doctors were overcome by waves of nausea, but Dora remained there day and night.
It was impossible to take food in these conditions, but she
swallowed sips of the patients' brandy. She took short spells to
change and rest, but for nine nights, although she was on duty
all day, she did not take off her clothes or go to bed. 'She was
with us night and day,' said one of the two survivors. He described
her going from bed to bed, talking, laughing, even joking with
the burnt men; sitting by their bedsides telling stories to divert
them, 'Sister's tales' as the patients called them. She never mini-
mized their pain, and always moved them with the tenderest care.
Nor did she try to conceal from them the approach of death. It
would have been impossible and she believed they were entitled
to know. Instead she talked very quietly and simply of her faith
in an after-life, and long after they had lost consciousness she
followed them with her prayers. One after another, in the ten
days after the explosion, ten men died. Sister Dora was with each

of them until the last. She felt herself the instrument of some spiritual force which bore her up, transcending human strength or skill. Without it she could hardly have lived through those ten days. Afterwards she was drained of emotion and totally exhausted.

Of the patients seriously burned in the explosion, only two survived, a Walsall man named Ward and an Irish labourer, Martin Cassity. They were both 'fillers', working at the top of the furnace, and as the explosion rocked their bridge, both had instinctively thrown up their hands, to protect their eyes from the sudden flaring of the flames. Both were burnt on hands, arms and feet. They stayed months in hospital, while the slow healing took place, and Dora watched them with anxious care, dressing their burns herself and coming down to check their dressings every night. 'There she went,' said Cassity, 'in shawl and slippers, silently going round at two in the morning, from bed to bed, smiling as she went. It did you good simply to look at her.' Sister Dora promised him a new pair of boots as a leaving present, but the bootmaker, after one look at his mutilated feet, said, 'You'll never wear boots again with those.' Cassity returned very downhearted, but Sister Dora burst out laughing. 'You'll wear out many a pair of boots yet, my burnty.' 'And,' said Cassity, 'she was right enough, but it was all along of her, who never left my burns a day, all those months. What we felt for her I couldn't tell you, for my tongue won't say it.' Exactly twelve months after his accident he was back at work.[29]

The explosion at the Birchills Furnaces had far-reaching effects, both for the hospital and for Sister Dora herself. A coroner's inquest on the dead men established the cause of the disaster. The foreman admitted that he had ordered the furnace to be over-filled, so that it would not need topping-up before he went off duty at the end of his shift. He had been in the habit of doing this and the wonder was that there had not been an accident sooner.[30] In fact, a similar explosion was to take place in the same iron works ten years later. The town, it was clear, was quite unequipped to deal with any major industrial disaster. Before October was out a large meeting was held at the Guildhall to open a fund for enlarging the hospital. Dr MacLachlan and Sister Dora wanted to emphasize the dangers of cross-infection and the urgent need for a new isolation ward. They found a spokesman in the town's Methodist minister, Mr Ridsdale, father of Sister Dora's young friend Eliza. He asked the meeting 'What could we give, in comparison with what was given by that heroic, great-hearted woman Sister Dora? What sacrifice could we make to compare with her hourly and incessant duty? I could not tell you of all I have seen and heard her do in the last ten days. You cannot and must not let the evening pass without showing Sister Dora her example has not been wasted, nor her labour given in vain'. There was loud and continued applause, a subscription was opened in the room and £600 was collected before the meeting broke up.[31] This was added to the £1100 already saved in the Building Account by Sister Dora's laborious economies since she took charge in 1868. The Mount, with its old-fashioned out-buildings, had served, more or less unaltered, as hospital for the last seven years; everyone agreed it was time to add a new wing. Sister Dora had already pointed out the shock to child patients of seeing dreadful mutilation and painful deaths.[32] The Secretary wrote to ten architectural firms inviting tenders.[33]

These plans were swiftly overtaken by events. When the last of the burns cases had died, Barnett ward was scrubbed out, with Sister Dora's usual homely thoroughness, and reverted to general surgical use. It is now known, of course, that such measures were quite inadequate to control the spread of a virulent infection in a hospital ward. The bacteria which cause such infections, for example the haemolytic streptococcus of erysipelas, may be carried in the throat or nose of nurses, to infect susceptible patients. Similarly, of course, patients, particularly when crowded together, may infect each other. A hundred years ago they threatened everyone inside the hospital walls with cross-infection. In December 1875 the first case of erysipelas appeared in the Walsall wards. Dr MacLachlan wrote for advice to two of the leading physicians of the day, Sir William Gull, F.R.S., of Guy's Hospital, and Sir James Simpson. In spite of anything they could suggest, the virulent infection spread from ward to ward. To Sister Dora's horror, Eliza, one of the young housemaids caught it and very nearly died.[34] The simplest cases were now liable to dangerous complications. Dr MacLachlan reported that one patient had been in hospital twelve weeks with a minor injury to his toe, another with a simple fracture of the arm, 'as had also a third with a slight scalp wound whose face was now in such a condition that his features could not be distinguished'. They thus found themselves, after eight years' hard work, in the same situation which had forced them to move from Bridge Street in 1868. He asked that 'Sister Dora should be empowered to refuse any fresh cases'.[35] This forced a decision; from January they admitted no new patients, but allowed the wards to empty gradually, while the Committee looked for a house to rent as a temporary hospital. At the same time they resolved to build in the grounds at the Mount, a completely new specially designed general hospital, of thirty-six beds, with room for expansion.[36] The out-patients department would remain open and Sister Dora would walk to it every afternoon from her temporary buildings, a ten minutes' walk uphill through heat, cold and wet, which she firmly insisted she enjoyed. 'Otherwise I shall get so lazy,' she said, 'that I shall never take to harness again.'

The Committee attempted as a temporary measure to rent the Epidemic Hospital, but were prevented because the Town Council had no legal power to let it. On 1st March 1876 as a last resort, they rented a house from the L. and N.W. Railway Company, which was clearly unsuitable in every way; they assured Sister Dora in all good faith that she would only have to endure it for a few months, until the new hospital was ready. In fact she was to stay there for more than two years. The temporary hospital stood in Bridgeman Place, a dark and narrow street which plunged sharply under an iron railway bridge and flooded with black and scummy water in every rainstorm. Close beside the railway bridge, so close that from passing trains one could see in at the first floor windows, stood a dingy three-storied house where every room seemed to open on a steep and narrow stair-case. It held ten beds for emergencies, but there was not a spare bed for another nurse, and Dora, rather thankfully, said goodbye to her 'lady pupils' whose emotional rivalries had been a perpetual worry. The Committee, saying 'she would kill herself with work', offered to engage a trained nurse to assist her, but this she obstinately refused. She was very fond of her old night nurse, Mrs Harrison, whom she had trained herself and knew to be, though uneducated, utterly reliable and very kind to the patients.[37] She stayed with Dora until the end of her life, and never complained of the difficulties at Bridgeman Place. Dora said that every passing train seemed to shake the house to its foundations, and the shriek of train whistles woke her feverish patients from their sleep. In the end, she went to the railway station and begged the engine-drivers, many of them former patients, not to let off steam near the hospital. 'You'd never believe how quiet they are now,' she said.[38] She dealt with the rats, if they ventured upstairs, by direct assault; her skirts gathered closely round her, and the kitchen poker in her hand, she could kill a large fierce sewer rat with one well-aimed blow. To the patients it was as good as a free show; all who could, left their beds and crowded in the doorways to watch, cheering her on with shouts of 'Give it him, Sister!'[39] Sister Dora flatly refused to take burns cases into this building; she said she would rather visit them daily and dress them in their own homes. The Committee realized that this entailed a vast amount of extra work upon the Sister and the surgeon, but promised that it would only be for a few months as they hoped to take possession of the new building in the autumn. During the year 1876 Dora visited 12,127 patients, and by ill fortune received an unusual number of hopeless crush injuries, of whom ten died, four of them being under fourteen years old.[40] Her one dread was another major disaster before the new hospital was ready.

Sister Dora and Dr MacLachlan were not cast down, whatever their difficulties. The prospect of a hospital built to their own specification was too exciting. They formed themselves, with the Chairman, into a special sub-committee to make detailed suggestions on the plan. They emphasized that no old materials must be re-used; the new hospital must be 'germ-free'. They wanted the wards to be wide and airy, with cross-ventilation. Sister Dora wanted the corridors much wider than usual, and glassed-in to form a sun-room for convalescents. Dr MacLachlan wanted an operating room, completely isolated, with a window from floor to ceiling. Finally, Sister Dora insisted, every ward must have its own bathroom, with hot and cold water, its own water-closet and sluice. The Committee members were stunned. 'If all these suggestions were carried out,' asked the Mayor, 'would the surgeon and the Sister be satisfied?' The Sister said they would.[41] Unanimously the Committee resolved to fit out the largest bedroom with a special grate, chimneypiece, bookshelves and fittings, 'to make it suitable for a comfortable private sitting-room for Sister Dora'. The Mayor of Walsall arranged for his own gardener at his own expense to lay out the grounds of the new hospital, while other Committee members presented turf, shrubs and trees. Their wives collected furniture and sewed linen. These hard-headed Midlanders had been totally converted to the idea that only the best was good enough for the sick poor, and the revolution in their attitude was largely the work of Sister Dora. To her the new hospital was the reward of her years of work; but she was never to see her patients in its wards or to occupy the sitting room prepared with such affection. The tall, dark house in Bridgeman Place, ringed with the flares of blast furnaces, and shaken night and day by passing trains, was to be the scene of the last drama in her life.

NOTES

1. Walsall H.M.C., *A Century of Walsall Hospital Services*, 44. The workhouse finally opened an infirmary with two trained nurses and four probationers in 1894.
2. *The Lancet*, 27th July 1872. See Appendix C.
3. Ibid.
4. F. W. Willmore, *History of Walsall*, 437. See Appendix C.
5. *The Lancet*, 3rd August 1872.
6. F. W. Willmore, *History of Walsall*, 431.
7. *Public Health Act*, 1848, Section 40, Duties of the Officer of Health.
8. *The British Medical Journal*, 26th June 1875.
9. *Walsall Observer*, 13th March 1875.
10. S. Welsh, *General Baptist Magazine*, 1889. He made a shorthand note of their conversation and could reproduce it verbatim.
11. Lonsdale, 140–41.
12. Ibid., 144. Sister Dora wrote a series of letters to the Cottage Hospital, but it is not clear to whom they were addressed.
13. Sister Dora was theoretically immune, having had smallpox in March 1865. Many exceptions have however been recorded, in which people have caught the disease twice.
14. See Appendix C.
15. Pattison, 57, ff. 69–71. The legacy was a small bequest under the will of Mrs Huntingdon, a cousin of their mother.

16. Lonsdale, 137, apparently felt she should have been left in charge. She believed Dora was jealous of a potential substitute, but it is much more likely that she simply expected to return to the Cottage Hospital after a week or two.

17. W.C.H.A.R., 1875.

18. *Walsall Observer*, 8th August 1875.

19. S. Welsh, *General Baptist Magazine*, 1889. Mr Postlethwaite was probably thinking of the riots in Lewes churchyard which had broken up the funeral of a young nursing Sister from the community at East Grinstead, some years earlier. He dreaded a similar scandal.

20. This did not necessarily prevent her from remaining, like her married sister Sarah Bowes, an Associate Sister of the Holy Rood. She certainly visited Sister Frances at the Middlesbrough convent in 1874, 1876, and shortly before her own death in 1878.

21. Ridsdale, xv.

23. Ibid., 36–7.

23. The tuyère is the hole at the base of the vertical furnace through which hot air is blown at high pressure to provide the 'blast'.

24. *Walsall Observer*, 16th October 1875.

25. This scene is illustrated in a relief of the Sister Dora statue.

26. E. J. L. Lowbury, "Infection of Burns", *The British Medical Journal*, 2nd April 1960.

27. Ibid.

28. *Walsall Observer*, 23rd October 1875.

29. Walsall H.M.C., *A Century of Walsall Hospital Services*, 21.

30. *Walsall Observer*, 30th October 1876.

31. Ibid., 22nd October 1875.

32. Ibid., 13th March 1874.

33. W.C.H. MS.

34. S. Welsh, *General Baptist Magazine*, 1889.

35. W.C.H. MS., 1876.

36. W.C.H.A.R., 1876. This forms the nucleus of the present Walsall General Hospital.

37. Lonsdale identifies her as Mrs R. The Hospital Committee paid for her mourning clothes after Sister Dora's death, since she was too poor to buy them herself.

38. Lonsdale, 179.

39. Ridsdale, 24–5.

40. W.C.H.A.R., 1876.

41. W.C.H. MS.

CHAPTER EIGHTEEN

The Flame and the Dark
1876–1877

❋

Sister Dora had lived through a year of concentrated and intense experience. For six months of it she had been alone, virtually a prisoner in the smallpox hospital, carrying single-handed responsibility for all its patients. She had known the pangs of Rachel's death, Mark's cold hostility, and the final parting from the Sisterhood which had once re-shaped her life. Finally after the blast-furnace explosion, she had endured the anguish of living among the dying. One might almost say she died with them, for she emerged to a new life.

This was revealed when during the 1930s a plumber and a decorator working independently in a large house at Highgate, Walsall, each found a packet of letters in Sister Dora's handwriting. Both men took the letters home, and each eventually, after an interval of more than twenty years, offered them to the local paper for publication.[1] When these two sets of letters are interleaved and read in order of writing, they tell a story of great poignancy. They are addressed to Kenyon Jones, of Cawney Bank House, on the hill above Dudley;[2] he was one of the two brothers who owned the blast furnaces where the explosion had taken place. At a casual glance they appear formal, for until almost the end they begin 'Dear Mr. Jones' or 'Dear Mr. Kenyon' and finish 'Sister Dora'. This impression is misleading; the Pattisons were old-fashioned people who followed the eighteenth-century usage of full names, even in family letters. These are the letters of the woman, not the nursing Sister, a revelation of the young Dorothy Pattison, quickening into life within the public figure of Sister Dora.

Kenyon Jones apparently first saw her on the day of the explosion as he helped to carry his men into the hospital. On that day, and the dreadful days which followed, she hardly noticed him, but during the next few weeks she came to know him well. He and his brother James came regularly to visit their workmen who were patients in the hospital,[3] bringing fruit, eggs, wine or any special comforts she needed for the convalescents. He won her approval by his care for the families who had lost their breadwinners in the disaster. He designed, and had made in his own workshops a set of overhead pulleys to lighten the work of lifting helpless patients. It was a practical gesture of thanks to the hospital and to Sister Dora for all she had done.[4] Kenyon Jones's visits to the hospital became more and more frequent. On New Year's Eve Dora put him off, because she always went to the midnight service, but on New Year's Day 1876, and many days after, he appeared in the wards. The patients, who observed their nurse closely, after the manner of patients everywhere, began to ask slyly at tea-time, 'Sister, are the visitors coming tonight?' Sister Dora was at a loss to answer them, and in January sent an ingenuous note by 'my faithful servant Murray', the porter. 'You didn't say when you should come again, but I do like to know when to expect you – for I should not like to be out or not finished my work. Now is not this very unlike a lady's letter!' Kenyon Jones replied that he would like to come every evening, but was sometimes prevented when the furnaces were working full blast. He suggested she should look out of her top-floor window in the direction of the ironworks, where the orange and crimson flames would act as a 'flamerometer'. This childish joke pleased Dora immensely. 'I look towards it the minute I get up in the morning,' she wrote. 'It is burning very brightly. Come on Monday, at what hour you like; you will be welcome and you are sure to find me at home.'

Kenyon Jones did not need any further encouragement; he called again and again. He was thirty years old, more than six feet in height and very handsome, a vigorous sportsman, fond of the open air and animals. A neighbour remembered him exercising two dogs regularly in his eighties, and sporting to the end of his life 'a fine pair of Victorian moustaches'. His niece remembers him as 'a dear, kind man'.[5] His masculinity swept like a fresh breeze through the closed world of the hospital in which Sister Dora had lived for so long. She was curious about this businesslike extrovert, so unlike the more reflective, intellectual men she had known in her girlhood. She enjoyed writing to him, but wanted to be sure her letters were private and would not be seen even by his brother. He assured her they would not. 'Then I can chat any kind of nonsense,' she replied, 'now that I know it is for your eyes alone.' To safeguard her reputation from gossip she always sent her letters by Murray, whom she could trust completely, and Kenyon Jones always posted his replies away from Walsall. Dora's letters were affectionate, playful, frank. If he had a cold, she fussed over it with brandy and hot water; if, schoolboy fashion, he attempted to send a kiss she teased him. 'Must I read the finish of your letter literally? It reads thus – your X (cross) friend!' Now do you find time to wonder how I can write all this nonsense to you?' She even took up a discarded game of her girlhood and on 9th January 1876 sent him a few lines of comic doggerel:

What has stirred the Poet's lyre
Which so long has silent been?
Is it flame or burning tuyere,
Is it love that ancient theme?
Surely it is not for gain.
Kenyon shall I tell you why?
All your guesses have proved vain –
It is cu-ri-os-i-ty!

'Are you not shocked,' she concluded, 'at my being so curious?'

There is no sign in these letters of the serious mental affinity which everyone had noticed ten years earlier between Sister Dora and the man who then wished to marry her. Kenyon Jones could teach her nothing about her work, and little about life in general, for she was a mature, experienced woman. To judge by what she wrote, she enjoyed his company and his frequent notes, without thought of any serious consequences. Secure in her work and her faith and accustomed to the discipline of everyday duty, she clearly did not realize how vulnerable a woman in middle life may be. She laughed at the young man's schoolboy jokes, forgetting how laughter disarms and leaves the heart open to deeper emotions. In the spontaneous pleasure of friendship, she was too light-hearted to see that she was skating on thin ice indeed. Her nature was incapable of shallow or guarded emotions; she knew no way of feeling except deeply. There must surely have been some half-remembered tide in the blood to warn her that she was falling in love with this decent, perhaps rather commonplace young man, yet she showed all the blind impulsiveness which MacLachlan had shrewdly noted as a dangerous feature of her character. As for Kenyon Jones, he was unable to resist her fascination. He did not realize she was some fifteen years older than himself. Her manner, which others found 'playful and winning', was innocently flirtatious towards him. His visits were spent in a happy dream, notes and letters passed to and fro, the weeks slid by uncounted by either.

On 5th February 1876, less than four months after their first meeting, affairs reached a crisis between them. Kenyon came to call and Dora, exempt from the chaperonage rules which bound other women,[6] received him alone in her little office-sitting room. They sat up till late into the night telling 'stories of older days', always an emotional subject. The long conversation ended in a love scene. Dora wrote with rueful amusement next day, 'If the Formidable Pastor[7] had walked in upon us two last night (when I was still his Sister) I should have had to bid farewell to Walsall the next morning.' Kenyon wrote her a letter so compromising she was forced to burn it, a prudent action which she immediately regretted. 'The resolution was never passed,' she wrote, 'that you would not write again. Besides if you had done, I should always break a rash vow. Your last letter was sufficient compensation for the one I was obliged to burn.' From this time onwards she was unquestionably in love with him.

Kenyon Jones was a Black Country man; he appreciated as no outsider could have done the difficulties of Sister Dora's position. Outwardly she appeared mistress of her own actions to an extent very rare for a woman of her times. Yet in fact she was the prisoner of her own legend, as conspicuous in Walsall as a reigning queen, and as circumscribed by duty. Especially since the smallpox epidemic and the blast furnace explosion of the previous year, she no longer belonged to herself, for she had become the guardian angel of all. 'Sister Dora was as like the Lord Jesus Christ as any human could be,'[8] said a grateful patient, and thousands echoed this opinion, without considering the burden they laid upon a very human woman. The doctors, the hospital committee and the clergy, all had a vested interest in her supposedly superhuman virtue. Because she was good, they insisted, she must be perfect. Her loneliness, like the loneliness of Agnes Jones at Liverpool, they believed to be ordained by Providence, which 'did *not make* these noble Christian workers happy wives, but set them apart, with their own full and joyful consent, as nurses of the sick and poor'.[9] Through this sentimentality ran, as so often, a streak of cruelty. No one seems to have considered, with the exception of Dr MacLachlan who knew her best, that she was growing older, often tired, lonely and herself hungry for the love she poured out on others. Dora accepted the burden; for the sake of her work there must be no scandal. She told Kenyon Jones that their meetings and their correspondence must be secret from all. Reluctantly, he seems to have agreed and a strange element in both their lives began.

She gave him her photograph and he gave her a locket which she wore on a chain, hidden under her Sister's black dress. She wanted a picture of him and hit on the old stratagem of cutting his face out of a group photograph. 'Get down among the group being photographed on Monday,' she begged. 'You would be lost in the multitude and I should so like to have you!' Once the hospital had moved to Bridgeman Place in March 1876 she had fewer in-patients and went out and about more than she had for years. Her letters are full of the innocent gaieties of Victorian provincial life, hand-bell ringing, yeomanry manœuvres, a Christmas tree for the children at a ragged school in Dudley, a harvest festival at church. Any public gathering formed an excuse to meet and exchange a few murmured words undetected by the crowd. The element of risk added zest to these occasions for Dora. 'You ought to be very careful what you are doing and with whom you talk if you do not want it to be known,' she wrote. Yet, eternally feminine, she did not want him to be too careful. 'You would not look at me in Birmingham last night,' she complained. She was adept at letting him know, in the most artless manner, where she was going to be on any given evening. 'I shall be at the meeting at the Agricultural Hall tomorrow night,' she wrote in February 1876, 'so if you should come here, it must not be till later – unless you will be tempted to come too. I should be very pleased to see you at the meeting, for I think I should enjoy it more.' A few months later: 'Tomorrow, if all is well, I am going to Birmingham by the 4.55. What will you think of me? Will you come to meet the train?' They travelled together to Dudley, to see his family home in 'its winter robe of snow', to Birmingham, to Ironbridge in Shropshire, and these carefully-arranged accidental meetings on the train, as she admitted, set her heart beating fast.

All witnesses agree that during 1876, the first year of her secret love, Sister Dora appeared youthful and radiant. She went for a short holiday at Saltburn on the Cleveland coast with the Ridsdale family, who had never seen her more pretty or more gay. 'Under her leadership,' said Eliza, 'we scaled fences, forded streams, wished at the Wishing Well, scaled Cat Nab, and enjoyed a scramble in the glorious breeze.' Dora swam every morning before breakfast, and took long solitary walks on the deserted shore. She went shrimping with the fishermen and boasted, 'I caught ten pennyworth – very fair for a first attempt.'[10] She took a rowing boat out to sea, with Eliza's sixteen-year-old brother, pulling on the oars as strongly as a boy. She walked as far as Marske, to see the village and the parsonage which would have been her home, if eighteen years earlier she had actually married James Tate. The young curate must have seemed a pallid and dim figure beside the reality of her present love. The Ridsdales, of course, knew nothing at all of this; they merely felt their staid family holiday transfigured by her fantastic vitality.

In hospital circles, colleagues must have noticed some change in her. She, who had been so gracious to all, was plainly irritated by the open admiration of Dr MacLachlan's junior assistant surgeon, whom she found too familiar. '*Please*,' she wrote to Kenyon, 'do not let Mr. Sharpe know that I am at home of an evening. Tell him I can see nobody – and that is final. I can only see Somebody.' She, who had always been on call twenty-four hours a day, was sometimes unavailable. 'I found something had happened during my absence,' she wrote in comic dismay. 'The Committee had come and gone!' The only record of a break in her work is a letter of July 1876 when Dora admitted that she was tired out and had spent three days in bed on Dr MacLachlan's strict instructions. 'I have felt so strong and well this last fortnight I could jump to the moon, so was very prodigal of my strength, and when some bad accidents came in on Monday, I thought I could work all night as well as all day and went on at that rate until Thursday when not feeling well I came to rest awhile and here I am. But the Doctor has given me leave to go down to-morrow, so I shall see you at the usual time . . . you must not disappoint me.'[11] Dr MacLachlan was a man of very few words; he put nothing in writing, but he must surely have been concerned for his old friend. He knew better than she did how dangerously she could swing from exaltation to depression, if circumstances changed. Dora herself insisted she had never been better, never happier in her life. 'The more I have to do,' she said, 'the stronger and happier I feel. You know I am as strong as ever I was – strong as a donkey!'[12]

The religious conflict of her broken engagement in 1866 was not repeated. There was no slackening in her ardent devotion. Kenyon Jones was sympathetic to her faith, though perhaps he could hardly realize its full intensity. He could not openly accompany her to church, but he attended services where he knew she would be, at St Paul's, Walsall, on Hospital Sunday and St James's Wednesbury, where he heard Mr Twigg preach. The presence of the rich young ironmaster must have caused some speculation in these humble congregations. Dora felt close enough to him in spirit to lend him one of her most treasured possessions, Rachel's prayer-book which Robert Stirke had sent her; 'the Prayer Book was my favourite sister's,' she explained, 'and she pasted in those little pictures to keep them safe. I do not know why, but I half expected you to bring it back last night.' She could never speak easily or glibly of spiritual things, but some letters to Eliza Ridsdale's mother hint at the depth of her feelings. 'I realized as I had never done before,' she wrote after a service for the prostitutes, 'God seeking the soul, even from the first moment man fell. The thought of my being so close – one has only to turn round, not to come even – makes one strong.'[13] She wrote about the meaning of her work; 'as St. Paul was a tent maker, so I am a tent repairer, always putting a stitch here and there to these earthly tents of ours'.[14] At the New Year's Eve of 1877, when she held her usual party for present and former patients, they sang Wesley's

watch-night hymn, which she greatly loved for its haunting
words:

Our life is a dream.
Our time as a stream
Glides swiftly away
And the fugitive moment refuses to stay

The arrow is flown,
The moment is gone.
The millenial year
Rushes on to our view and eternity's here.

Come let us anew
Our journey pursue.
Roll round with the year
And never stand still till the Master appear.

It found an echo in the letter she wrote the next day to the
Ridsdalse. 'The old year is rolling round with all its joys and
sorrows, trials and temptations. We cannot help sitting down by
the milestone and remembering how much of our journey is
done.'[15] To one of the young Ridsdale girls she wrote with
understanding about a disappointment in love. 'My dearest, do
not think because some people don't write that they forget or do
not care. Life is very full if one does faithfully what God gives to
be done in the present. Take it and every circumstance as direct
from Him. Our lives would be so different, I believe, if we were
living with God at the heart of things.'[16] For the present, she
herself took her love, like her work, as a circumstance direct from
God and gloried in it. Both she and Kenyon Jones were living as
though neither past nor future existed; but this could not continue. Many things combined to make the idea of marriage impossible: Dora's public work, which he could not share as her
former fiancé had done, the scarcely veiled doubts of the Jones
family, the fourteen years' difference in their ages, and her own
hereditary instability of temperament. The relationship threatened
to cause scandal damaging to the hospital, just when it most
needed the public's goodwill.[17] Finally, Dora was reminded
sharply of the agonizing decision to break her engagement and

her strange illness ten years before; the reminder came in an unmistakable form. 'I went to sleep last night,' she wrote to Kenyon on 3rd January 1877, 'hoping to dream of my lost ward keys, but instead I had a most frightening dream. I actually dreamt I lost my leg. Oh how thankful I was to awake and find it only a dream!'

The connection with the events of 1866 was clear, and to her impressionable temperament the nightmare had all the force of a warning. This impression was confirmed a few days later by an event which caused her the deepest self-reproach. She was summoned to a patient far outside the town, promised to go to him after seeing all her out-patients, and, in the pressure of work, forgot. Next day she remembered, but as she walked over the field paths 'feeling', as she wrote to Kenyon, 'awfully dejected, a woman rushed up to me and said, "Too late, Sister Dora, too late!" He was dead. My moral courage failed me more than ever. I thought of retiring on the spot from public life.' Abruptly, as always with her temperament, she plunged from exaltation to the depths of despair and self-blame. Love, she thought, had made her selfish. Her instinct, shrewdly noticed by Edith Simcox, was always to run away from herself, to bind her unruly temperament by an implacable discipline. She knew by now that the answer for her could not be found in a convent, but it was still to religion that she turned for help. Shortly afterwards, when Walsall's Roman Catholic priest was visiting his parishioners in the wards, she asked him for a private interview. They went into her little office, scene of so many happy and affectionate evenings with Kenyon. There she made a full, though informal, confession, and asked, 'Is it my duty to become a Roman Catholic?'

Father Joseph McCarten was a Doctor of Divinity and a parish priest of long experience. No one had done more than this plump and genial man to make Catholicism respected in the town. He was a good musician, a lively preacher, a warm-hearted friend and a generous opponent. Dora both liked and trusted him. She spoke to him freely, and something which she now revealed convinced him that she could never be received into the Catholic Church. He was not of course at liberty to say where the difficulty lay, except that 'the obstacle was quite unconnected with religion'. She became so distressed during the course of their discussion that, as he wrote, 'I was obliged to insist that the question should never be revived in our intercourse.'[18] The difficulty was perhaps connected with various hints of a burden which lay upon her conscience. Mr Postlethwaite wrote of 'another matter', about which they had long corresponded. Louisa Twigg wrote of her 'woman's faults', Margaret Lonsdale of her 'desperate battles against an ambushed enemy'; Edith Simcox remarked that in her, as in many saints, 'there are the makings of a sinner'. Sister Dora seemed sometimes to despair of herself. 'Oh don't talk about my life,' she wrote to a woman friend. 'If you knew it you would be down on your knees, crying for mercy for me, a sinner. How God keeps silence so long is my wonder.'[19] Nothing in Sister Dora's conduct seems to justify this despairing self-reproach; she was to all the most generous and loyal of friends. The truth will never be known, but she was perhaps ashamed of her passionate sexuality, at a time when she was no longer young, and decent women were authoritatively said to be incapable of sexual feeling. 'Love of home, children and domestic duties,' wrote Dr William Acton in 1857, 'are the *only* passions they feel.' Dora herself read an article on the growing freedom of women which suggested 'the animal is practically extinct; the soul and mind are dominant. In fact civilization obliterates sex'.[20] Significantly, she told Kenyon Jones that this had not been her experience. To Margaret Lonsdale she said she felt a sense of failure at falling in love, and it had taught her humility. It is tragic that she should have felt so. In love she understood and shared the deepest feelings of ordinary people, and it was from this that she drew her profound compassion. Nevertheless the burden of guilt lay heavily upon her at this time.

She could not avoid meeting Kenyon Jones so long as they both lived in the same town. As late as 14th July 1877, when she was summoned as witness in a law suit at Stafford Assizes, she sent him a note begging for moral support – 'it seems so natural to turn to you. Do come tomorrow evening. I have just met your brother and told him of my misfortune. I shall need you so much. *Do come.*' Perhaps James Jones disapproved of this urgent summons. Soon afterwards Kenyon Jones made a business journey of some months to South Africa. When he returned, in the winter of 1877–8, he neither wrote to Dora nor came to see her. Evidently he had decided, or had been convinced, that their equivocal relationship must end. Dora was convinced that they would never meet again. Restless and dissatisfied, she confessed, 'I have such a longing to travel this year.' She played with the idea of going to Rome with some friends for a holiday, or of joining Louise MacLaughlin's Red Cross unit in Serbia;[21] but in the end it was always Walsall and work which held her.

The hope of the new hospital buoyed her up. She petitioned in September 1877 for the new out-patients' department to be built first, since crowds of eighty to a hundred patients waited for her every afternoon. With the help of the architect, she arranged a public exhibition of plans to interest and attract subscribers. Mr Henman, the architect, who modestly described his plans as 'of the Brick-o-logical Order' was surprised by the response.[22] Sister Dora followed every detail of the building programme with a precision worthy of Florence Nightingale. The machinery for the hospital laundry and drying rooms, the hot-water pipes for the corridors, the kitchen ranges, the gas-fittings, the bell-pulls by each bed, the speaking tubes, the glazed tiles for the antiseptic operating room, the sinks for cleansing wounds, and the wide doors to permit moving helpless patients in bed were all planned and installed to her exact requirements. Nothing was too large or too small to escape her notice, from the revolutionary idea of 'a recovery room near the theatre for persons operated on and unfit to be removed to a ward', and a day sitting-room for convalescents, to door-scrapers at every entrance 'to reduce dirt on the floors'.[23] The committee voted unanimously that she should be invited to lay the foundation stone of the new building, but she refused. The Jones family would be present and perhaps she feared emotional strain; in any case she cared more for the reality than the trappings of achievement. The Chairman and the Mayor 'waited on Sister Dora with a view to inducing her to accept', but as so often found the tables adroitly turned upon them. Before they left, the Chairman found himself agreeing to deputise for her at the foundation ceremony.[24]

The future of the hospital looked brighter than ever before, and this gave Dora hope. She needed it, for, apart from private griefs, she was working under unspeakable conditions at Bridgeman Place. The hospital and her nursing had become famous throughout the Black Country. The committee received continual applications from doctors wishing to join the consulting staff, which was now considered a mark of professional distinction.[25] They also wished to send her their serious cases, but with only ten beds, Dr MacLachlan would admit only desperately injured. The nursing of these helpless patients, particularly two railway shunters, who had had both legs severed on the line was heavy on body and mind alike.[26] Sarah Watts and Mrs Harrison, the night nurse, were both elderly women and Dora would not allow them to carry heavy weights up the steep, winding stairs. Instead she herself ran up and down with buckets of water, hods of coal and rolled up mattresses. The staircase was too narrow to admit a stretcher, so she carried helpless patients up to bed in the wards in her own arms. She improvised a sling for carrying the bodies of patients who died, down to a room in the damp rat-haunted basement, which served as a temporary mortuary, since she would never allow a body to remain in the ward. Burns cases she flatly refused to admit to the temporary hospital, fearing the spread of infection to surgical patients with open wounds. She preferred to visit them in their own homes, though, as Dr MacLachlan warned the Committee, this entailed 'a vast amount of extra work upon the Sister'.[27] Every evening at six, when old Mrs Harrison the night nurse came on duty, Dora harnessed the pony and set out on a round of visits to towns and villages within a ten-mile radius of Walsall. She called at the camps and shanty towns where labourers on the railway line lived and in these brutal surroundings found several seriously injured men. She paid for their board and lodging at an inn, where she visited them every evening during the winter of 1876–7. She was seldom home before ten, but defended her 'owlish habits' by saying she enjoyed the drive under the stars. She was once attacked on a lonely road, but came to no harm. During these expeditions in 1877, she successfully treated more than three hundred burns cases in their own homes, as well as nearly fifteen and a half thousand patients in the out-patient department.[28]

In spite of these mental and physical strains, she wrote cheerfully to the Ridsdales at Easter 1877. 'This is a glorious day and we are all busy preparing for laying the foundation stone of the new hospital. I am very well indeed and working hard.' Not long after this, she began to find difficulty in lifting heavy patients. She had always delighted in her own strength of body, and impatiently dismissed this as a passing strain. Yet it did not pass, and after the departure of Kenyon Jones she found herself increasingly fatigued by any physical effort. For weeks, stretching into months, she fought it off. In the end, at some unknown date in 1877, she consulted a doctor.

Some clinical instinct born of long experience, must have warned her, for she did not turn to Dr MacLachlan, or to any of the Walsall consultants. She drove herself in the pony carriage to Sutton Coldfield to consult the physician to whom she had sent, at her own expense, poor women patients in the past and whom she looked on as a personal friend.[29] He examined her carefully, formed an opinion and referred her to Dickinson Crompton, F.R.C.S., consulting surgeon to the Birmingham General Hospital. Crompton was one of the leading Midland surgeons and, as Sister Dora herself said, 'From his opinion on a surgical case, there could be no appeal.'[30] He confirmed what she already suspected; she had cancer of the breast. He advised an immediate and radical amputation, but she asked for time to consider the alternatives. After a few days she came back. She had nursed many cases of mammary cancer, she said; she knew from personal observation how mutilating the operation, as then performed, was likely to be and how uncertain the final result. This was true. 'Repeatedly,' wrote a nineteenth-century surgeon, 'one must weigh the possible gain to the patient against the hazard of increasing her suffering.' Breast cancer was at that time considered an inevitably fatal form of the disease. 'Once cancer of the breast becomes widely disseminated,' read a standard authority, 'the patient's days are numbered.' Sister Dora, who had studied surgical text-books under MacLachlan's direction, certainly knew this. An operation might prolong her life for months or even years, but it might also leave her without the strength to continue her work, which, since the end of her love affair, was what she lived for. 'After a short struggle,' she wrote, 'I made up my mind to allow the disease to run its natural course, and I am firmly resolved that no one shall know of my condition.' She knew that her illness would be a professional secret with the two doctors, and that she could continue to lead a normal

life for as long as her strength lasted, without well-meaning interference from friends and relations. This was all she wanted. It is
striking that neither man seems to have attempted to over-
persuade her, or to conceal the fact of her inevitable death.
Crompton considered her fortitude and self-control exceptional
in his long experience of cancer patients; it was, he later said,
'more than mortal'. Sister Dora went back to the temporary
hospital in Bridgeman Place. She was thankful to live alone there;
although for many months there was no sign of illness or suffering about her, it was easier to keep her secret with no other
woman to observe her close at hand. She began to work with an
intensity and urgency greater than ever before. Later, someone
remembered her saying, 'There seems so much left undone,
so many opportunities lost, so much time wasted.' She was
determined to make the most of every day that remained to her.

From now on she showed special affection to everyone she
had loved in the past. She mourned the loss of a friend of
Middlesbrough days, old Sister Mary who died in autumn 1877,
still at work in a home for incurables which she had founded.[31]
In August 1877, Dora took her five nieces for a seaside holiday.[32]
Mary, Jane Anna, Dora, Rachel and Philippa Stirke were as
dear to her as their mother had been, but there was nothing
cloying in her affection. On this holiday she taught them all to
swim, striking out through the waves with the greatest vigour
and enjoyment. She gave them a croquet set, and suggested tennis
for the following summer. Only later, they recalled, 'she did not
walk quite so far or fast as in earlier years'. She went to London
to stay with Louise MacLaughlin, who had returned with Emma
Pearson from the Serbian war to a triumphant reception. 'I
dropped in for their being feted,' wrote Dora, 'and it was very
pleasant to meet so many nice people, but the entertainment did
not send me to bed so glad as work among patients.' She understood the feeling of the two girls that after such an experience
they could not return to being ladies of leisure. Instead, with their
joint capital, they were planning to open one of the first private
nursing homes in London, where patients could receive trained
nursing under their surgeons' personal supervision. Sister Dora
promised to visit them in the new nursing home if it materialized.

By September 1877 she was back at Walsall, to find that during her absence Richard Twigg had been very ill. She drove regularly over to Sutton Park, where he had been sent for the usual remedy of hopeless cases in those days, 'a change of air'. He was already suffering from the disease which was to kill him within three months of her own death. He was lonely and grateful to see her. Perhaps he had felt hurt by her comparative neglect during recent months, for he said pathetically to Margaret Lonsdale, 'I had rather be beaten by Sister Dora than caressed by anyone else.' This remark has such astonishing unconscious implications to modern ears that it seems unfair to attempt any interpretation out of context. Another, more intimate, relationship had lain neglected for much longer. Dora was reminded of it when she saw in the newspaper that her brother Mark was to lecture on 29th October 1877 at the Midland Institute in Birmingham, on the subject of 'Modern Books'. She attended the lecture as an ordinary member of the audience, and after it was over went up to Mark to speak to him. They had not seen one another for eleven years, and she appeared to him 'full of life and energy, a striking contrast to myself faded and worn away to nothing'. The old resentment, the old contempt for the work she had chosen came to the surface and he greeted her with frosty jocularity. 'What, Dora, still cutting off little Tommy's fingers and little Jemmy's toes?'[33] They exchanged a few minutes' desultory conversation in the public hall before she went away. It was their last meeting; the figure so 'full of life and energy' was already a dying woman.

By contrast, the happiest reunion of 1877 was on Christmas Day, when Sister Dora gave at her own expense a Christmas dinner party to as many former patients and nurses as could come. She said later that as it was likely to be her last Christmas on earth she had wanted them all to remember it happily after she was gone. The challenge of putting up trestle tables, of decorating the dingy house to look cheerful, of cooking and dishing up a meal for so many people in the pokey little kitchen, called up all her gift for improvisation. It was a good party. 'There was a large gathering,' wrote one of the guests, 'and much merriment. Old and young, rich and poor, patients and nurses, met together to be welcomed by their dear Sister Dora, and hear her talk to them as she alone could speak. None of her family, or of her

317

friends, nor a single soul in Walsall, had the slightest idea that that she was not in robust health.' She hurried to and from the kitchen to wait on them, laughed and talked with the adults, played games with the children and sang carols until it was time to say good night. No one who attended that last Christmas party ever forgot it.[34]

NOTES

1. *Walsall Observer*, June 1952 and April 1966. As the originals are now missing, all subsequent quotations from this correspondence come from these two issues.
2. Post Office Directory of Birmingham Hardware District 1870.
3. *Walsall Observer*, 19th June 1875. Messrs. Jones Brothers were a well-known Staffordshire firm. Their furnaces in Birchills were among the largest in the Black Country, and they also owned the Buffery furnaces and the Eagle Iron Works. Their head office was at Tansley Hill, Dudley.
4. W.C.H. MS., 1875.
5. Mrs Howard, formerly Jones, in her eighty-eighth year, kindly wrote personal reminiscences of her uncle.
6. In 1866 when Elizabeth Garrett, L.S.A., became London's first practising woman physician at the age of thirty-four, it was considered necessary for a school friend to share the house where she had her consulting rooms.
7. This was her nickname for the Rev. John Postlethwaite, in real life a far from formidable figure.
8. Lonsdale, 196.
9. Ridsdale, ix.
10. Ibid., 23–4.
11. Lonsdale, 202, describes this illness as 'a return of the acute inflammation' of 1866, but there is no record of this in letters or hospital minutes. Nor is there any suggestion that 'the old doctor', John Burton, Sen., was consulted. Lonsdale's account of the broken engagement, 76–8, and subsequent illness, may confuse two incidents, one in 1866 and one in 1876.
12. Ridsdale, 22 and 40.
13. Ibid., 51.
14. Ibid., 50.
15. Ibid., 52.

16. Ibid., 68.
17. Shorthand note by the Secretary, Samuel Welsh.
18. *Walsall Observer*, 28th December 1879.
   The conversion of Sister Dora would have been a triumph, so the objection must have appeared grave.
19. Lonsdale, 152.
20. 'The Coming Woman', *The World*, 28th June 1876.
21. Ridsdale, 67.
22. W.C.H. MS., Building sub-committee, 1876–7.
23. Ibid., Building sub-Committee, 1877 and *Walsall Observer*, 2nd November 1878.
24. Ibid., 1876–7.
25. Ibid., 1877–8.
26. W.C.H.A.R., 1877.
27. W.C.H. MS., 1877–8.
28. W.C.H.A.R., 1877.
29. He is never identified by name, but was possibly Thomas Chavasse, gynaecologist and member of a famous Birmingham medical family, who lived at Wylde Green House, Sutton Coldfield.
30. Lonsdale, 207.
31. H.R.C.
32. Lonsdale, 214, says 'in the Isle of Man'. Other evidence suggests Saltburn.
33. J. Sparrow, *Mark Pattison and the Idea of a University*, 40.
34. Lonsdale, 204.

CHAPTER NINETEEN

The Furnace
1878

❋

In the spring of 1878 Sister Dora received warning that she had not many months to live. At this time she was nursing three women with her own disease, two as out-patients and one who was near to death in the temporary hospital.[1] She therefore knew what to expect when, about March 1878, her own cancer began to develop rapidly, the skin broke down and the growth began to suppurate. She went back to Birmingham to receive her surgeon's directions for the daily dressing which would now be necessary, and which she said 'she was firmly resolved to undertake herself'. Crompton pointed out that she must eventually need nursing, but she replied that she hoped this would not be necessary. Secretly, she now longed and prayed for death as never before.[2] Nothing in her religion or character admitted for one moment the possibility of suicide, but she hoped for some sudden illness or accident to deliver her from the lingering death which she knew lay ahead. In March 1878 she took into the hospital, as an emergency case, a small child with diphtheria. The child was breathless and choking with the characteristic membrane of the disease, its fingers and lips slowly becoming blue. As a last hope Dr MacLachlan performed an emergency tracheotomy, and inserted a tube through which the patient could breathe. Sister Dora had nursed so many of these cases for him that he had no need to give her the standard instructions; she must sit by the child's cot, watch its breathing constantly and clear the mucous from the tube with a feather, to maintain a free airway.[3] Sitting alone, by the light of a single nightlight, Sister Dora knelt on the floor, put her mouth to the tracheotomy tube and deliberately cleared it by sucking the diphtheric mucus.[4] All she got was a severe sore throat and a severer scolding from Dr MacLachlan. Both she and the child recovered, though to her grief, the child died soon afterwards of another disease.

As so often before she tried to lose herself in work. Since she could not die at once, her one wish was to live long enough to nurse in the new hospital. The year 1878 began with a series of disappointments about the building; the work was months in arrears, in spite of solicitors' letters to the architect and threats to terminate the builder's contract.[5] On the building sub-committee there were resolutions, rows, and finally resignations. One thing at least was accomplished. The new out-patients department, for which Sister Dora had petitioned, was finished and opened in March 1878; it offered a waiting hall, where formerly patients had been forced to stand out of doors in all weathers, surgeon's room, clerk's office, and separate dressing cubicles, with sinks and running water.[6] Sister Dora was very proud of it. By contrast, responsibility for the in-patients at the temporary hospital caused her the deepest anxiety. No deaths occurred there for seven months, a tribute to her skill, but the confident Annual Report for 1877 by no means reflected her private fears. Dr MacLachlan wrote to the Committee early in 1878, with his habitual bluntness. 'The condition of wounds has been very unsatisfactory, inflammation showing itself in the simplest cuts, although every precaution has been taken to avoid it.' The patients were no safer in the temporary building than they had been in the old hospital, now demolished at such trouble and expense, for the mysterious 'hospital disease' had followed them. Many medical men, including Simpson,[7] believed that hospital buildings themselves bred disease; they proposed 'that large hospitals should be abolished, and in their place there should be congeries of cast-iron cottages, capable of being taken down',[8] regardless of disturbance or discomfort to the patients. Dr MacLachlan himself at first thought this, when he insisted that no materials from the old hospital should be incorporated in the new building,[9] but later his opinion changed.

In the early months of 1878, he apparently studied the published papers of his old chief, Joseph Lister, now Professor of Clinical Surgery at King's College Hospital, London. Lister maintained, in the teeth of medical tradition that 'a very large hospital, by enforcing strict attention to the antiseptic principle' could be an environment as healthy for patients as 'the best private houses'. He gave, as a telling example, his own former ward, the male surgical ward on the ground floor at Glasgow Royal Infirmary, hemmed in by tall buildings and abutting on a burial ground. He described the stench in the ward, the ineradicable infections, from which, he wrote, 'my patients suffered in a way that was sickening and almost heart-rending.' Yet, in spite of the unfavourable conditions, 'after nine months in which the antiseptic system had been fairly in operation in my wards, not a single case of pyaemia, erysipelas or hospital gangrene had occurred in them'.[10] Of twelve amputation cases, he wrote, 'before the antiseptic period, no fewer than six died, a frightful mortality. . . . Very different was the result of corresponding amputations during the antiseptic period, for eleven of the twelve cases recovered. In short, hospital gangrene, pyaemia and erysipelas may be said to have been banished by the antiseptic system'.[11] Moreover, he added, 'anyone duly impressed with the importance of the subject and devoting to it the study and practical attention which it demands, will securely obtain the results which he desires'. In 1875 Lister published another set of reports on recent modifications and refinements of his method, which make plain the intense self-discipline and attention to detail it demanded. 'It were far better,' he wrote of the many failures which had occurred through slovenly technique, 'that the antiseptic method should not be employed at all, than that it should be used improperly. Such attempts only end in disappointment and they bring discredit on the system.'[12]

Sister Dora was completely convinced by Lister's evidence. Since she had only a limited time left to her in life, she resolved to take this great step forward in her work while strength still lasted. She determined, with all the force of her indomitable will, to master the principles and practice of antiseptic surgery before she died. Against all the odds, she was to succeed.

Dora's emotions were no less potent for being hidden under these urgent practical concerns. She was forcibly reminded of them on an evening in March when she went to a concert and found herself sitting next to Kenyon Jones. He neither looked at her nor spoke to her. The meeting could have formed a scene in a novel by Thomas Hardy, the gaslit Agricultural Hall, the amateur performers, the audience in Sunday broadcloth, and two lovers sitting silent in the crowd with their secret relationship, an uninvited third, between them. By now, they must have looked incongruous, the stalwart young businessman and the middle-aged woman who carried the seeds of death within her. Yet their love was still alive, for Kenyon went home to write a letter, asking to see her again. Dora let fall the pride of a lifetime, and answered without reserve.

Do you not think you call largely on faith and friendship when you tell me 'not to think that you have entirely forgotten me?' Why, I should have to be an angel to go on hoping against hope! I am only a frail, weak woman and cannot live on trust but am obliged to judge by facts. When a quarter of a year has gone and your friend has neither written nor called to see you, when he actually sat by your side and never spoke to you, what has friendship, I ask you, to live on? Why nothing.

I did expect you would have spoken to me the concert night. I too, took out my pen to write and ask if you had forgotten me, but I thought you would think me silly, so did not. You know how you stand with me, and I am afraid, so loving a creature as I am, that nothing can alter my feelings towards you. You will always find a loving welcome, come when you will. . . . Send me word if you can come and stay longer, or come earlier, for I will not receive you for that short time. I cannot sign myself your friend but yours very faithfully, Sister Dora.

He came next day to see her. Dora, who could be so feminine and yielding, could also be like iron. She was determined he should never know of her condition; she could not bear to receive pity, where what she desired was love. From this time onwards her determination to conceal the true nature of her illness was absolute. She yielded to Kenyon's desire that she should come to Dudley to visit his family. 'I shall like to see your home in all its summer beauties,' she wrote bravely. 'I was delighted with it in its winter robe.' She loved the old house, with its large garden and echoing rookery, 'on the top of your hill enjoying the breeze and sunshine'.[13] Yet when she entered the large, solid ironmaster's household, she felt that Kenyon's widowed mother, his brother James and his sister Lizzie disapproved of their relationship.

'I have been thinking of you all this morning,' she wrote a few weeks later. 'What will you think of me when I tell you that it was cowardice, not patients, that kept me away yesterday? I could not screw up courage to face the party. Do not think when I say this that they are anything but kindness itself to me, but I thought your sister might think me intruding too much. You must be forgiving as I have made a full confession to you, with no excuse as to work etc.'

Dora was deeply conscious of the difference in their ages; Kenyon was thirty, while she was forty-four. It was bitter to recall the wasted years of her girlhood, imprisoned at Hauxwell, now she no longer had youth to offer a lover, and so little time left in which to love.

Yet with determined courage, she kept her letters light, selecting characters and incidents to amuse him just as she had long ago in letters to her brother Mark. She told him about her child patients. 'So you have heard of my family; three under three years old. And all so good – never was such a good baby! I have three other children besides all the men, so you can fancy my hands are full. Now do you wonder I can find time to write all this nonsense to you?' When Kenyon complained of toothache, she rallied him. 'It is very fashionable here and dentists are in great requisition. I cannot tell you how many teeth I have drawn this week!' She told him about one of the Walsall ladies who was said to admire him. 'I hope you will not be too cruel to her!' Sometimes he seems to have protested at her teasing, for she answered, 'Many a one gives me credit for having no heart'. Their carefully-contrived meetings began again, and now she was tenderly frank about the pleasure they brought. 'You *did* look so nice yesterday,' she wrote on 6th May. 'I do not think I ever saw you look better. I wonder if I shall have the pleasure of a peep at you at the concert tonight? If I did, I should enjoy the evening more.' If he looked pale, she worried over him. 'You must promise me,' she wrote, 'not to be ill without sending for your doctor.' He invited her to come to see the blast furnace tapped, an invitation which she accepted on 10th May, with a wry joke at her own expense. 'So you want me to come and see the furnace – I do not think I should be sorry to see the flame again. They say a burnt child dreads the fire, but I think I am an exception. Certainly, if love and good wishes will keep it burning, it has them. What a famous cast you get with it!'

They discovered a method of seeing one another, in spite of their busy working lives, almost every day. Kenyon travelled regularly from his home at Dudley to the Walsall iron foundry and the Dudley trains passed within a few feet of a ward window, on the first floor of the temporary hospital.[14] If Dora stood in the window as his train went past, her face, framed in white cap and collar, showed up clearly against the dark house. 'The face in the window' became part of his daily round, while she had just time to catch a glimpse of him in the lighted carriage, as the train rumbled slowly over the bridge. Soon she knew his time-table by heart. 'Yes, I did see you pass yesterday morning,' she wrote, after a night when she was called out to attend a casualty. 'I only awoke at 8.15, but after a hasty toilette continued in the ward window until the train went out. I could not see you come back this morning, though I looked out as all the Dudley trains came in.' Sometimes she was disappointed. 'I have peeped today, to see you return from your dance last night, but all in vain.' Sometimes she had to explain her own absence. 'The reason you do not often see me at the window on Sunday mornings is that I am at early Service, except once a month, like last Sunday, when Holy Communion is at mid-day.' The only thing better than to see her, he replied, would be to travel together. Into these snatched glimpses was compressed all the love of her remaining life.

She did not complain. The renewal of their love brought an exaltation of happiness, which was all the greater because she knew that death must cut it short. She had no conflict between love and duty, no anxiety about decisions concerning their joint future; the ultimate decision would be taken for her in its own time. She seems to have accepted her situation with unflinching courage. As always, love heralded a period of joy and gratitude in her faith. Every day seemed precious to her and full of meaning. During this summer she wrote to Mrs Ridsdale of 'happy times frizzling in the close air of the Bridgeman Place house. I go forward in exceeding joy, for a little while; we can never tell how long, only we know we must work while it is day.' Sometimes, she added, it seemed 'as if she spoke with Jesus face to face while about her daily duties'.[15]

Sister Dora, who had seemed never to change for many years, was beginning to look frail. Her face was thinner, the powerful bones of nose and jaw showing prominently. In the last year of her life she began to show a family likeness to her brother Mark, which had lain hidden beneath the changing play of colour and expression in her face. Her auburn hair was flecked and streaked round the temples with white. Kenyon Jones, young and inexperienced, was easy to deceive in matters of health, but James MacLachlan was anxious about her, and she felt uneasy under his shrewd and penetrating glance. 'Doctor was here,' she told Kenyon, 'but I kept well out of his way.' At midsummer 1878 an unexpected decision was forced on them all. The house in the hollow under the railway bridge was liable to flooding whenever the sewers overflowed with storm-water. Probably a pipe was fractured somewhere in the nightmare plumbing; at all events by June the first cases of typhoid appeared in the wards. The weather suddenly grew hot, so hot that Sister Dora felt faint and giddy as she went about her work in 'the frizzling house'. The typhoid outbreak spread rapidly and Dr MacLachlan issued a characteristic ultimatum to the committee. 'As these are not the first cases (of typhoid) we have, nor likely to be the last, I suggest you close the hospital at once.'[16] The committee agreed, but Sister Dora protested. What would become of the patients? He had already arranged for urgent cases to be admitted to Birmingham and Wolverhampton. What about the out-patients? He said he would see them without charge at his own house. Sister Dora, he told the committee, was 'overworked and very tired, with all the marks of fatigue exposure and anxiety upon her.' She must go away for a holiday.[17]

Perhaps Dora feared to be questioned more closely about her health, for she agreed with unusual meekness. She had plans to use this unexpected freedom, not only for a rest as Dr MacLachlan ordered, but to get practical training in antiseptic surgery. For the sake of this she was prepared to forgo seeing Kenyon Jones for some weeks or months if necessary. She did not suggest in any way that this might be a final parting, but made it plain that the demands of work must take first place in her life. 'This will be the best plan,' she wrote firmly. 'I am very well and happy, not a silly child, to waste my life just because I could not have what I wanted.' She went on to write about her patients and her work.

Dora spent the second week of June 1878 in clearing up all her private possessions, and packing them separately from the hospital's property. She burnt a great many private papers, and a journal which she is known to have kept disappeared, probably at this time. 'Oh that I had no possessions – in theory at least!' she was heard to say.[18] The staff watched her with some curiosity. 'Why, Sister, anyone would think you were never coming back!' said the Secretary. Sister Dora was not to be drawn and replied casually, 'One can never be sure; it's just as well to be prepared for anything.'[19] When the clearing up was finished, she took the night nurses and the servants for a day's outing to Lichfield. They remembered her afterwards 'talking and laughing with us in the train', serving them with her own hands at lunch, taking them round the Cathedral and showing them everything herself, with individual care for each one's enjoyment. A few days later, on 21st June, the Secretary saw her again, at Walsall station where she was running to catch a train. 'Goodbye,' she called, 'I'm off on my holiday.' It was a lovely day; his last sight was of Sister Dora laughing and waving from the carriage window as the train steamed out.[20]

She went for a few days to the Stirkes, and wrote Kenyon Jones a long letter, which she was careful to make light-hearted and lively. They were still getting in the hay and one of Robert's labourers cut his hand in the mowing machine. Dora sutured it; the man went to the nearest doctor, nine miles away, who refused to believe the dressing had been performed by 'a lady', and made an excuse to drive over and look at her. 'It was so amusing,' wrote Dora, 'I dare not tell him I could set limbs etc., . . . I now have quite a fame down here with this (to me) very small accident!' She boasted of getting 'quite clever at croquet' and promised 'to try my hand with you some day' at lawn tennis.

'I really am so glad,' she wrote more seriously, 'that you miss the face in the window, but I do not fancy you miss it so much as the face misses you. I actually pull out your photograph and look to make up for it. I wish I had a small one of you to put into a locket, then I could look at you very often. I showed my nieces the locket and photo of self, they were charmed with it.'

Next she visited the convent at Middlesbrough, to see Sister Frances and inspect the hospital where she had taken her first steps in nursing. She was delighted to find in the kitchen an old bread-cutting machine, which she had presented many years before, and which still gave good service.[21] It is a profound mercy that Dora and Frances were able to have this last meeting; it also tends to support the view that Dora was still an Associate Sister of the Community whose good work she often praised to the Ridsdales. While in Yorkshire she could have gone to see her sisters at Richmond, though the coolness between them was marked and she chose always to stay in Robert Stirke's house rather than with them. There is no written record of a family meeting. She saw Kenyon Jones again briefly, 'making some excuse to call' on her way through Walsall, when she received a subpoena for a case at the Staffordshire Assizes.[22] From 20th July she was free of all other obligations and could go where she liked. By temperament and conviction she was determined to live life fully to the last possible moment. She took this chance to go abroad, for the first and last time, and chose to spend some weeks in Paris. She is said to have nursed in a Paris hospital[23] and to have studied the surgical instruments at the great International Exhibition on the Champ de Mars, but there is no firm evidence for this. The city of Paris had long fascinated Dora by its surface brilliance and the profound seriousness of thought which lay beneath. Now, briefly, while she could, she saw it for herself.

Sister Dora returned from Paris and went straight to stay with Louise MacLaughlin and Emma Pearson, at the Medical and Surgical Home, 15 Fitzroy Square, a house in the handsome Greek revival terrace on the north side.[24] Here among the Italians and artists of Fitzrovia the two friends had opened one of London's first private nursing homes. Apart from friendship, Dora had a purpose in visiting it, for the greater number of its rooms housed Lister's patients. He operated there, with his own

assistants, and visited his cases every morning on the way from
his home in Park Crescent to King's College Hospital, where he
was Professor of Clinical Surgery.[25] Sister Dora applied and
received permission to observe him at work, with the surgical
team which he had brought from Edinburgh; eventually she
herself was trained to attend them in meticulous detail. It was a
tremendous experience for her, so near the end of her own
working life, to witness the making of medical history. She left
no written impression of Lister's character and had probably little
personal contact with him; yet to see him at work was enough to
be inspired by his total dedication. Although weakened and tired,
she still had the intelligence to respond; she felt it a privilege to
share the nursing of the great surgeon's patients. 'I am busy with
wonderful cases,' she wrote to Margaret Lonsdale on 27th September, and again later, 'I have the privilege of seeing Mr. Lister
do some wonderful operations.'

She grasped the central fact which Lister explained so lucidly.
'It has been shown by the researches of Pasteur that the septic
property of the atmosphere depended not on any gaseous con-
stituent but on minute organisms suspended in it.' The essential
principle of antisepsis lay, he wrote, 'In the destruction of any
septic germs which may have been introduced into the wound,
either at the moment of accident, or during the time which has
since elapsed.'

This was more than a profession largely untrained in science
could swallow. 'I cannot see the disadvantage of a little suppuration,' wrote an elder surgeon plaintively. 'To mention antiseptic
surgery was to elicit a scoff or a sneer,' wrote a junior doctor at a
London teaching hospital. Enthusiastic students who advocated
antisepsis in examination papers were liable to fail. The germ
theory eluded the great Simpson to the end of his life, and his
pupil Lawson Tait of Birmingham never fully accepted it. As
late as 1870 textbooks of surgery ignored it. Florence Nightingale, with her immense prestige, pooh-poohed the existence of
germs to the last, and the rank and file of the medical profession
took many years to grasp the theoretical basis of antiseptic
surgery. It is remarkable that where so many were ruled by
prejudice, an obscure provincial nursing sister should have been
eager to explore new methods to the very end of her working life.

Sister Dora was trained at Fitzroy Square in Lister's rigorous routine.[26] She was particularly interested in the dressing of accidental wounds, including compound fractures, where dirt had already been driven deep into the tissues. These were irrigated with antiseptic lotion, or cleaned with carbolized lint, held with a pair of forceps. Sutures were of carbolized catgut, and dressings of antiseptic gauze, both previously unknown and both needing special preparation. Sister Dora was able to see for herself that 'the severest forms of contused and lacerated wounds heal kindly under the antiseptic treatment'.

She stayed for some weeks[27] at Fitzroy Square, being trained and ordering the equipment for an antiseptic operating theatre in the new hospital at Walsall. She might have stayed longer, but towards the end of September her own health began to deteriorate rapidly; it grew steadily harder to hide her increasing weakness from so many skilled observers. She was losing weight every week, her hair was turning white, and a cough, which had troubled her for some months, increased so that by the evening she was exhausted. One of the doctors tentatively offered to examine her chest, and this kindly-meant suggestion threw her into a panic. She said later she was 'terrified at the sudden prospect that a stranger might discover her long kept secret'.[28] He insisted that if she would not see him, she must see her own doctor. On 25th September the hospital committee wrote from Walsall asking her to come and inspect the building operations. Accordingly on 29th September she travelled to Walsall.

She spent the day going round the building site in exhaustive detail. She had kept in close touch with the building sub-committee by letter; the three separate blocks linked by well-ventilated corridors to minimize cross-infection, the seven wards, the forty-two beds, the three hundred yards of tiled corridor, the glazed operating theatre, were all just as she had approved them.[29] The detailed inspection of plans and buildings lasted until it grew dark. Dora had refused all offers of hospitality, fearing to offend some by accepting others. She intended to look for lodgings, but by the evening she was too exhausted to walk any further. She took the train to Birmingham and had herself driven to the Queen's Hotel, meaning to rest there and return to Walsall after a few days. During the night she collapsed with a massive haemorrhage. A messenger was sent for Dickinson Crompton, who at first believed she had only a few hours to live, and wanted to remove her to his own house. She refused, and next day, at her plea, he telegraphed for Dr MacLachlan, who came at once. The truth could no longer be hidden.[30] She told him it was twenty months since she had noticed the first unmistakable symptoms and begged, 'Let me go back to Walsall, that I may die among my own people'; he promised that she should. She also asked 'How long?'; he replied, to the best of his judgment, 'Perhaps a fortnight.' Dr MacLachlan went back to Walsall and on the train saw the hospital Secretary, whom he beckoned into an empty carriage. 'When do you intend to open the new hospital?' he asked and Welsh replied, 'On the fourth of November.' 'Then,' said the doctor, 'that is just about the date Sister Dora will be buried.' 'You're joking!' said Welsh. 'I had a most cheerful letter from her only a week ago!' 'No, I am not joking and I thought it best to tell you at once.' 'Are you sending her home to Yorkshire?' 'No, she wishes to die in Walsall, and if she is to be moved she must be moved immediately.'

Next day was Sunday, but for the hospital Chairman and Secretary it was no day of rest. Within a few hours they rented a cottage in the Wednesbury road. On Monday morning they moved in Sister Dora's own furniture and telegraphed for Sarah Watts to take charge of the housekeeping. By noon everything was ready; Welsh's daughter had even filled the little parlour with flowers. In the afternoon James MacLachlan drove his own carriage over to Birmingham, and brought the patient home with slow care.[31] The committee wished to pay all her expenses, but this loss of independence caused her such distress that they allowed rent and other bills to be paid on her behalf by her solicitor, James Slater. They also wished to engage trained day and night nurses for her, but Dora insisted she would only have Lucy, a cheerful girl who was one of the housemaids, and at nights Mrs Harrison, for whom she had a deep affection. Mac-Lachlan was forced to agree to her wishes, and to her desire for secrecy about the cancer which he later described as 'almost frantic'. Above all, she would not let Kenyon Jones know her true condition. The voluminous hand-smocked nightgowns of the day hid her surgical dressings from ordinary visitors, and she was commonly believed to be suffering from 'consumption'. The news spread like wildfire, but the poor could not believe Sister Dora was going to leave them. 'Her'll get well,' the women in the market were heard to say. 'Her never can be going to die; her's *strong*.' Her sisters had no idea at first that her illness was serious; later when they heard she was worse, two of them made the cross-country journey from Richmond to visit her. They stayed for a week, but she insisted that she 'needed nothing' and would not allow them to do anything for her. The two elderly women went home, puzzled and saddened, while Sister Dora sent reports that she was 'getting better'[32] to forestall further intrusions. Her insistence on secrecy was so absolute that within a fortnight of her death the Committee were waiting 'until Sister Dora could be consulted', about some administrative decision.[33]

Dr MacLachlan watched all this with sympathy but regret. Later he and Margaret Lonsdale agreed, 'There was a wilfulness about her determination, which neither her own lonely agony nor the distress she must have known she was causing her own family, could shake. She showed on her deathbed the same proud and wilful reticence, the same determined following of her own way at all costs which marked her character so strongly in days of health and strength. In this part of her nature good and evil were strangely mixed; it is impossible for any human observer to separate them.'[34] She was too proud to endure pity from anyone, least of all from the man she loved.

There was no hope of any lasting improvement in Dora's condition, but with rest and relief from strain, she was granted three or four weeks of remission. On her 'best days', as she called them, she was her old self and kept visitors in constant laughter. She made a general rule that no one who genuinely wanted to see her should be turned away from the door, and the little cottage near the hospital gates was the scene of continual comings and goings. Many old patients went away saying 'Sister was that cheerful and jolly they were sure she would pull round'.[35] Edward Fitzgerald was, as always, a more perceptive observer; he had not met Dora for four months and his first sight of her darkened skin and haggard, gaunt features against the pillow reminded him of a bronze bust of Dante.[36] He could not believe she had long to live, and either he or Richard Twigg brought her the Sacraments regularly. Her neighbour Father McCarten asked Dora whether she was satisfied with her communion and the absolution she had received. According to him she answered, 'Yes, perfectly.'[37] The *Dictionary of National Biography* asserts that 'On her deathbed Monsignor Capel visited her and vainly attempted to persuade her to be baptized into the Church of Rome'. This repeats a mis-understanding which Monsignor Thomas John Capel, Rector of the Catholic University College of Kensington and a well-known writer, indignantly denied. He said he had called on Sister Dora, because he happened to be in the diocese, for which he had in any case no faculties; he had wished to thank her for her kindness to the Catholic poor. Her next visitor was a Non-Conformist minister, the Rev. F. Willetts, whom she greeted with the words 'Aha! You are just in time! I have had a narrow escape, for Monsignor Capel has been here and he was *fascinating*!'[38] Greatly excited the poor man rushed round Walsall spreading the scandalous news; he was to be the last victim on earth of Sister Dora's wayward sense of humour.

Dr MacLachlan also endured some teasing when the fortnight he had given her to live was at an end and she still survived. He said 'her eyes used to dance with all their old brightness as he entered the room', and as the days passed and she still lived on, her enjoyment of his mistake became keener. She was delighted that she had, as she put it, 'done the doctors again!'[39] He took it in good part and defended himself by saying, 'We all know you are an exception to every rule.' It was an absorbingly interesting day for them both when the new surgical equipment was delivered. She had it unpacked and laid out on her bed, as they went through it together piece by piece, discussing and demonstrating the process of sterilization 'after Mr. Lister's principle' which she wanted to enforce 'as soon as soon as possible' in the new hospital. She also dictated the orders for china, linen and household stores, and discussed with Dr MacLachlan and the Chairman the question of her successor as Sister-in-Charge. The appointment went to 'an old friend and fellow worker' Sister Ellen, perhaps the same Ellen who had been an Associate Sister with her at the Children's home at Coatham.[40] She had nursed at the North Ormesby hospital and the Hospital for Children, Broad Street, Birmingham, and seems to have been an excellent nurse. 'I *did* think we should have had some working days together in the new hospital,' said Dora, but she knew this was impossible. She said she would be satisfied even to see it. 'Could I not be carried even to the door.' Dr MacLachlan replied, 'You would be dead before you got there.'[41] It was opened by the Mayor of Walsall in her name, with a silver key which she had put into his hands. Sometimes she said 'she longed to go back to nursing', but more often she was content to lie and listen to minute details of the new patients. One of the nurses told her that a man who had broken his back had been brought in. 'Then look here,' she said, 'and I will show you how to move him in bed without hurting him.' She doubled up a corner of the sheet and laid her finger in the fold to represent the patient; they noticed that 'her short, concise professional manner' had not deserted her. During this period of respite she put her business affairs in meticulous order. Her solicitor James Slater drew up her brief and simple will, signed Sister Dora, on 17th October. She left 'in priority to all other payments' three hundred pounds to the hospital, her few personal possessions to her nieces and any remaining capital in trust for her sisters jointly.[42] Slater arranged for the pony and its carriage to go to the farm for the enjoyment of the Stirke girls, and paid all her bills. She wrote him a grateful little note of thanks.

Extreme weakness is so painful to me; every now and then little bills crop up and I fear they will do so, to your annoyance, after I am gone. What a great deal of trouble I have been to you! But I keep praying God will reward you, and that you and yours will find such a friend when you need him. Yours very gratefully, Sister Dora.[43]

She was pleased that her disease was, as she said, 'Hopeless – I use that word merely technically – so they don't tease me with medicines and remedies and there is no fluctuation of hopes and fears.' She enjoyed books, and the flowers which made her room 'almost a garden'. 'I am so happy,' she wrote to one of her former nurses. 'I have so longed to go home.' This was long believed to be her last letter, but there was one more. From the time of her return to Walsall, she had one faithful visitor. Every evening, when his work was over, Kenyon Jones came to sit by her bedside. There is no hint of what he felt when he saw her ravaged face. At the end of October she grew suddenly much worse, and saw that the emotional strain of these meetings was more than he could bear. The habit of sparing others pain was ingrained in Sister Dora by years of practice. Propped up against her pillow, she wrote her last letter, to release the young man to more than fifty years of healthy, normal life which still lay before him.

The Hospital, Walsall, October 30 1878.

My dear Kenyon,

I have got propped up to write this to you. See how boldly I commence! I was so sorry you should have had a useless walk last night particularly in the snow – I pictured you walking up Green Lane facing it. My darling I shall not see you again for it agitates me so much I feel almost it might kill me. I am sure it distresses you to see me in such a state yet I cannot prevent it, so I am writing to hinder you coming tonight – for I am so weak, although I slept better that I am obliged to rest at every line.

Oh Kenyon, you must not fret for me or grieve. I think I shall soon lay down the cross and I trust exchange it for a crown. Yours very faithfully, Sister Dora.

To write this had frayed the last strands of her will-power. 'I look back on my life,' she said wearily, 'and see nothing but leaves.' Her hearers, in a Bible-reading age, recognized the reference to the barren fig tree of the gospel, doomed never to bear its natural fruit.[44] A time of great darkness followed, when this proud woman, who had refused to admit to weakness or suffering, was humbled to the level of common humanity. In cancer of the breast, lying so near to the centre of circulation, metastases are widespread. Dora's lungs were already affected; incessant cough, thick expectoration and terrible sweats exhausted her. 'My cough is terrible, it will not cease, and the nights are so distressing,' she confessed.[45] Dr MacLachlan believed her right lung to be 'almost consolidated'. She had to be propped almost upright in order to breathe. Blockage of the veins caused her right arm and hand to swell until they lay helpless on a pillow; from pain and weakness she could no longer write, though she still liked to have letters read aloud to her. Towards the end of November it seems likely that the metastases reached the brain, for she began to suffer from headache and persistent vomiting. 'I am so troubled by sickness,' she confessed. 'I care for nothing except water, which is my one cry all day long. I think I cannot live long.'[46] A terrible depression overwhelmed her, as she felt 'the cold waters of death closing round me . . . with a horrible dread'. She had calmed the dying so often by talking to them of God as a merciful father, but now in place of this beloved figure, appeared the God of her childhood's dread, preached by the wrathful tyrant of the Hauxwell nursery. 'I cannot pray, I cannot think, I fear I shall be lost; I can only trust.' She asked for a large crucifix to be placed on the wall exactly opposite her bed. On this her eyes were continually fixed, although she said, 'I feel sometimes I dare not look there, I cannot bear the sight of His sufferings. My own sink into nothing by the side of them, yet I am so impatient.' She could no longer bear to be left alone at night for a moment, but clung to the hand of her old nurse, Mrs Harrison, crying, 'I am not half so good or so patient as many of those I have nursed.' The kind, simple woman protested, 'Why, Sister, only think of the good you have been to us poor folk. Where should we have been without you?' Dora interrupted her with a gesture of despair. 'Don't talk of what I have done; I have never done half what I might. I am not nearly so good as you are.'[47]

At the end of November she appeared to the relief of all who watched her to be dying, but her immense vitality dragged her back to consciousness. She had still nearly four weeks to live. Now she moved into the calm of total exhaustion. She seemed hardly to recognize James MacLachlan when he came every day to measure out her graduated doses of opium. She was now completely helpless, so Sister Ellen came from the hospital to change the dressings and make her as comfortable as possible; once she was touched to hear Dora murmur, 'If my patients can only be nursed like this, I shall be more than satisfied.' For much of the time she neither moved nor spoke. She appeared resigned, though Fitzgerald was honest enough to say, 'I do not think she had the times of extreme happiness which some people have felt near death.'

His frankness was unusual for the time. Florence Nightingale, in her incomparable *Notes on Nursing*, condemned the 'unwise exertions' of friends who try to force the religious emotions of a

sick person. In her opinion, 'Friends are apt to judge most un-
fairly of the spiritual state of the sick from physical manifesta-
tions.' Sister Dora's despondency had a likely physical cause in
brain damage. She had not forgotten her friends, for she gave
Fitzgerald her Bible, and asked him to distribute thirty pairs of
warm gloves, which she had ordered, to the railway cabmen and
porters in his parish, 'as a Christmas remembrance'. To other
friends she gave small keepsakes, her thimble, her chatelaine, her
scissors. She requested 'the plainest possible funeral' and 'no vain
eulogy upon me when I am gone'. The Bishop of Lichfield came
to visit her, and asked her not to forget the poor of Walsall, whom
she had so deeply loved. She whispered, 'I will never forget you;
I shall always think of you, and pray for you all.'[48]

The days passed; she lay while her intense vitality slowly wore
away and consciousness ebbed and flowed through her wasted
body. If she attempted in waking moments to weigh up the profit
and loss in her life there must have been much to put in the
credit balance. She had suffered all that the conflicts and conventions of her time could inflict, but she had never lost the intensity
of moral vision which gives such distinctive quality to Victorian
life. Her force of character had triumphed over warped heredity
and a baneful home. She had experienced the long fight for freedom, the crisis of faith, the urgent challenge of work, the sacrifice
of personal love, all with the full force of her nature. Nothing
had been shallow, nothing trivial or meaningless. She was dying,
but she had truly lived. By 21st December it was clear that her
end must be very near. She dreaded the last pangs of death, which
she believed would seize her during a paroxysm of coughing, yet
she longed to be gone. 'Oh I do hope,' she said, 'I can sing my
Christmas carol in heaven.' As each day passed, her hope of
release before Christmas grew fainter.

Yet she was too experienced to mistake the signs of death when
they came, and too courageous to evade them. Early in the morning of Christmas Eve, she said, 'Run for Sister Ellen; I am dying.'
The women of the house stood round her bed, trying to relieve
the distress of her breathing, and to remind her of the joys of
heaven. 'I have lived alone,' she said between laboured breaths.
'Let me die alone.' They hesitated and she cried sharply, 'Let me
die alone.' They were forced to leave her, and to stay, watching

anxiously through the half-open doorway. For some hours she lived on, but said no more. It was only by a slight movement at about two o'clock that the watchers in the doorway knew Sister Dora had died.

NOTES

1. W.C.H. MS., 1878.
2. Lonsdale, 203. She later confessed this, probably to Richard Twigg.
3. C. Heath, *Manual of Minor Surgery*, 24.
4. Lonsdale, 208, says she intervened at the operation, but Mac-Lachlan denied that she had ever acted in so unprofessional a manner.
5. W.C.H. MS., Building sub-committee, 1877–8.
6. Ibid., 1878. Building sub-committee.
7. J. A. Shepherd, *Simpson and Syme of Edinburgh*, 200.
8. *The Lancet*, 8th January 1870.
9. W.C.H. MS., 1876.
10. *The Lancet*, 1st January 1870.
11. Ibid., 8th January 1870.
12. Ibid., 15th March and 3rd April 1875.
13. The house has now been demolished and a number of small houses built on the estate.
14. The house has been demolished, but entering Walsall station by train from the south, one can still see that it stood almost within touching distance.
15. Ridsdale, 70.
16. W.C.H. MS., 1878.
17. W.C.H.A.R., 1878. It is impossible to calculate how much Dr MacLachlan sacrificed in time and income to poor patients, but after thirty years' hard work he left little more than £3000.
18. Ridsdale, 34.
19. Lonsdale, 213, dates this at the end of August, but Welsh, who kept shorthand notes, places it around the middle of June 1878.
20. S. Welsh, *General Baptist Magazine*, 1889.
21. Ridsdale, 37.
22. Reynolds *v.* L.N.W. Railway, 18th–19th July 1878. Dora gave evidence that Mrs Reynolds, who claimed damages for a fall at Pelsall station, was drunk when admitted to hospital.
23. S. Welsh, *General Baptist Magazine*, 1889. Redfern Davies had been a post-graduate student at a hospital in Paris.

24. *Medical Directory*, 1878. As Lonsdale, 215, omitted the name and address of the home, it has long been a mystery how Sister Dora came into contact with Lister. It was simply through a personal recommendation from Louise MacLaughlin.
25. R. Godlee, *Lord Lister*, 408.
26. *Recent Improvements in the Details of Antiseptic Surgery, The Lancet*, 13th March 1875. See Appendix E.
27. The exact date of her return from Paris is not known.
28. Lonsdale, 216.
29. W.C.H. MS., Building sub-committee, 1878.
30. *Walsall Observer*, 17th October 1878.
31. S. Welsh, *General Baptist Magazine*, 1889, 268, dates this 4th October; Lonsdale, 8th October.
32. Pattison, 131, f. 57. Mark Pattison's diary: 'the reports made from time to time by her own direction had been that she was better.'
33. W.C.H. MS., 1878.
34. Lonsdale, 223.
35. Ibid., 227.
36. W.P.L. Album. The bust, by an unknown fifteenth-century master, is in the Museo Nazionale at Naples.
37. *Walsall Observer*, 4th January 1879.
38. Ibid.
39. Lonsdale, 231.
40. H.R.C. Register of Associate Sisters. Sister Ellen is elsewhere described as a complete stranger who volunteered for the work; the contradiction here cannot be resolved.
41. W.P.L. Album.
42. P.P.R., 1879, Lichfield, f. 38.
43. Lonsdale, 221.
44. Mark: xi: 13.
45. Lonsdale, 230. Margaret Lonsdale was helping in the hospital at this time; hers may be accepted as first-hand evidence.
46. Lonsdale, 231.
47. Lonsdale, 228.
48. W.P.L. Album.

A Day in 1886

The winter after Sister Dora's death was hard; the canals of the Black Country froze for seven weeks; lacking raw material, colliers, brickmakers and furnacemen were thrown out of work. School attendance officers reported that many children could not go to school from 'want of food and clothing, frost bite and general distress'.[1] Everything conspired to remind the poor of the friend they had lost. The medical and lay committees of the hospital, meeting for the first time since her death, felt they faced 'an irreparable loss, the greatest misfortune that has befallen our Institution since its establishment'.[2] They voted as one man 'to place on record our deep and grateful sense of the self-denying services, which for fourteen years she rendered with the rarest Christian love and almost unequalled devotion to Walsall Cottage Hospital'.[3] Their loss was greater than they knew, for without Dora's tact and charm to hold the balance, laymen and doctors could no longer work in harmony at the administration of the hospital. Before two years were out the lay committee and the new matron found themselves locked in conflict with the medical staff, who demanded, successfully, 'that the duties of the Sister shall be limited to the nursing and domestic departments.'[4] At the same time, in spite of protests from clergy and former nurses, the Sunday afternoon services which Sister Dora had held in the hospital for patients and their families had to be discontinued; a member of the public wrote a formal complaint to the Committee that these were 'sectarian in character' and therefore violated the hospital's articles of incorporation.[5] It also became more difficult to attract voluntary 'lady nurses', and in the end the hospital had to resort to paid probationers.

Edward Fitzgerald, taking up the work of his hard-pressed

parish, wondered how he and his people would manage without Sister Dora. He turned to one of his most valued possessions, her Bible, which she had given him on his last visit, shortly before her death. He opened the fly-leaf and read again her well-remembered writing, black and angular, with the square-cut characters which are said to show executive ability. She had written:

> God's intention in the creation, He himself has declared, is that man should be in His image and likeness. This intention appears to me to be the keystone of life's work, to help restore and build up what is ruined in ourselves and others, to love and help others and to have the blessed life originally intended for us.

He copied this and sent it to the local paper as Sister Dora's last message to her people. He found in it the clue to her life's work, and an inspiration to all who came after her.[6]

Great as their loss was, Sister Dora had left the people of Walsall a new hospital, and a steadily growing fame.[7] The committee members were surprised, in the years which followed her death, to find their hospital well known all over the world. Lawson Tait went out of his way to praise the excellence of its casualty work in a presidential address to the British Medical Association.[8] The Princess Imperial of Prussia, eldest daughter of Queen Victoria, wrote asking for a copy of its rules, as she intended to open a similar hospital for industrial casualties in Berlin.[9] Visitors with a professional interest in the casualty department arrived from America, Australia and the Far East.[10] Walsall people had always looked on Sister Dora as belonging to them alone; after her death the national press began to set her work in a wider perspective. A church paper wrote of her religious inspiration and influence. 'All her great gifts, her personal beauty and strength, her charm of manner, her cultivated mind, her wit and humour, were dedicated to one end, the glory of God. She never preached, but a look from her was a sermon, and her whole life preaches now that she has entered into her rest.'[11] A national daily paper compared the effect of her work with Florence Nightingale's. 'What Florence Nightingale did for military hospitals, Dorothy Pattison accomplished in civilian duty.'[12]

For Black Country pride was mixed with chagrin, for too often praise of Sister Dora's achievement was expressed in terms very wounding to their own feelings. 'At Walsall in the Black Country,' ran an article in a London review, 'with its wastes of charred scenery, its smoke-vomiting pits, its wild and degrading surroundings, its brutal population, Sister Dora worked with self-denying love. Her courage was undaunted, she visited the vilest haunts, won the hearts of the most abandoned characters and was in all, the most generous and tender of friends.'[13] It is hardly surprising that a series of articles along these lines reinforced the determination of Walsall people to raise their own memorial to the woman who, they knew, whatever the outside world might think, had loved them even above her own happiness. An open meeting for the whole town was held in the Guildhall of the Borough. Walsall's Member of Parliament, Sir Charles Forster, who was in the Chair, spoke for all present when he said he would like a memorial 'to be raised by the subscriptions and to be the property of all classes'. When it came to the form this memorial should take, however, agreement was at an end. Open rivalry broke out among Sister Dora's relations and friends, each claiming to know what her own wishes would have been.[14]

The hospital committee wished, as a first step, to re-cut the lettering on her tombstone, which, only two years after her death, was already obliterated by the malignant atmosphere of the Black Country. The Pattisons, regarding this as a slight on their family pride, took umbrage; with much tact James Slater arranged to set the work in hand at the family's expense. In February 1882 Mr Postlethwaite wrote demanding to know what the memorial to 'Sister Dora's noble work' would be. One feels he was not altogether sorry to have a grievance against the people who had taken her away from him.

Next in the field was the Vicar of Walsall, the Reverend Prebendary William Allen, who suggested beautifying the parish church with a memorial window and opened a fund for this purpose. He received subscriptions from all over the Midlands and beyond, with the proposal that the window should illustrate the corporal works of mercy. These are traditionally seven in number: feeding the hungry, giving drink to the thirsty, clothing the naked, harbouring the stranger, visiting the sick, ministering to prisoners and burying the dead. All had been performed by Sister Dora and are depicted in the excellent Victorian East window of St Matthew's, Walsall, to commemorate her work.[15] Other people, however, particularly the staff and committee of the hospital, wished for a more personal memorial. They collected privately among themselves, and commissioned the portrait by Henry Munns of Birmingham, a watercolour copy of which forms the chief decoration in the Boardroom of Walsall General Hospital. Sister Dora's appearance was so well known and so striking that Munns had no lack of descriptions, as well as photographs, from which to work; his portrait has vanished but the copy remains the only picture of her in colour.[16]

The memorial which would undoubtedly have appealed most to Dora herself was a fund to send convalescents to the seaside. In the early years at Walsall she had regularly sent cases to Coatham, but after she broke her connection with the Homes she felt unwilling to ask their help. Instead, she herself began a seaside holiday fund and had already invested £200 by the time of her death. Yet even this straightforward proposal ran into difficulties. Sister Ellen had 'a little plan' for a house on the coast of North Wales.[17] Margaret Lonsdale, who had been gathering material during the last months of Sister Dora's life, brought out her memoir in 1880 and, with sincere generosity, offered to donate the entire royalties to building and endowing a Sister Dora Home, which should be '*her* Convalescent Home'.[18] Meanwhile Walsall had read the book with mounting fury; as one man the Town Council and the Hospital Committee members 'refused to touch a penny' from the writer who, as they said with unconscious irony, had 'blackened them in the eyes of the world'. Miss Lonsdale retaliated by writing to *The Guardian*, 'stating that it is now two years since the death of Sister Dora. No public memorial has been raised to her and since no one else seems disposed to do it, she proposed to erect at her own expense a small convalescent home to be called by Sister Dora's name.' The Rev. John Postlethwaite wrote to the Committee, with a certain complacency, enclosing this press-cutting.[19] The hospital committee, wisely refusing to be drawn, continued to add subscriptions to Sister Dora's existing convalescent fund until it stood at £700. This, carefully invested, produced a yearly income large enough to send twelve or fourteen of the most severe cases to existing seaside convalescent homes. Dr MacLachlan, in particular, believed this to be a useful service, and the memorial subscriptions after his own death were added to the fund's capital.[20]

None of these schemes, stained-glass window, official portrait or the two rival convalescent funds really satisfied the largest group in Walsall – Sister Dora's former patients. From the first they wanted her to live, not only in their hearts, but in the minds and eyes of their children for all generations to come. No one knows who first put forward the proposal, but at some time during 1879 a group of working men came to see Samuel Welsh, who had more than once represented them during strike negotiations. They told him that what the working people of the town really wanted was a statue of the Sister, and that they would willingly collect money to meet the cost. A railwayman put the point well. 'Nobody knows better than I do,' he said, 'that we shan't forget her. No danger of that! But I want her to be there, so that when strangers come to the place, and see her standing up, they'll ask us "Who's that?" Then we shall say, "Who's that? Why, that's *our* Sister Dora!" '[21] Several points told in favour of the idea. A correspondent of the *Walsall Observer* wrote an article maintaining that this would be the first statue in Britain to a woman not of royal birth; the appeal of this to local pride was powerful. Dr MacLachlan, when asked for his opinion, revealed that he had spent Christmas Day 1878, the day after Sister Dora's death, alone at the hospital. Working all day, he had taken plaster casts of her face and her powerful, maternal hands.[22] He would be willing to make these casts available to a sculptor. Both Hospital and Borough Committees agreed, and the work of raising the money began.

It took seven years to collect twelve hundred pounds, mostly in very small sums from works collecting-boxes, although larger sums came from London and an anonymous donor sent a hundred pounds from Cincinnati, Ohio.[23] During this time the Corporation chose a site on The Bridge, which is the central square of Walsall,[24] removed a public clock and a drinking fountain, apparently without opposition, and constructed a granite plinth to receive the statue. The sculpture itself was commissioned from Francis Williamson, who had carved the much admired memorial to Dean Milman in St Paul's Cathedral. He selected a block of white Sicilian marble and Samuel Welsh, who travelled to his studio at Esher to see the work in progress, returned quoting:

Ne'er did Grecian chisel trace
So pure a form, so fair a face.[25]

In October 1886 Williamson despatched the finished statue by rail, to a committee already heavily involved in the planning of the unveiling ceremony. Local pride demanded royalty: failing that Florence Nightingale, or, if the worst came to the worst, Mr Gladstone to unveil Sister Dora's memorial. However, a small Midland borough lacked pulling power. Royalty was unavailable. Miss Nightingale declined as 'a prisoner through illness', though she did send her greetings to 'those noble, rough fellows, the workmen of Walsall'. Even Mr Gladstone sent a telegram, 'Regret cannot undertake public celebration. – If any it would be this as I profoundly revere Sister Dora.'[26] In the end they decided that the statue should be unveiled by the Mayor of Walsall on 11th October 1886, the twenty-third anniversary of the hospital's opening. It was thus a purely local occasion, a family affair, and Sister Dora was once again, as she had wished to be 'among my own people'. 11th October was a murky autumn day, with a lowering sky threatening to pour rain on the forty thousand people packed densely round the swathed statue on The Bridge. A series of curiously touching press photographs records the town *en fête* for 'the day of Sister's statue'. The square and every window around was filled with a sea of faces. All Sister Dora's Walsall friends were there: a choir of school children, with drum and fife bands, the police, the railwaymen, the fire brigade, who had constructed a triumphal arch of ladders and looped hoses, the strangely named workmen's friendly societies, Free Gardeners, Good Templars, Caledonian Corks. Every black façade of warehouse or factory was strung across with fluttering many-coloured bunting; engineers stood at the ready in each workshop to greet the statue with hooters and steam whistles at the moment of unveiling.[27]

The circle of people, who had been closest in life to Dorothy Pattison or to Sister Dora, was now broken. Not many of them were present to see her statue unveiled. Her sisters, all elderly women, did not make the cross-country journey from Richmond. They had been hurt by her refusal to tell them her true condition at the last, and by the knowledge that they had played a very small part in her life. Only Rachel, twelve years dead, had been really near to her heart. Mark, too, was gone; he had died in 1884 of cancer, a long, hard death, for he had shared the stubborn vitality of his sister Dorothy and their father. Mother Frances, so reticent and sensitive, had been wounded by repeated attacks in print on Mother Theresa and the Community of the Holy Rood. Now she herself was Mother Superior, directing the affairs of a busy convent, hospital and orphanage, and she preferred to draw a veil over the past by destroying many early records of the Order.[28] Frank, the cheerful schoolboy and prosaic young man, had grown into the mainstay of the dwindling Pattison family. He travelled from London to represent them at the unveiling and declared the statue 'a speaking likeness' of his sister.

The Coatham Homes, the original sponsors of Sister Dora's work in Walsall, sent no representative. Mr Postlethwaite had died three months earlier, and his Sisterhood, never established on any firm constitutional basis, apparently scattered at his death.[29] The convalescent home, though it continued as a charity, passed into the hands of a secular management,[30] which lasted well into the present century. Of the men in Dorothy Pattison's life, Purchas Stirk and Redfern Davies were both long since dead. James Tate, the shadowy clerical suitor, had been for years rector of the Kentish village where he was to remain until his own death. Kenyon Jones married a daughter of the Town Clerk of Walsall and continued to live in the town until the 1930s. His father-in-law was one of the promoters of the memorial, but there is no means of knowing if he saw Sister Dora's statue unveiled, or what his feelings may have been on that October day. He kept her letters until the day of his own death.

Of Sister Dora's friends, Richard Twigg had died within a few months of herself. The working people of Wednesbury, in recognition of his devoted service among them, raised a fund to complete the education of his orphan children.[31] The Ridsdale family had moved with their father's appointment to a Methodist church at Stockton-on-Tees; the boy who had rowed in the boat with Dora became one of Middlesbrough's leading industrial chemists.

Dr Burton was old and living in retirement; his son, for ever 'young John Burton', was serving with his regiment. Louise MacLachlan, Dora's best pupil, was a leading figure in the developing profession of nursing, with a high reputation in the medical world of London; she was too much in demand to make the journey to Walsall. Margaret Lonsdale was present, but invisible. The people of Walsall were still, after six years, so enraged by her book that she had been warned not to show herself in the streets for fear of insult. Dr MacLachlan, who issued the warning, kindly offered to hide her at an upper window in his own house. There, peering between drawn curtains, she watched the unveiling from afar.[32] She had used the entire profits of her memoir, translated into several languages, to found the Sister Dora Memorial Convalescent Home which opened in April 1884 at Milford, on the heights of Cannock Chase, and she herself had trained as a nurse at Guy's Hospital in order to qualify for the duties of matron.[33] Her entire life was now devoted to Sister Dora's memory, and she still claimed to be the true interpreter of her wishes and character. It is not too much to say that her whole rather pathetic destiny had been shaped by one chance schoolgirl encounter. She was the most extreme case among many men and women who fell victim to Sister Dora's charm.

Perhaps the best, certainly the most clear-sighted, of Sister Dora's friends, was there, though a shadow of his old self. James MacLachlan had suffered a major and disabling illness two years earlier. He was nursed for three months by Sister Ellen and recovered, though, to his great regret, he was not strong enough to return to full time work. Like Dora, he had hoped to die in harness; he did not enjoy retirement and lived only until 1888.[34] Perhaps illness had softened his taciturn Lowland character, for, as he stood looking at the statue after the unveiling, an acquaintance was astonished to hear this least sentimental of men say, 'But Sister Dora looked younger than that, and besides, the waist is not small enough.'[35]

Three o'clock was the hour fixed for the ceremony of unveiling Sister Dora's statue. The clock struck from the Town Hall. As the Mayor pulled the cord and the covering slipped slowly to the ground, wrote Samuel Welsh, 'the soft outlines of chaste marble were revealed and a hushed murmur ran through the crowd'.

It was followed by long applause and the boom of factory hooters from far and near. The statue of white marble gleamed against the blackened house fronts of the town, standing eight feet high on a plinth of the same height, so that Sister Dora looked out over the crowd with her old air of easy command. It showed her in the cap and apron, familiar to so many who stood watching, rolling a bandage with deft hands. The sculptor had captured the spirited and lively turn of her head. It was a long time before the crowd was satisfied with looking and began to ebb quietly away.[36]

The rain held off and the rest of the day was given over to celebrations. The gates of the hospital were decorated with an archway of evergreens and the trees in the grounds illuminated with fairy lights. The wards and departments planned and furnished by Sister Dora were open to the public and so many thousands came that 'all that could be done was to keep the people moving to prevent a deadlock'. The hospital gained greatly, both in gifts and goodwill.[37] The Corporation and the memorial committee attended a collation at which predictable speeches were made by the Town Clerk and the Mayor. There was probably more enjoyment when seven thousand children of all ages, many from poor and needy homes, sat down to a free tea served by the ladies of Walsall. Afterwards there were balloons for all, and when darkness had fallen, a firework display. Children from the Roman Catholic parochial schools were also invited to the tea-party, and this seems to have been the first occasion on which Catholic and Protestant children in the town shared a school treat. If so, Sister Dora even in death had kept her healing touch.[38]

The Black Country's debt to her has been faithfully repaid. Social change has incorporated her most revolutionary ideas, new medical techniques have made her practice old-fashioned and secular philosophy has questioned the religious inspiration of her work; but her personality refuses to grow stale. Every year her birthday, 16th January, is greeted with a ceremony at the statue. Generations of mayors and hospital chairmen, of matrons, young nurses and school children, even of representatives of remote Hauxwell, have laid flowers at Sister Dora's feet. When so many Victorian statues have an air of forlorn and dusty neglect, she still seems to live at the heart of the crowded, noisy hardworking town. White marble proved an over-optimistic choice for the

Black Country; by the middle of this century atmospheric pollution had eroded the outlines of her features and the four relievos illustrating her work. Among all the competing economic pressures of post-war reconstruction and the welfare state, a fund was 'readily subscribed', says the hospital history,[39] to cast a complete replica in bronze. The bronze statue was unveiled on 16th January 1957, the hundred and twenty-fifth anniversary of Dorothy Pattison's birth, in its old position, dominating the centre of the town. It did not seem out-of-place, unnecessary or a waste of money, because it symbolized a continuing tradition. Sister Dora had changed a world, simply by living in it.

NOTES

1. *Report of Board of Guardians: Walsall Observer*, 13th February 1879.
2. W.C.H.A.R., 1879.
3. Ibid.
4. *The Lancet*, 1st May 1880.
5. W.P.L. Album, and for letters of protest, W.C.H. MS., 1879.
6. Reprints, 3.
7. Her name is now incorporated in the title of Walsall General Hospital.
8. W. J. S. McKay, *Lawson Tait*, 409-10.
9. Reprints, 23.
10. W.C.H.A.R., 1883.
11. *The Guardian*, 1st January 1879.
12. *Daily Telegraph*, 8th October 1879.
13. *The Westminster Review*, April 1880.
14. The negotiations which followed form the subject of an additional chapter in Lonsdale, 2nd edn., 1887.
15. Lonsdale, *Sister Dora*, 2nd edn., 1887, Appendix.
16. W.P.L. Album. Extensive inquiries failed to trace the original.
17. W.C.H. MS., 1880.
18. Lonsdale, *Sister Dora*, 2nd edn., 1887, Appendix.
19. W.C.H. MS., 1882.
20. W.C.H.A.R., 1888.
21. Lonsdale, 245.
22. Reprints.
23. W.C.H. MS., 1880-81.

24. The river flows beneath it in a culvert.
25. Walter Scott, *The Lady of the Lake*, canto I, xviii, misquoted.
26. *Christian Age*, 8th October 1886.
27. *Daily Mail*, 11th October 1886.
28. C.H.R. The Community much regrets the loss of these unique documents.
29. *The Guardian*, 28th July 1886.
30. T. H. Bulmer, *Directory of North Riding*, 1890.
31. F. W. Hackwood, *Religious Wednesbury*, 128.
32. W.P.L. Album.
33. M. Lonsdale, *Care and Nursing of Children*, 1885, Preface.
34. *Walsall Observer*, 15th December 1888.
35. W.P.L. Album.
36. *Walsall Observer*, 15th October 1886.
37. W.C.H.A.R., 1886.
38. Reprints.
39. Walsall H.M.C. A Century of Walsall Hospital Services, 25.

Case Summary for 1872

Abscesses	4
Amputations	5
Burns and Scalds	16
Burned and crushed	24
Burned by Gunpowder	4
Cut Throats	2
Concussion	7
Dislocations	2
Dog Bites	3
Excision of Elbow Joint	2
Fracture, simple	39
„ comminuted	2
„ compound	7
„ of skull	2
Injuries to joints	43
„ „ eye	3
„ „ head	3
„ internal	2
Kick by horse	3
Lock Jaw	1
Pig bite	2
Poisoned	1
Ruptures	2
Sprains	7
Tumours removed	6
Ulcers	4
Wounds to flesh	10

17 deaths

Extract from Annual Report 1877

A table showing the different towns and occupations from which accident cases were admitted to the temporary hospital in Bridgeman Place. No accident case was accepted unless it was 'very severe'.

Wednesbury – Collieries, heavy iron-casting for girders, railway wheels, axles and tubes.

Willenhall – Collieries, iron casting for locks and keys.

Wolverhampton – heavy iron forging, steam hammering.

Birchills, Pelsall, Coal Pool, Great Barr, Rushall – Collieries and ironstone pits.

Bloxwich – edge tool making, pressing and die stamping.

Darlaston – iron casting for nuts, bolts and gun locks.

Potteries – clay mining.

Lichfield – railway work, especially shunting and linesmen's duties.

Total of serious injuries admitted as in-patients   102, 8 deaths.

Dorothy Pattison and George Eliot

In May 1870 the novelist George Eliot had been working for ten months on the early stages of *Middlemarch*, which then consisted, in her own words, of 'the Vincy Featherstone parts'.[1] During 25th–28th May she broke off to stay at Lincoln College as the guest of Mrs Mark Pattison, with whom she had been corresponding since January 1869. During this visit Francis Pattison drove her in a pony carriage round Littlemore and to a cottage which she kept as a 'country refuge' at Headington.[2] Francis became one of George Eliot's 'spiritual daughters' or 'God-daughters', addressed as 'Dear Figliuolina' in letters signed 'Your affectionate Madre'. During the months after the Oxford visit, George Eliot began to write 'a story called Miss Brooke', which in December 1870 she decided to incorporate, as the Dorothea and Casaubon narrative, in the framework of *Middlemarch*.[3] It had been, she wrote, 'among my possible themes ever since I began to write fiction, but will probably take new shapes in the development.'

The Oxford visit, the fact that the Pattisons were, like the Casaubons, separated by twenty-seven years in age, the physical contrast between them, the Rector, as Lord Rosebery wrote, 'looking wizened and wintry by the side of his blooming wife', gave rise to gossip and speculation among readers of *Middlemarch* when it was published, and indeed ever since.

The relationship between the character of Casaubon and the Rector of Lincoln has been endlessly discussed and has produced some fascinating difference of learned opinion.[4] There is no need to add to them here. The theory that his wife Francis may have provided the novelist's inspiration for the character of Dorothea remains problematical. Her future husband, Sir Charles Dilke, contradicted himself on the subject. At one time he claimed that a number of passages from Francis's intimate letters are repeated in George Eliot's account of Dorothea;[5] at another he said the attempt to find a likeness was 'never made by any but a simpleton'.[6] Francis, like Dorothea, had married a man much older than herself whose intellect she revered, though, unlike Dorothea, she never ceased to admire him. 'I think,' she said, 'he is the only truly learned man I know.' Nevertheless, in spite of intellectual sympathy and a distinguished social life, both parties to the marriage were deeply unhappy; Francis's letters and Mark Pattison's diary make no attempt to conceal the fact. Francis found herself as disillusioned in marriage as Dorothea was.

In appearance and personality Francis was far from the ardent simplicity of Dorothea. She was described by H. A. Sayce as 'worldly and brilliant'. As an art student she had lived independently in London, and shocked friends by her 'fearless advocacy of the necessity of drawing from the nude'.[7] Her youthful religion involved a somewhat ostentatious ritualism. After her marriage, she became increasingly elegant and sophisticated. Her frocks, like her special hand-made cigarettes, came from Paris; her witty conversation, wrote R. C. Jebb, 'affects a certain specially Oxford type of feminine fastness'. During George Eliot's visit in 1870 another guest described Francis as 'a brilliant apparition. . . . The pale, pretty head blond-cendrée; the delicate smiling features and white throat; a touch of black; a touch of blue; a white dress; a general eighteenth-century impression as though of powder and patches'.[8] This stylish portrait does little to suggest the heroine who is introduced with the words 'Miss Brooke had that kind of beauty which seems to be thrown into relief by poor dress', and who is to be compared with St Theresa. Conversely, as a critic points out, it is difficult to imagine Dorothea growing into the 'plump, bejewelled Lady Dilke' of a surviving portrait.[9]

Yet the appearance and character of Dorothea does show haunting, apparently inexplicable resemblances to another member of Mark Pattison's family, his sister Dorothy. The nearness of their names need not, taken alone, mean anything.[10] Yet Dorothea's hair, dark brown like Dorothy's, was likewise 'flatly braided and coiled behind so as to expose the outline of her head in a daring manner', contrasting with the frizzled curls of the period. As a young girl, Dorothy shared the love of fresh air and country pursuits with Dorothea, of whom we read 'her eyes and cheeks glowed with mingled pleasures'; Dorothea enjoyed riding, and her social successes, like Dorothy's, were in the hunting field. 'Most men thought her bewitching when she was on horseback.' Later, as a widow, Dorothea wears, like Sister Dora, a plain black dress and a white cap which frames her face. More significant for character, is the description of Dorothea's hands, 'powerful, feminine, maternal hands', capable, like Sister Dora's, of much devoted work for others.

Indeed, devotion, 'an ardently willing soul', was the keynote of Dorothea's character; the devotedness which was so necessary a part of her mental life, could also be found at the core of Dorothy Pattison's compelling personality. Dorothy was driven by what George Eliot calls in Dorothea 'the fanaticisms of Sympathy'. She might almost have spoken Dorothea's words – 'How can we live and think that anyone has trouble – piercing trouble – and that we could help them and never try?' Dorothea, like Dorothy, cared personally and practically for the poor; she 'knelt suddenly down on a brick floor by the side of a sick labourer and prayed fervidly' as Sister Dora did every day in her work. Like Sister Dora she was austere towards herself and had 'strange whims of fasting like a Papist, and of sitting up at night to read old theological books'.

Dorothea, like Dorothy, was 'remarkably clever', she had 'a passionate desire to know and think', and like Dorothy, had suffered 'the strain and conflict of self-repression in woman's conventional life'. Dorothea, indeed, 'used to despise women a little for not shaping their lives more and doing better things', or as Dorothy put it in a letter of 1873, 'When they have faithfully fulfilled their home duties, instead of spending their time in dressing, novel reading, gossiping, let them "spend and be spent". There would be more real work done and less talk, if we laid it on this sure foundation,'[11] Edith Simcox, reviewing the memoir by Miss Lonsdale for the *Fortnightly Review*, provided the most intelligent and perceptive contemporary account of Sister Dora.[12] She noted that Dorothy 'thought meanly of the feeble minds and bodies of women'.

Dorothea, like Dorothy, was unable to settle to the conventional domestic round because 'the idea of some active good within her reach haunted her like a passion'. This recalls Dorothy's poignant confession, in a letter to Mark, of her fight 'not to waste my life in useless regrets. God grant my yearning for good may be carried into *action*'.[13] The comparison of Dorothea with St Theresa in the Prelude to *Middlemarch* involves, as a critic has noted 'not mysticism, but the opportunity for practical work as the reformer of a religious order'.[14] He traces this, not to Francis Pattison's Tractarianism, but to George Eliot's own Evangelical upbringing; the same might be said of Dorothy's early training. Both Dorothea and Dorothy are reckless in devotion, Dorothea 'enamoured of intensity and greatness and rash in embracing whatever seemed to her likely to have these aspects; likely to incur martyrdom'. In just the same way, Dorothy gave the impression to Edith Simcox of 'a passionate love of her work', because it alone fulfilled her 'need to lose her own consciousness in the whirl of action, and the scarcely veiled longing for some hope forlorn enough to throw away her life upon'. She even confessed her deep longing 'that God would find me fit to lay down my life in his service'.

How did Edith Simcox gain her insight into Sister Dora's powerful and, as she noted, enigmatic character? Even the face in which most people saw only beauty, struck her as 'somewhat unfathomable'. Certainly her understanding went deeper than anything she could have learnt from Miss Lonsdale's *Sister Dora*, which was the occasion of her article. She questions 'whence came the intense pathos' of Dorothy's solitary life, and states frankly that 'there were shadows' in her conflict with her family and her deliberate refusal to marry, though the love of men was 'a serious temptation' to her. Among much rather shallow adulation, she speaks with real understanding and sympathy of the cost in human terms of Sister Dora's career. She hoped 'future heroines would have less to cool and sadden their generous ardour'. It is not unreasonable to ask, did this deeper insight come from conversations with someone who had heard Sister Dora's story at first hand? From 1872 Edith Simcox was a frequent caller upon George Eliot and G. H. Lewes. She became, like Francis Pattison, a member of the circle of George Eliot devotees, centred on the Lewes's London house in Regent's Park. On several occasions, as Edith Simcox's journal records, she and Mrs Pattison were present together as callers in the Lewes's drawing-room.[15] Did Edith Simcox learn something of Sister Dora's real character and history from conversations there, either with Francis or with George Eliot herself, who already knew it?

Written evidence on this interesting possibility is unpromising. The correspondence of George Eliot and Mrs Pattison survives only in fragments, after what Professor Gordon Haight justly describes as 'the mutilations of Sir Charles Dilke's notorious scissors'.[16] The manuscript of *Middlemarch* has been exhaustively studied by Professor Jerome Beaty, who found the deletions in the original draft of *Miss Brooke* largely illegible, though the gist of five lines deleted on page 96 'appears to be contrast between the effort to seem and Dorothea's inner ideal standard'.[17]

What is certain is that Francis Pattison knew well the tragic history of her husband's sisters. Writing years later on the question of women's employment, she stressed the bitter resentment of wrong which women feel under 'the suffering inflicted by unjust rule'.[18] She seems never to have met Dorothy in nearly twenty years as her sister-in-law, but Jane, Mary, Fanny and Eleanor all stayed with her at Oxford; Fanny in particular had intimate knowledge of Sister Dora's work. Francis visited Richmond, and there met Sarah and Rachel who had been the closest companions of Dorothy's troubled youth. The Pattison letters show how often Dorothy was a subject of anxious conversation, and what an indelible impression she made on every member of the family circle. If Francis, in conversation with a great novelist, chose to describe this remarkable sister-in-law, she was certainly in a position to do so. She may even have described Sister Dora's work in reply to a question from George Eliot herself, who in 1869 was asking friends for information on 'provincial hospitals' and compiling 'Notes from a letter on Hospitals', dealing with the duties of the house-surgeon and staff.[19] The relation between Dorothy and Mark was first close and trusting, later cold and distant, like the relationship of Dorothea and Casaubon. The respect of the young wife for a much older husband resembles Dorothy's admiration of the brother twenty years older than herself. Both sister and wife failed to find in this relationship the inspiration they had hoped for.

No one, of course, would suggest that George Eliot's methods of composition involved crude copying from life, though, as a critic points out, it is difficult to distinguish in her work between

Sister Dora

what the nineteenth century called 'judgment' and 'inspiration' and what the twentieth calls the 'conscious' and the 'unconscious' mind.[20] Striking personal characteristics could inspire her; thus Mordecai in *Daniel Deronda* owes his learning to the Talmudic scholar, Emanuel Deutsch, and Romola her golden hair to Barbara Bodichon. Dorothea is in no sense a portrait of Dorothy Pattison. Yet their characters do have enough in common to suggest a line of inquiry about the novelist's inspiration.

NOTES

1. G. Haight, *George Eliot*, 420.
2. Ibid., 428.
3. J. Beaty, *Middlemarch from Notebook to Novel*, 3.
4. G. Haight, *George Eliot*, Appendix II, cf. J. Sparrow, *Mark Pattison and the Idea of a University*, 9–18. Contrary to what one might expect, Pattison scholars have tended to accept a connection between Casaubon and Pattison, while George Eliot scholars deny it. For Mark Pattison's later years, see Appendix D.
5. J. Sparrow, *Mark Pattison and the Idea of a University*, 14.
6. G. Haight, *George Eliot*, 449.
7. J. Sparrow, *Mark Pattison and the Idea of a University*, 43.
8. G. Haight, *George Eliot*, 427. The writer was eighteen-year-old Mary Arnold, the future novelist Mrs Humphrey Ward.
9. G. Haight, *Notes and Queries*, May 1968.
10. G. Haight, *George Eliot*, 448, relates the name Dorothea to the heroine of Bulwer Lytton's *Pelham*.
11. Quoted, Lonsdale, 115. 'Spend and be spent' is a quotation from a hymn by Charles Wesley.
12. E. Simcox, 'Ideals of Feminine Usefulness'. *The Fortnightly Review*, May 1880.
13. Pattison, 65, f. 188–91.
14. G. Haight, *George Eliot*, Appendix II.
15. K. A. McKenzie, *Edith Simcox and George Eliot*, 15.
16. G. Haight, *Notes and Queries*, May 1968.
17. J. Beaty, *Middlemarch from Notebook to Novel*, 7–9 and facsimile pages.
18. Lady Dilke, Introduction to *Women's Work in Social Questions of Today Series*.
19. J. Beaty *Middlemarch from Notebook to Novel*, 22, 39, 57.
20. J. Beaty *Middlemarch from Notebook to Novel*, 114–5.

The Walsall Smallpox Epidemic

The Walsall Smallpox Epidemic of 1875 was one of a number of 'considerable local outbreaks', which followed the international epidemic of 1871–3. This had been, said Dr Seaton in a report to the Local Government Board 'of world-wide diffusion, marked wherever it occurred by an intensity and malignancy unequalled by any previous epidemic of the disease within living memory'. The epidemic had been a sudden explosion, killing more people in two years than the epidemic of 1837–41 did in four, while the population increase had been 'between a third and a half'. At its height the proportion of deaths in 1871–3 had been, as in the classic smallpox epidemics of the eighteenth century, one in six of all cases.[1] Mortality increased from 35% to 47% among cases admitted to one fever hospital. The disease showed its malignancy in a variety of ways; 'great diffusiveness', a high proportion of deaths in infants under one year, even among those supposed to have been vaccinated, and the frequent occurrence of the fatal haemorrhagic type. It was noticed that 'the mortality in all mining districts was exceptionally high'.[2] In Walsall itself during 1872 there were 502 deaths from smallpox, among a population of roughly seventy thousand.[3] Against this sombre background the threat of another major smallpox epidemic in Walsall caused general alarm. Questions were asked in the House of Commons early in 1875 about the 'unusual mortality in the Walsall Union and inquiries were made of the Sanitary authorities on the subject',[4] since it represented a menace to the public health of the whole Midland region.

In the event the total deaths from smallpox for the whole of Staffordshire in 1875 were only 24, far fewer than the deaths from measles, infantile diarrhoea or for that matter from violence, which accounted for 869 inquests in the county.[5] Most of these smallpox deaths occurred in Walsall; the surrounding towns and villages were not affected. The number of deaths in two great

Sister Dora

Staffordshire outbreaks were, in 1837–40 1325 and in 1871 3050. Thanks to the isolation of all new cases deaths during the Walsall epidemic of 1875 were fewer than they had been in 1872, 20.5 per thousand in 1875 as against 28.9 per thousand in 1872. An important factor of course is that the smallpox infection itself was on the wane, but nevertheless evidence confirms the tradition, always maintained in Walsall, that Sister Dora's personal courage in taking charge of the smallpox hospital in 1875 averted a second major epidemic.

NOTES

1. C. Creighton, *A history of Epidemics in Britain*, II, 615.
2. *The Lancet*, 23rd October 1875.
3. Annual Report of Registrar General, 1874, lxix.
4. *The British Medical Journal*, 26th June 1875.
5. Annual Report of Registrar General, 1876, 187.

Mark Pattison

*Some notes on his private papers from his last meeting with
Sister Dora to the time of her death*

The years had not brought happiness to Mark Pattison in his
private life, since he last saw Dorothy in 1866, although his
scholarly reputation stood high. Francis, his wife, spent a large
part of the year in the South of France for her health. 'She is never
to winter in Oxford, perhaps not in England,' wrote her husband.[1]
From Nice she had written in 1876, admitting 'a physical aversion
which always existed, though I strove hard to overcome it, and
which is now wholly beyond control'. She was already corresponding regularly, sometimes every day, with her future husband, Sir Charles Dilke, 'reserving', wrote Mark, 'all her interest
for the other man and his affairs'.[2] After Mark Pattison's death his
widow censored his private diaries by vigorous circular crossing
out, by scratching with a penknife, and by snipping out whole
passages with scissors. This recalls Dilke's technique for 'reducing
the bulk' of his used engagement books, which caused such
unhappy consequences for himself in the Divorce Court. The
hollowness behind the façade of the Pattison's marriage must
have been obvious to the sharp eyes of Oxford society. Mark's
one rather pathetic autumnal love affair did not begin until after
Sister Dora's death and was, in its turn, the subject of much ill-
natured gossip. Everything conspired to depress and irritate him.
The College, which as a young man he had served so devotedly,
was now a source of annoyance. 'Undergraduate (Clark) to breakfast,' he wrote. 'How dismally ignorant these schoolboys are!'[3]
The dons were no better. 'Bothered by Bursar,'[4] he wrote testily.
'College meeting with the usual vexations'; or 'Chapter day with
more than its usual botherdom'.[5] College festivities were, if anything, more vexatious than College business. 'Day spoiled by the
shadow of the coming Gaude,' he wrote, and added, the morning
after, 'though I neither ate nor drank yesterday the effort of

talking and listening in that Babel of voices unhinged me.'[6] Hypochondria, which in earlier days had been a refuge from more urgent worries, steadily gained the upper hand over him; his later diaries were a melancholy catalogue of visceral embarrassments. 'Weak, fagged, depressed and overflowing with gout. East wind continues making me quite ill,' is a typical introduction to the day's events. A fine day in April could be even more depressing. 'This almost the first summerlike day,' he wrote, one golden Oxford evening, 'and many strangers down from town, Parks full of strollers. Had constantly to stop and greet or chat with someone, which, ill as I am feeling, was very trying.'[7] His dislike of society became an obsession. 'Last night a dinner party at home and people staying in the house,' he wrote in November 1873, 'it upsets the house, strains and exhausts the service and makes a demand on my nervous powers which anticipates their reserves for several days,' or, more succinctly, 'Dinner party of stupid people.'[8] Dining out offered the added torture of unwanted partners. 'I very unfit to go and bored to death by sitting between two idiotic women.'[9] To Mark's morbid sensitivity, Sister Dora's brains and character, her enjoyment of people, her refusal to let circumstances interfere with her work, must have seemed a calculated insult. She had achieved her purpose in life, unworthy though it seemed to him, while he was haunted day in, day out, by the ghost of the great work of scholarship, his History of European Learning which he knew he would never complete. 'My devouring anxiety now,' he wrote in his private diary, 'is grown to be to live to complete my book. It is the only thing which now really interests me. But a despair comes over me when I find myself this day 60 and still face to face with a chaos of materials to which my feeble memory affords the only clue.'[10] Reading this, it is impossible not to pity him. He professed to be contented in his agnosticism. The Pattisons, from their provincial upbringing, were all old-fashioned; Mark seems to have held an eighteenth-century conviction that holy orders were an occupation for a gentleman, whatever his private opinions. Yet preaching, praying, celebrating, week after week, a faith in which he no longer believed must have overshadowed his life with a sense of falsehood. It was one more burden to carry. An acquaintance of his last years received an impression of bitterness, an overwhelming physical depression, 'wearied with vexations as if he might sink into an exhausted sleep at any moment.'[11] Mark felt the contradictions in his own temperament, but was powerless to control or resolve them. 'By whatever name you call it,' he wrote bleakly, 'the unconscious is found controlling each man's destiny, without, or in defiance of his will.'[12] Ironically, the unconscious drove him during his last years in his father's footsteps. His meanness over money increased; he greeted a niece's illness when on a visit, with the remark, 'costly to me who have to pay . . . she will not be fit to move for another week, another unforeseen outlay!'[13] He brooded over his life savings; one entry in his diary could have been written by the Rector of Hauxwell. 'Have now at last settled the two codicils to my will, which I have so long meditated. I have left away from F[rancis] above £3,000 by a 3rd codicil which I keep separate from the rest as I might still destroy [erased with knife].' Like his father and sister, Mark Pattison died of cancer, and died hard, slowly, in days of anguish and terror. Reading the private papers of this gifted, most unhappy, man, one appreciates the stresses Sister Dora had to overcome in her own character.

NOTES

1. Pattison, 130, f. 116.
2. J. Sparrow, *Mark Pattison and the Idea of a University*, 45–7, calls attention to significant dates in the Crawford divorce case.
3. Pattison, 133, f. 1.
4. Ibid., 130, f. 124.
5. Ibid., 130, ff. 154, 133.
6. Ibid., 151.
7. Ibid., 130, f. 1.
8. Pattison, 130, ff. 72, 94.
9. Ibid., 130, f. 82.
10. Ibid., 130, f. 71.
11. L. Tollemache, *Memoir of Pattison*, 32.
12. Pattison, *Memoirs*, 330.
13. Pattison, 130, ff. 168–9.

The Listerian Technique

The technique was set out and related to its underlying principles in a series of characteristically lucid papers by Lister himself.[1] His nephew and biographer, Rickman Godlee, also left a first-hand account of his duties as a member of the operating team. The method demanded rigorous self-discipline and attention to detail. Its object was to 'destroy once and for all any septic organisms that may have been introduced', and thus to prevent infection from ever starting in an incision or accidental wound. Every source of bacterial infection was eliminated in a step by step routine.

Before operation the staff had to select the instruments the Chief preferred, wash and polish them, and lay them for half an hour in a 1 in 20 solution of carbolic. Surgical sponges, which were elsewhere used to mop blood off the floor, were similarly washed and sterilized. The operating table, of scrubbed deal, was covered in towels wrung out in the solution. Next the nurse set a bowl of antiseptic lotion for the surgeon to scrub his hands, and pinned a clean huckaback towel over his waistcoat; cap, mask or gloves were still unknown. While the patient inhaled the chloroform, she purified the skin round the site of operation with carbolic lotion, and covered it with towels wrung out in carbolic. If any instrument, sponge or towel was laid aside, even for a moment, in the course of the operation, it could not be used without re-sterilizing. Sterile catgut ligatures eliminated a prime source of infection. The most famous piece of Listerian apparatus was the high-pressure spray, 'for providing an antiseptic atmosphere' around the incision. In practice its effect was described by an assistant with barely suppressed emotion. 'A huge cloud of fine spray could be produced, enveloping the patient and all those engaged in the operation and capable of filling a room with a dense, damp and pungent mist, so that the occasion often became a trial of physical endurance.'[2] Mercifully a smaller model was available for dressings, which were also carried out with full antiseptic precautions. Lister refused to hand over a surgical case to a general practitioner until healing had taken place and all danger of infection was past. By the use of this method dressings could safely remain unchanged for as long as a week, with great saving of fatigue and pain to the patient.

In skilled and experienced hands the method fully justified Lister's claim that 'Putrefaction *never* occurs, provided of course that all the proceedings have been in every respect conducted antiseptically'.

NOTES

1. 'Recent improvements in the details of antiseptic surgery,' *The Lancet*, March-April 1875.
2. R. Godlee, *Lord Lister*, 283.

BIBLIOGRAPHY

I. Manuscript or Privately Printed Sources

Pattison Manuscripts, Bodleian Library, Oxford.
Community of the Holy Rood, Registers, Draft Rule, Correspondence and Chapter Minutes, Convent of the Holy Rood, Middlesbrough.
Walsall General (Sister Dora) Hospital, Manuscript Minute books of management Committee, and privately printed Annual Reports, Walsall Group Hospital Management Committee.

II. Newspapers and Periodicals

MacMillan's Magazine. April 1867
    Volunteer Hospital Nursing. E. Garrett, L.S.A. August 1879
    A New Vocation for Women. Jane Chesney
The Contemporary Review. May 1880
    Miss Lonsdale on Guy's Hospital. Walter Moxon. August 1884
    Christianity and the Equality of the Sexes. J. Llewelyn Davies
The Nineteenth Century. April 1880
    The Present Crisis at Guy's Hospital: Margaret Lonsdale
    Replies to above article. May 1880 ⎱ William Gull, S. Haber-
       „   „   „   „   June 1880 ⎰ shon and A. Henriques, O. Sturges
The Fortnightly Review. May 1880
    Ideals of Feminine Usefulness. Edith Simcox
British Medical Journal. 1880 Vol. I
    Correspondence on nursing at Guy's Hospital, pp. 525, 605, 670, 706
The Saturday Review. May 1 1880
    Review of M. Lonsdale, *Sister Dora*. Anon
The Westminster Review. April 1880
    Review of M. Lonsdale, *Sister Dora*. Anon
St. Paul's Magazine. August 1871
    Nursing as a Profession for Ladies. Charlotte Haddon

The Birmingham Medical Review. 1872–92.
The British Medical Journal. 1880. Vols. I & II
The Lancet. 1880. Vols. I & II
The Wensleydale Advertiser
The Walsall Observer. 1868–89
The General Baptist Magazine. 1889
The Birmingham Post. 1867
The Birmingham Sunday Mercury. 1963
The Christian Age. 1880
The Guardian. 1886
The Church Times. 1886
The World. 1875–6
Album of miscellaneous press cuttings in the Local History Room
of the Walsall Public Library.

III. Printed Books: A Selection

ABEL SMITH B. *A History of the Nursing Profession*, 1960; *The Hospitals, 1800–1948*, 1964

ALLCHIN, A. M. *The Silent Rebellion*, 1958

ALLEN, G. C. *Industrial Development of Birmingham & the Black Country* (1929), 1966, 2nd edn.

ALLEN, WM. *Three Sermons on the life of Sister Dora*, 1879.

ANON. *Hospitals & Sisterhoods*, 1855.

ANSON, PETER, *The Call of the Cloister*, 1955.

BARING-GOULD, S. *Virgin Saints and Martyrs*, 1900.

BEANEY, J. G., MRCS *Conservative Surgery*, 1859.

BEATY, JEROME *Middlemarch from notebook to novel*, 1960.

BENSON, R. M. *The Religious Vocation*.

BRIGGS, ASA *Victorian Cities*, 1965.

BROCKINGTON, C. FRASER *Public Health in the Nineteenth Century*, 1965.

BRISTOW & HOLMES *The Hospitals of the United Kingdom*, 1864.

BROWN, FORD K. *Fathers of the Victorians*, 1961

BURDETT, H. C. *Cottage Hospitals*, 1896, 3rd edn.

BURLEIGH *Sister Dora*, n.d., *circa* 1890.

BURNS, W. L. *The Age of Equipoise*, 1964.

BURRITT, E. *Walks in the Black Country & its Green Borderland,* 1868.

COPE, SIR Z. N. *Almroth Wright,* 1966.

COPEMAN, W. S. C. *A Short History of the Gout and the Rheumatic Diseases,* 1964.

CULLINGWORTH, C. J. *The Nurses' Companion,* 1876.

CURTEIS, E. A. *In Memoriam,* 1878.

CURTEIS, G. H. *Bishop Selwyn,* 1889.

DAVIES, HORTON *Worship & Theology in England, Vols iii & iv*

DRABBLE, P. *Black Country,* 1952.

EDE, J. F. *History of Wednesbury,* 1962.

ELLIOTT-BINNS, L. E. *Religion in the Victorian Era,* 1936.

FRAZER, W. M. *English Public Health, 1834–1939,* 1950.

GALE, W. K. V. *The Black Country Iron Industry* *Iron and Steel,* 1969.

GODLEE, RICKMAN *Lord Lister,* 1917.

GREEN, V. H. H. *Oxford Common Room,* 1951.

Hauxwell Church, 1961.

GRIFFITH, G. *Hospitals & Asylums of Birmingham,* 1861.

HACKWOOD, F. W. *Religious Wednesbury,* 1900.

HAIGHT, G. S. *George Eliot,* 1968.

HARTLEY, M. & INGILBY, J. *Life and Tradition in the Yorkshire Dales,* 1968.

HEATH, CHRISTOPHER *A Manual of Minor Surgery,* 1861.

HOMESHAW, E. J. *Corporation of the Borough & Foreign of Walsall,* 1960.

HUNTER, R. & MACALPINE, I. *Three Hundred Years of Psychiatry, 1535–1860,* 1963.

JONES *Memorials of Agnes Jones* – with introduction by Florence Nightingale, 1871.

KAMM, JOSEPHINE *Hope Deferred: Girls Education in English History,* 1965.

KITCHEL, A. T., ed. (George Eliot's notebook) *Quarry for Middlemarch,* 1955.

LONSDALE, MARGARET *Sister Dora,* 1st edn. 1880 and 2nd edn. 1887; *Care and Nursing of Children.* 1885.

LUCKES, E. C. E. *Lectures on General Nursing.* 1884.

MANNING, B. L. *The Hymns of Wesley & Watts.* 1942.

MAYER-GROSS, W., SLATER, E. & ROTH, M. *Clinical Psychiatry*, 2nd edn., 1960.

MCKAY, W. J. S. *Lawson Tait*, 1922.

MCKENZIE, K. A. *Edith Simcox and George Eliot*. 1961.

MONTAGUE, F. C. *Some Early Letters of Mark Pattison*. 1934.

MORRISON, J. T. J. *William Sands Cox and the Birmingham Medical School*. 1927.

NEWSOME, D. *The Parting of Friends*. 1966.

NIGHTINGALE, F. *Notes on Nursing*, 2nd edn., 1860; *Notes on Hospitals*, 1863; *Introduction to Memorials of Agnes Jones*, 1871.

PATERSON, R. *James Syme*. 1874.

PATTISON, MARK *Memoirs*, 1885; *Essays*, ed. Nettleship, 2 vols.

PONTEFRACT, ELLA *Wensleydale*, 1935.

Post Office Directory of Birmingham Hardware District. 1865–9.

Post Office Directory of the North Riding of Yorkshire. 1872.

POYNTER, F. N. L., ed. *Medicine & Science in the 1860s'*

PRICE, MILLICENT *Inasmuch as . . .*, 1957

RIDSDALE, E. *Sister Dora*. 1880.

ROBINSON, W. H. *A Guide to Walsall*. 1889.

ROYSTON PIKE, E. ed. *Human Documents of the Victorian Golden Age*, 1967.

Human Documents of the Industrial Revolution. 1966.

SPARROW, J., *Mark Pattison and the Idea of a University*.

SWETE, H. *Cottage Hospitals*. 1871.

The Wellesley Index to Nineteenth Century Periodicals, 1824–1900. 1966.

THOMPSON, E. P. *The Making of the English Working Classes*. 1963.

TIMMINS, S., ed. *Birmingham & Midland Hardware District*. 1866.

TOLLEMACHE, L. *Recollections of Pattison*. 1885.

WALSALL HOSPITAL *Annual reports of the Committee to the Subscribers*. 1866–97.

Walsall Red Book. 1879.

Walsall Hospital Services, 1863–1963: an illustrated centenary History. 1963.

Walsall Historical Association Proceedings. 1922–31.

Walsall Observer – 'Sister Dora' [reprints]. 1886.

WARING, E. J., *Cottage Hospitals*. 1867.

WHELAN, T. D. *York & the North Riding.*

WHITAKER, T. D. *History of Richmondshire.* 1823.

White's Directory of Birmingham, Wolverhampton, Walsall, etc. 1869.

WILLIAMS, R. & FISHER A. *Hints for Hospital Nurses.* 1877.

WILLIAMS, T. J. *Priscilla Lydia Sellon.* 1950.

WILLMORE, F. W. *History of Walsall.* 1887.

Index

Index

Page, Rev. R. L., appointment to Christchurch living and chaplaincy of convent, 213
Paine, Tom, 277
Parish churches, 15, 17
Pasteur, Louis, 232
Pater, Walter, 106
Patients, types, 116; increase in number, 185
Pattison, Anna, sister of D.P., 34, 41, 58, 117, 123, 125, 141
Pattison, Dorothy Wyndlow, Sister Dora; infancy, 28–9, 32, 35, 37; childhood, 40; opens voluntary school with sisters, 41; first nursing, 42; influence of brother, 46, 50; end of childhood, 59, 62, 63; education, 62; 67, 69; meets Tate family, 71; tyranny of father 77, 81, 83, 85, 87; relationship with Purchas Stirk, 88; James Tate, suitor, 90; nurses mother, 99; first holiday with brother Mark, 100, 101; breaks and renews engagement to James Tate, 104–5; religious discussions, 108–11; tied to Hauxwell, 116, 118, 120; death of mother, 124, 125; finally breaks engagement, 126; self-discipline, 128; leaves Hauxwell for Little Woolston, 133–6, 138; nursing, 139; engagement to James Tate again, 142; Sisterhood at Coatham, 149–60; sent to Cottage Hospital, North Ormesby, 163; scarlet fever, 164; sent to Cottage Hospital Walsall, 168, 171, 173; death of father, 174; holiday, 178; smallpox, 181; Murphy riots, 184; opthalmic

work, 187; relationship with Redfern Davies, 197; broken engagement, 199; pyaemia, 200; smallpox epidemic, 206–8; 'Sister-in-Charge' at Walsall, 214, 216–19; patients, 223–5; learns anatomy and dissection, 230–1; surgery, 232; performs tracheotomy, 233; ability, 234–235; people of Walsall, 244–6; trains pupil nurses, 251, 259; colliery disaster, 271–2; discipline, 276; religion, 278; takes charge of epidemic hospital, 284, 287–90; ironworks accident, 294–7; Kenyon Jones, 310; cancer, 315; visits London, Paris, 328; trains in antiseptic techniques of Lister, 320, 329–30; last days in Walsall, 330, 332–3; death, 15–17, 337–8; cult of Sister Dora, 341
Pattison, Eleanor, sister of D.P., see Mann, Eleanor
Pattison, Elizabeth, sister of D.P., 34, 41, 132
Pattison, Frances, sister of D.P., see Sister Frances
Pattison, Frances, née Strong, wife of Mark, 131–2, 272
Pattison, Frank, brother of D.P., 72, 83, 123, 173–4
Pattison, Grace, sister of D.P., 28, 34, 57
Pattison, Jane, sister of D.P., 34
Pattison, Jane, née Winn, mother of D.P.; background, 25, 27; anxiety over husband, 32, 35, 40; religion, 48; children, 56, 59; illness, 77, 93, 99; invalid, cared for by daughters, 113, 117; death, 124

377